The Medical Delivery Business

The Medical Delivery Business

Health Reform, Childbirth, and the Economic Order

Barbara Bridgman Perkins

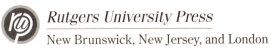

Rutgers University Press

New Brunswick, New Jersey, and London

Library of Congress Cataloging-in-Publication Data

Perkins, Barbara Bridgman.
   The medical delivery business : reform, childbirth, and the economic order /
Barbara Bridgman Perkins.
   p. cm.
   ISBN 0-8135-3328-7 (hbk. : alk. paper)
   1. Health services administration—Economic aspects—United States.
2. Health planning—Economic aspects—United States. 3. Medical economics—
United States. 4. Medical policy—United States—History. 5. Health care reform—United States—History. 6. Maternal health services—Economic
aspects—United States. I. Title.
   RA395.A3P47 2003
   338.4'33621'0973—dc21

                                      2003005986

British Cataloging-in-Publication information is available from the British Library.

Material that appears in chapter 2 was based on the original article, "Shaping
Institution-Based Specialism: Early Twentieth-Century Economic Organization of
Medicine," in *Social History of Medicine*, 10(3): 419–435, 1997. Pearson Education,
Ltd.: Essex, UK.

Material that appears in chapter 4 was based on the original article, "Economic
Organization of Medicine and the Committee on the Costs of Medical Care," in
the *American Journal of Public Health*, 88(11): 1721–1726, 1998. Copyright 1998
by the American Public Health Association.

Material that appears in chapter 5 was based on the original article, "Re-Forming
Medical Delivery Systems: Economic Organization and Dynamics of Regional
Planning and Managed Competition," in *Social Science and Medicine*, 48: 241–
251, 1999. Marcel Dekker, Inc.: New York.

Material that appears in chapters 6 and 8 was based on the original article,
"Rethinking Perinatal Policy: History and Evaluation of Minimum Volume and
Level-of-Care Standards," in *Journal of Public Health Policy*, 14(3): 299–319, 1993.

The publication program of Rutgers University Press is supported by the Board
of Governors of Rutgers, The State University of New Jersey.

Manufactured in the United States of America

Contents

Preface and Acknowledgments

In October 1983 hospital administrators throughout the United States were anxiously preparing Certificate of Need applications to purchase nuclear magnetic resonance imaging machines—a brand-new, multimillion-dollar technology.[1] As a health planner for the state of Washington, I staffed the advisory committee convened to develop standards for reviewing the applications. This experience of trying to rationalize the introduction of a new clinical technology, subsequently renamed "magnetic resonance imaging" (MRI) as a better marketing term, encapsulates some of the issues in this book. It illustrates the strength of the business model of medicine and how this model has contributed to medical intervention in ways unrelated to people's health.

The radiologists on the committee insisted that every major radiology group in the state had to have an MRI to keep up with their specialty. Business consultants were bullishly advising hospital administrators that clinical imaging units offered them recession-proof financial growth.[2] On the paying side of this growth, insurers advised strictly limiting the number of machines approved, recognizing that every new major technology caused the price of health care and health insurance to rise. Entirely missing the point that the populace ultimately pays for medical care, one radiologist maintained that MRI costs were not a problem because "these things pay for themselves." From the vantage point of individual providers, MRIs would indeed pay for themselves. They would enhance radiology's professional status by expanding the number of procedures it produced and the revenues it generated for doctors, hospitals, and academic practice plans.[3] Hospital administrators accused the Certificate of Need process of abrogating their property rights to buy all the equipment they wanted. In fact, however, recognizing that the very existence of the technology upped the ante of competition, most administrators wanted to purchase an MRI in the first round only if their direct competitors were doing so.

By 1990 the United States had installed over 22,000 MRI scanners (and abolished health planning). This figure meant there were 8.4 MRI machines for every million people at the time, compared with 1.5 per million in Sweden and 0.9 in the United Kingdom.[4] Such a large supply mandated heavy utilization of the machines in order to amortize their costs. Some providers saw the four million pregnant women and fetuses each year as a "huge potential market" for MRI and a way of helping them achieve the necessary use levels.[5] MRI was from the beginning a business proposition for hospitals and radiologists. Although some patients undoubtedly benefited from its diagnostic capabilities, the vast growth in number of machines and the need to use them at capacity rapidly led to MRI use far beyond its known efficacy.

Aside from truly impressive pictures, there was little evidence of the technology's efficacy or safety. The U.S. Food and Drug Administration (FDA) would not require safety evidence, deeming it "economically impractical" for manufacturers to conduct the necessary research.[6] Some investigators would later circularly argue that MRI's rapid acceptance and wide utilization themselves demonstrated its efficacy.[7] Yet others would claim that there had been no good evidence demonstrating MRI efficacy at the time of its widespread adoption.[8] The providers on the committee even had to deny that the technology was still investigational—six months before the FDA would grant premarket approval to the first clinical device—so that insurers in the state would reimburse it as standard medical practice.

There was no question that MRI represented a fascinating and useful tool. From my graduate studies in Medical Sciences / Pathology at Harvard Medical School and my work experience in electron microscopy, I knew the allure of visualizing the body's internal structures. At Harvard I had absorbed both the science and the scientific explanation of medicine. Subsequently, I joined a women's group in the early stages of preparing a course called "Women and Their Bodies," which became the book *Our Bodies, Ourselves.* The purpose of the course and the book was to provide sufficient information for women to participate in medical decision making concerning their bodies, including their reproduction, their pregnancies, their labors, and the care of their babies. I was particularly struck by the fact that group members questioned the necessity for much of the medical intervention they had experienced and were continuing to experience during childbirth.

Yet I could not accept the assumption that the male and medical dominance they experienced in the doctor's office and hospital adequately explained excessive medical intervention. I would also find the consumer-oriented approach to be an insufficient model for medical reform. Feminist and other populist health reform movements can too easily fall into the classical economic role of the individual as consumer. This role is in fact—but not in theory—an unequal relationship in which the producers and sellers hold considerably more power. Yet many feminists, finding the subject boring or alienating, ignore the economic aspects of medical care. In so doing, they yield a significant arena of control to the very men and institutions they accuse of dominating the field.

I looked to the national health planning program gearing up at the time to offer a more systemic strategy for health care reform. One baby and two jobs later, I became a health planner, first in a regional health systems agency, followed by a stint in a state office of health planning and development (where I worked with the MRI committee). But I would find that planning didn't get it entirely right, either.

Health planning developed as a quintessentially progressive program to control costs and excessive growth in medical care while equalizing access to it. I believe in planning's values of equity and allocation of society's resources according to social benefit as defined by integrating scientific evaluation with democratic process. Such an allocation contrasts with the laissez-faire approach of leaving production and distribution to the market. Even market advocates admitted that the ethic of providing "a single standard of medical care for all" was not compatible with market-based reform.[9] Yet (paradoxically?) planning itself promoted business models of health care that were not consistent with its own values. I questioned health planning's implicit assumption of a progressive evolution in economic organization from individual entrepreneur to corporate enterprise. This book is my analysis of why such business models cannot fulfill planning's expressed values. I offer it as a feminist critique of progressive health care reform and a progressive critique of feminist health care reform.

The extensive endnotes reveal the extent to which this book is a conversation with and builds on the work, expertise, and inspiration of many before me. For their incisive critique and other more direct contributions to my learning, writing, and confidence, I would like to thank Rita Arditti, Paul Edelson, Elizabeth Fee, Jeanne Hahn, Ed Leibson, Penny MacElveen-Hoehn, Helen Marieskind, Robert Massey, Helena Meyer-Knapp, Elizabeth Minnich, Regina Morantz-Sanchez, Ed Morman, Karen Reeds, Jean Richards, David Smith, Hugh Wilder, and Tom Womeldorff. People I regret I did not sufficiently thank while they were alive include Fontaine Belford, David Cogan, Arthur Hertig, Irwin Miller, Esther Rome, and Mildred Selzer. As an independent scholar, some of my most important colleagues have been the many anonymous reviewers who have carefully scrutinized drafts of my published (and unpublished) papers. Janet Bronstein, Cheri Lucas-Jennings, and Camilla Stivers deserve special credit for reading the entire manuscript in draft. I appreciate the Union Institute & University for its service to interdisciplinary scholarship and the help from countless librarians at the American College of Obstetricians and Gynecologists, American Hospital Association, British Medical Association, Countway Library of Medicine, King's Fund, Lane Medical Library at Stanford University, New York Academy of Medicine, Royal College of Obstetricians and Gynaecologists, The Evergreen State College, University of California Berkeley School of Public Health, University of Washington, and the Wellcome Trust. Rutgers University Press science editor Audra Wolfe provided invaluable editorial advice and encouragement. I particularly thank John Perkins for paving the way and a sophomore named Robin who asked if I could be a little more specific.

Abbreviations

ABC	alternative birthing center
ACOG	American College of Obstetricians and Gynecologists
ACS	American College of Surgeons
AHA	American Hospital Association
AHEC	Area Health Education Center
AMA	American Medical Association
AMC	academic medical center
CCMC	Committee on the Costs of Medical Care
COTH	Council on Teaching Hospitals
CQI	continuous quality improvement
DRG	diagnosis related group
ECMO	extracorporeal membrane oxygenation
EFM	electronic fetal monitoring
HMO	health maintenance organization
HSA	health systems agency
ICU	intensive care unit
IPA	independent practice association
IQMS	industrial quality management sciences
JCAHO	Joint Commission on Accreditation of Healthcare Organizations
MRI	magnetic resonance imaging
NBER	National Bureau of Economic Research
NHS	National Health Service (U.K.)
NICU	neonatal intensive care unit

NYAM   New York Academy of Medicine
ob-gyn   obstetrics and gynecology
OBICU   obstetric intensive care unit
OTA   Office of Technology Assessment
PHS   Public Health Service (U.S.)
RMP   regional medical program
TQM   total quality management

The Medical Delivery Business

One

Introduction

Business Models and Medical Interventions

The United States was in an uproar in the late twentieth century over whether medical care was or ought to be a business. The prestigious *New England Journal of Medicine* made the Health Policy Advisory Center's earlier warning about the rise of a "medical-industrial complex" a mainstream concern.[1] Political scientist James Morone advised that medicine was suddenly and rapidly becoming a "corporate enterprise organized and run along business principles."[2] Group practices, promoted for decades as progressive reform, took on a new business identity as health maintenance organizations (HMOs) in what sociologist Donald Light called perhaps the "greatest rhetorical reversal in the history of American health care."[3] HMO and other managed care supporters declared that the cottage industry of medicine was finally having its industrial revolution.[4]

Identifying cottage industry as the problem mandated an industrial and corporate development as the solution. So-called market reformers sought to transform medicine into a "modern corporate system, featuring the sophisticated financial and managerial controls associated with big business."[5] They advised that such a system offered "economies of scale and scope through mass production manufacturing techniques."[6] Critics pugnaciously described the same developments as an "invasion of commerce into medical care" and an "epic clash of cultures between commercial and professional traditions."[7] Medical care did reproduce industrial, corporate, and commercial models of organization, but it was not so sudden. Ray Lyman Wilbur defined medicine as an industry when he was chairman of the 1927–1932 Committee on the Costs of Medical Care (CCMC). The committee defined its purview in terms of reforming the economic organization of medicine, defining it as the "methods of producing and financing" medical services.[8]

What This Book Is All About

In contrast to most historical and policy studies that focus on financial aspects of medical reform, this book investigates the production side of the economic organization of medicine. It is compatible with an approach that historian Louis Galambos called "organizational synthesis."[9] This interdisciplinary method combines scholarship from history and the social sciences to describe how a wide range of social institutions adopted similar forms of economic organization. It allows an integration of individual actions and beliefs with institutional momentum and systemic dynamics as motors of change. Like other organizational synthesis approaches, this book identifies functional specialization and the building of complex production units as significant structural developments in the early part of the twentieth century.[10] In rejecting the hypothesis that doctors at that time looked to business for their organizational strategies, historian Donald Madison held that the "immediate commercial interests of medical practitioners steered them on an opposing course," leading them toward individualistic rather than bureaucratic organization.[11] This patently successful continuation of individual entrepreneurial practice led historian Thomas Goebel to reject the pertinence of organizational synthesis to medicine, even as he acknowledged that the rise of specialties and bureaucratically managed, large-scale institutions "reconfigured American medicine."[12] I specifically address that reconfiguration structurally and clinically.

Conventional medical as well as historical explanations of medical care organization and its therapeutics have assumed that both are driven by scientific and/or technologic development. Two spectacularly successful approaches to fighting disease—immunization and antibiotics—supported a positive view of scientific and technologic progress in medicine. Investigators increasingly questioned, however, the extent to which medicine was a "structure shaped by an inexorable and laudable accretion of scientific insight," as historian Charles Rosenberg put it.[13] Much that twentieth-century medicine had to offer was not nearly so effective as immunization and antibiotics. Experts acknowledged the inadequacy of evidence to support existing intervention levels and that the evidence that was available sometimes contradicted practice patterns. Joseph Califano, former secretary of the U.S. Department of Health, Education, and Welfare, answered "certainly" to his 1988 query, "Is it possible that in this era of high-tech medicine we just don't know with any precision whether many procedures truly affect the medical outcome?"[14] This book examines how widespread use of medical procedures came about in the face of insufficient evidence of their efficacy.

My first thesis proposes that many medical care developments and reforms throughout the twentieth century applied contemporary elements of economic organization to the structure of medical care. In examining this thesis, I use health administration scholar Avedis Donabedian's framework defining structure in terms of characteristics of medical providers, their tools, and their organizational settings.[15] The thesis does not merely draw an analogy between business and medicine; it examines how medical occupations and institutions incorporated elements of business organization into the foundation of medical care. This process created institution-based specialties, academic medical centers, and (somewhat later) multi-hospital regional systems. Medicine did not exactly "escape" the corporation prior to 1965, as Paul Starr maintained in *The Social Transformation of American Medicine,* using the prevalence of organized groups as his measure[16]—medicine *became* the corporation. This first thesis stands alone: medicine did apply business models; the second thesis builds on the first.

My second thesis links the economic organization of medicine to its clinical content, practice, or what Donabedian called "process"—the sets of diagnostic, treatment, and interpersonal interventions that providers use on patients. The business elements built into medical care had a powerful impact on shaping its clinical interventions. Without denying that clinical process development also entailed many other factors, this thesis means that the economic organization of medicine shaped the clinical activities and the theories that we know as twentieth-century medicine. It means that the business elements are not neutral tools that merely enhance efficiency without impinging on medical science itself; rather, the science, the practice, and the business of medicine are intertwined at the most fundamental level. What exactly are these elements, and where did they come from?

Twentieth-Century Economic Order

A new kind of enterprise boomed in the American economy in the late nineteenth and early twentieth centuries, creating organizational changes that some would call a second industrial revolution. This new enterprise changed the workplace, the nature of work, and its products. Its productive features included concentration in large plants, labor specialization, process standardization, monopoly of technology, and professional management.[17] Extending the division of labor of Adam Smith's pin factory, Frederick Winslow Taylor further subdivided and managed labor processes, publishing *The Principles of*

Scientific Management in 1911.[18] Incorporating such a labor division, managers designed production processes to achieve the most efficient and intensive use of their highly capitalized facilities.[19] The assembly line, which added a flow of material to scientific management's task differentiation, grew up in Chicago's slaughterhouses (where they were actually disassembly lines) and came to maturity in Ford Motor Company plants. Corresponding with the new production systems, the new economic order valued uniformity, control, and efficiency.[20] Initially referring to mechanical efficiency, that is, the energy output-input ratio of productive machinery, efficiency came also to mean financial efficiency, or the "output-input ratio of dollars."[21]

The corporation emerged as the major organizational strategy for integrating and managing the new production, its finances, and its markets. Organized into divisions with their own accounts, the corporation applied bureaucratic management methods, centralized financial control, and accumulated capital.[22] The new mass production required mass consumption, which necessitated marketing products on regional and national scales, creating demand, and designing products for their salability in the marketplace.[23] Corporate combines integrated vertically and horizontally, seeking economies of scale and scope as well as control of competition.[24] Their leaders tried to order industries as a whole with regional organization and monopolistic market structures.

These elements of economic organization—scientific management of functional division of labor, assembly line production, corporate organization, horizontal and vertical integration, and regional marketing—formed the business model that spread across the economy. With varying degrees of success over the course of the century, medical leaders and reformers tried to apply the same model to medicine. All of its elements will appear in this book—as professional and institutional accomplishments and as reform strategies. But, first, it is necessary to define my terms and discuss some difficulties in using them. There is no single best term to characterize medicine's model of economic organization, in part because its features changed over time. In addition, existing terms carry disciplinary and philosophical baggage that I do not mean to imply.

Medicine conventionally portrayed its organizational model as *professional,* and scholars contributed to viewing it through the lens of professionalism.[25] Like the critics who perceived a sudden invasion of commerce into medical care, doctors often used the concept of profession as an antithesis of economic organization. They emphasized medicine's service over self-interest and its production of knowledge over commodities. Sociologist Eliot Freidson, however, defined professions as structurally similar to other occupational groups. To Freidson the key difference—an important one—was that professions retained control over their work. He used the term *professional dominance* to refer to medicine's continued control over its division of labor, its skills, its technology, and its "production standards."[26] Assuming an evolutionary development of a corporate model of medicine, Freidson saw professional dominance as a developmental lag for which stronger management was the solution.[27]

Some reformers in the early part of the century called their efforts to organize medical providers *cooperative* and/or *progressive*.[28] The concept of cooperation offered both anti-business and pro-business tactics. To consumers cooperative meant collective ownership and/or collective decision making. To managers cooperation meant workers co-operating machines and scientific management's "integration of differentiated labor."[29] To barons of industry cooperation meant cartel and monopoly. Progressive reform often used the language of cooperation and, for the most part, enacted its forms of business. A common progressive view accepted the rise of big business as an "inevitable product of capitalism's continuous tendency toward the concentration of capital and production into larger and larger units."[30] As part 2 discusses in more detail, progressive reforms tried to mitigate the social upheavals of corporate industrialism, but they also spread its organizational model throughout society.

A number of investigators perceived models of professional organization constituting specialized divisions of labor, teamwork, and managerial hierarchies as "industrial."[31] Freidson accepted an *industrial* organization of professions as the "commonsensical model of what an organization 'really' is."[32] Business school professor Theodore Levitt called functional specialization and professional concentration in managed institutions an "industrialization of service."[33] While noting the power of industrial analogy, historians were apt to dispute the extent to which its forms of organization were actually applied to medical care. Among those accepting some level of application, George Rosen held that medical care organization was "intimately linked" to economic, political, social, and cultural factors.[34] Morris Vogel and David Rosner each demonstrated how hospital administrators in the early part of the century expanded revenue-generating services and adopted other business management techniques.[35] To be sure, methods of business and scientific management were not applied as rigorously in hospitals as in factories,[36] and hospitals' "multifaceted historical mission" also shaped their managerial practices.[37] Rosemary Stevens attributed the popularity of an industrial vision of medicine to the "pervasiveness of industrial imagery in American culture."[38] Stevens concluded, however, that there was "no single trajectory of change."[39] I agree that there was no single trajectory in the sense that scientific and professional models also shaped medicine. In addition, medical care development and reform did not apply the same forms of economic organization over time. But there was a single trajectory in the sense that medical care did selectively apply forms of economic organization prevailing at any one time.

Bureaucratic or *managerial* were other common adjectives describing organizational models in medicine. Organizational theorist Charles Perrow used the term *bureaucratic* to identify the combination of "specialization, formalization, and hierarchy."[40] These elements became accepted early in the century as the "normal human condition," Perrow observed, as they "spread from the factory to the farm, government agency, research lab, hospital, university, and church." Organizational theorists tended to portray bureaucratic features of twentieth-century economic organization as fundamental principles of organization per se, principles that governed the "entire social order."[41] But an earlier edition of *The Principles of Organization*—with "Onward Industry!" in the title—and other works demonstrated that organizational innovators Frederick Winslow Taylor, Chester Barnard, James Mooney, and Alfred Sloan identified and developed the components of the new organization in particular corporations manufacturing particular products.[42] The corporations represented the United States's largest industries: Midvale Steel, American Telephone and Telegraph Company, and General Motors.

Developed within large corporations, some of the organizational components of modern medicine can be called *corporate.* This was the label that the American Medical Association derisively applied to contract medicine in the 1910s and to the forms of group medicine recommended by the Committee on the Costs of Medical Care in the early 1930s. Later leftist critics portrayed medical care development as a progression from entrepreneurial craft work to differentiation of labor, concentration in factory-type institutions, hierarchical management, capital intensification, mass production, and horizontal and vertical integration, some calling this process a "corporatization" of medicine.[43] I describe similar structural developments, but I do not assume that they were necessarily driven by profit or a motive to advance capitalism—although I think both were the case in some instances. Starr also called this kind of organization in both profit and nonprofit hospitals "corporate medicine" but only when it happened later in the century.[44]

Superimposed on similar developments throughout the century, providers and insurance companies further consolidated providers and expanded managerial processes in the 1980s and 1990s. They called the whole package "market reform." To justify this somewhat contradictory use of the term *market,* leaders attributed the bureaucratic growth and vertical and horizontal integration in medicine as well as in industry to strategic adaptations to the market.[45] Most market reformers at the end of the century, however, did not really mean a laissez-faire market. They were actively engaged in rationalizing medical care as industry. In so doing, they consolidated and managed hospitals, organized regional markets, integrated production with finance, mobilized capital, and promulgated professional as well as governmental regulation.

Twentieth-century models of medical organization can also be called *capitalist,* the label with the most baggage of all. Medical care did to a certain extent employ organizational elements that economist Robert Heilbroner as well as business school professor Thomas McCraw identified as characteristics of capitalism. These elements included division of tasks according to a tiered labor structure, factory-like institutions, accumulation of fixed capital, and market regulation of production and distribution.[46] (Partially) excluding the role of the market, however, these elements also developed in what was called socialist medicine both in Britain and in the Soviet Union. The other important distinction was that these countries removed medical care from the private, investor-profit system. The term *capitalist* in the sense of being dominated by finance capital was particularly pertinent in the United States at the end of the century, when insurance and finance companies tried to restructure medical care as a rewarding place to invest capital. The financial restructuring of that time was said to have transferred billions of dollars from providing medicine to the wallets of investors and executive management teams.[47]

There is obviously considerable overlap in the features I have identified as progressive, industrial, bureaucratic, managerial, corporate, market, and capitalist. Each term represents a wide complexity of organizational forms, processes, and motives, and any choice among them is bound to oversimplify. I have chosen *business* as the most generally applicable term. Historian Thomas Cochran grappled with the same dilemma and made the same choice in *The American Business System.*[48] A 1998 book identified market development, capacity consolidation, service integration, risk assumption, and clinical process industrialization as key factors in *The Business of Health Care.*[49] Within what I am calling a business model, I identify production elements as industrial, their administration as managerial, their funding as financial, and their overall organization as corporate. Finally, I conform to the terminology of the 1980s and 1990s in identifying the changes of those times as market-oriented reforms.

My naming choices for my thesis that medicine adopted forms of economic organization are solely descriptive; in calling structural elements business, industrial, or corporate, I am trying to identify the nature of medical care components, not attribute their cause. I do not reify the terms by using them as economic, social, or historical "forces" that determine certain developments. While I agree with Marxist scholar Vicente Navarro that models of production and distribution in medicine—including specialization and concentration—replicated characteristics of capitalist industry, I am not using his argument that this replication was necessarily determined by capitalist economic development.[50] Nor do I accept the capitalist version of necessary stages of development.[51] Not accepting a determinist development of medical care organization leaves room for the possibility of fundamental structural reform—although it does not make such reform more feasible politically.

Supporters as well as critics of reforms at the end of the century tended to single out profit making as the crucial characteristic of business, capitalist, or market models of medicine. Profit was far from new to medicine at that time, however. Private physician practices, proprietary hospitals, and the pharmaceutical, insurance, and supply industries had always been for-profit. Profit making did loom larger, to be sure, when previously nonprofit hospitals and Blue Cross health insurance plans "converted" to for-profit status. Yet, contrary to market economic theory, I do not infer that financial self-interest necessarily drove either individual or institutional behavior. Although profit incentives did have an impact in medical care, they do not sufficiently explain its professional or institutional developments or its clinical activities. Most hospitals and physicians were committed to developing their services and their interventions as science, as service, and as progress. I am questioning the validity of these assumptions, not the beneficence of their intentions. Irrespective of intentions, however, the business elements in medical care had clinical consequences.

Excessive Procedures and Inappropriate Practice Patterns

Although the dominant policy issue had long been paying for (and not paying for) health care, consumers and corporate purchasers at the end of the century were finally asking what they were actually paying for. Closely related to their functional divisions of labor and institutional developments, many acute care specialties—followed by their subspecialties—concentrated their clinical work on the performance of technological and surgical procedures. Specialists had faith in these procedures and took pride in how well they could perform them. Their procedural emphasis was also consistent however, with an end-of-the-century view that the U.S. health care system had evolved "to deliver line-item, billable medical services."[52] The annual market basket of surgical and technological procedures in the mid-1990s included seven million MRI examinations, nearly a million and a half cardiac catheterizations, and over a half-million (each) of coronary artery bypass grafts, hysterectomies, and gall bladder removals.[53]

But what did these numbers mean in terms of people's health? Were these procedures the best way to spend so many billions of health care dollars? For much of the century the medical profession assumed that its scientific knowledge about the body and about disease had driven its use of procedures. Patients also generally accepted the procedures, assuming that they had been scientifically validated. But for many procedures this assumption simply was not true. The deputy director of the Rockefeller Foundation estimated that only 10–20 percent of all clinical interventions used in 1980 were based on demonstrated efficacy and safety.[54] Although medicine had competed with other healing professions on the grounds that it alone was scientific, it had neglected to apply the scientific method to evaluating its own work.

Ernest Amory Codman was a significant and early exception to the neglect of clinical evaluation. He made the radical proposal in 1914 that the hospital standardization movement look into whether patients lived or died after hospital discharge.[55] But the standardization movement quickly came to focus on structure rather than outcome. Excoriated by his colleagues and forced to leave his position at the Massachusetts General Hospital, Codman was rehabilitated by evidence-based medicine in the 1990s. The remarkable and rather appalling implication of the popularity of evidence-based medicine at that time was the extent to which medicine throughout the century had not been evidence-based.

After Codman, accusations of excessive procedures and unnecessary surgery rumbled within the profession, albeit at a low level. By the last third of the century it was accepted in some medical as well as planning and payer circles that the use of many medical procedures vastly exceeded scientific evidence of their benefit. While recognizing that many procedures did offer life-enhancing intervention under certain circumstances, patients, purchasers, managers, and researchers were increasingly questioning the nature of and the necessity for medical procedures. Califano charged in 1988 that at least 60 percent and perhaps as many as 80 percent of all coronary artery bypass graft operations, over 50 percent of cardiac pacemaker implants, and at least 50 percent of cesarean sections performed in the United States were unnecessary.[56] Researchers estimated that the money spent on excessive procedures equaled or exceeded 20 percent of the national medical care bill.[57] At the end of the century feminist scholars identified overuse of "costly, ineffective technologies" to be a continuing problem.[58] Citing international data demonstrating higher mortality rates along with the higher intervention rates in the United States, payers and other reformers made evidence-based medicine a national policy issue.

From my experiences in medical research, the women's health movement, and health planning, I welcomed evidence-based medicine. I see the growth in surgical and technologic intervention without adequate supporting evidence as bad medicine. It is difficult to distinguish the good that medicine does for some people from the erroneous, the unnecessary, and the frivolous. I also recognize that excessive intervention is in large part a middle- and upper-class issue. The other side of the (same) coin is a seriously inequitable access to medical care and inadequate intervention levels for some populations. Excessive procedures siphoned off resources that could have (which isn't to say they would have) gone to improving equity, fostering caring, and developing less intensive, less invasive, and less costly interventions. Perinatal medicine became a favorite target for accusations of inappropriate medical intervention.

Connections between Organization and Practice: Perinatal Medicine

From sharing personal experiences as well as information from the childbirth movement, members of the *Our Bodies, Ourselves* group came to recognize that we were putting up with weeks of pain and disability from the incisions of episiotomies that may not have contributed anything to our health or that of our babies. The International Childbirth Education Association subsequently published Doris Haire's *The Cultural Warping of Childbirth,* which documented her charge of inadequate evidence to support much of the routine technological intervention practiced in birth at the time.[59] On the heels of the Haire report, feminist activists and academics continued to challenge birth intervention in books with titles such as *Forced Labor, Immaculate Deception,* and *Alternatives to Medical Control.*[60]

The U.S. Senate and the U.S. General Accounting Office then got into the act, making unnecessary birth intervention an overt political issue.[61] Senator Edward M. Kennedy charged at his 1978 Senate hearing that technology was used in obstetrics as in other areas of medicine far beyond any scientific assessment of it. Haire more forcefully testified that the "aggressive practices which have become routine in most American obstetric care have made childbirth a traumatic event, often detrimental and, at time, destructive for both the mother and her infant."[62]

My participation in the *Our Bodies, Ourselves* group was the first but by no means the last time I was to witness the dawning outrage among women—including obstetric nurses—as they found out for themselves that routine birth intervention was not necessary or beneficial. The women's health and childbirth movements contributed significantly to growing skepticism concerning medical intervention in general. Ironically dependent on medicine's own research, questioners were repeatedly astounded at the lack of available evidence to defend prevailing obstetrical practices and beliefs. They frequently became more knowledgeable about the perinatal effectiveness literature (and its deficits) than many practicing obstetricians.[63] The first systematic medical approach to assessing perinatal efficacy was obstetrician Iain Chalmers's work in Britain's National Perinatal Epidemiology Unit. The unit's studies and re-search analyses empirically demonstrated the inadequacy of evidentiary sup-port for many routine perinatal practices. Chalmers's work supported the critics' accusations that birth intervention levels were excessive (although to different degrees) both in Britain and in the United States.[64] But growing pro-fessional recognition of the lack of evidence did not necessarily change clini-cal practices or even attitudes about them.

In their outrage about medical practices birthing women often expressed fear and concern about a lack of control over what was happening to their bod-ies. Some of this lack of control, of course, was due to the nature of the bio-logical process of childbirth itself. But much of it was also due to physician attitudes and hospital rules. One obstetrics chief pronounced it "simply inap-propriate for lay people to dictate the modalities and circumstances under which they receive *medical* care."[65] Doctors use the term *modality* to refer to a type of diagnostic or therapeutic intervention; the term distinguishes surgical, me-chanical, chemical, and psychological treatments. Doctors use the term also to maintain medical mystique and authority. One obstetrician even called sexual intercourse a medical modality when he suggested it as a potential means of initiating labor past the due date.

Pointing to controlling obstetricians, the women's health movement theo-rized that male dominance drove inappropriate birth intervention. Feminist activists and scholars blamed excessive intervention in birth on patriarchal doctors and/or patriarchal systems and continued to do so up to the end of the century. But British sociologist Sally Macintyre had cautioned both sup-porters and critics of birth intervention against oversimplified analyses that supported their own paradigms.[66] Although dominance (gender and profes-sional) does play an important role in patient-doctor relationships and there-fore has a strong impact on personal birth experiences, it does not sufficiently explain medical practices.

A generation after the publication of *Our Bodies, Ourselves,* women like Naomi Wolf in *Misconceptions* were still voicing outrage about their high-tech childbirth experiences.[67] Women were still telling birthing stories that "pro-viders exerted control through the application of various procedures," and they were still asking to be "partners in the process of giving birth."[68] They were still asking whether their suffering from the pain of episiotomy and cesarean section incisions was necessary.[69] They still emphasized that, while they per-sonally sought a more satisfactory birth experience, their babies' health was paramount. Social scientists interviewing women over the decades found a wide consensus against excessive intervention in birth.[70] The vote was not unani-mous, however. From her sample (and disagreeing with it) interviewer Robbie

Davis-Floyd concluded that "American women do not rise up in protest against technocratic birth because it is in fact what most of them want."[71]

Whether or not most women wanted it, intensive medical intervention remained part of the birth experience of four million American women (and babies) a year in the 1980s and 1990s. Although different procedures waxed and waned at different times, at least one was always classified as standard procedure. The annual perinatal market basket in the mid-1990s included a million and a half episiotomies, over a million neonatal circumcisions, and close to a million cesarean sections.[72] Put another way, for every 100 live births in the year 2000 there were 84 electronic fetal monitoring procedures, 67 ultra-sounds, 26 episiotomies, 23 cesarean sections, 20 labor inductions, 18 labor accelerations, and 7 vacuum or forceps extractions.[73] Birth intervention crit-ics at that time claimed that the emperor was still scantily dressed and that a large gap remained between evidence of efficacy and intervention practices in perinatal medicine.[74]

With potential consequences for the health of every person in the nation, perinatal medicine—obstetric and pediatric services delivered to women and infants "around birth"—offers an excellent perspective on interactions between the business model of medicine and its practices. Reasonably accurate data are available concerning nearly every birth, providing an all-important population-based denominator not available in other specialty areas for determining in-tervention and outcome rates as well as disease incidence. Low-birthweight and mortality rates provide outcome measures across a range of population and geographic scales. While the U.S. infant mortality rate declined continu-ously after the mid-1930s, its international ranking fell from third in 1950 to twentieth in 1964, plateauing at that level until the 1990s, when it sank to twenty-sixth in 1996.[75] The United States's low international ranking exposed a "peri-natal paradox," which family medicine professor Roger Rosenblatt defined as "doing more and accomplishing less."[76]

Constituting a large sector of the U.S. health care system, perinatal medi-cine was an industry in its own right. It accounted for around one-quarter of all hospital admissions for much of the century (and that was not counting the babies). Maternity care played a significant role in keeping underutilized, and perhaps superfluous, hospitals operating. Normal delivery remained the num-ber one reason for hospitalization at the end of the century.[77] This was doubly ironic in light of the childbirth movement's failure to move normal birth out of the hospital, when highly invasive procedures such as cardiac catheteriza-tion did shift to outpatient settings. In the late 1980s perinatal care cost—or generated revenues of, depending on one's perspective—nearly $30 billion a year. This averaged out at $7,000 per birth.[78] By 1993 the national expenditure on pregnancy, birth, and neonatal care was $40 billion, or around $10,000 per birth.[79] The $40 billion figure compared with $49 billion spent on all cancer treatments and $80 billion spent on treating cardiovascular diseases, the major causes of death. Obstetric procedures and neonatal intensive care accounted for large portions of the perinatal costs.

My study of perinatal medicine fills in some of the details for women's health scholar Sheryl Burt Ruzek's proposed connection between birth intervention and the academic, social, and economic organization of the health care industry.[80] It investigates how business models of medical organization contributed to birth intervention practices and patterns. Gender discrimination, one of the key alternative interpretations, may explain why many investigators deemed the study of perinatal care less important than other medical areas better than it explains its interventions. There remained a notable sex bifurcation at professional meetings: perinatal sessions were attended primarily by women, and medical economics sessions were attended primarily by men. In using perinatal care to exemplify connections between medical intervention and economic organization, I am challenging feminists to take business models seriously and mainstream investigators to take the health of women and children seriously. We cannot fundamentally reform childbirth practices without changing the business model of medicine, and we may not be able to do this without women's participation.

Outline of the Book

The chapters in this book weave together threads of different colors and textures. The thread representing the various forms of economic organization provides the framework for every chapter. The thread that connects the organizational forms of medicine with its clinical practices appears in selected chapters. While the organizational threads pertain to specialty medicine in general, the clinical connections draw from the perinatal specialties in particular. The weaving process selects strands from different times during the twentieth century and from two levels of organization, the institutional and the systemic.

The book is divided into three parts. Part 1 examines organizational and clinical impacts of the economic organization of hospital specialty departments, particularly academic ones, in the early decades of the century. Although an economic model of production was only partly assimilated in medical care at the time, certain of its elements formed the fundamental structure of twentieth-century specialty medicine and played an important role in shaping its therapeutics.

Chapter 2 investigates the adaptation of a Tayloristic type of scientific management in medicine. Clinical departments in the grand new academic medical centers built the framework for a functional division of labor in medical care and provided the necessary managerial structure for coordinating the divided tasks. This form of organization enhanced the hospitals' revenue-generating capabilities. Its fragmentation of tasks reconfigured the work of doctors and nurses and required a multiplicity of ancillary and managerial staff working in a form of group practice. Some leaders described their new departments in industrial terms, although most saw them as scientific and/or professional models of organization.

Studying this scientific management–like departmental development in a particular specialty, chapter 3 explores how obstetrics and gynecology developed and managed its own functional division of labor. Its academic departments divided medical as well as childbirth labor into a sequence of technical procedures performed in a sequence of work stations, reminiscent of factory assembly lines. These divisions shaped the specialty's clinical practices and its clinical paradigms, as did its market-oriented stratification of services. Obstetric leaders frequently accused their profession of unnecessary intervention in birth, but they used their concerns to denigrate their competition and to further their institution building, rather than to question it.

The massive specialty department growth and the costs engendered prompted reform efforts to rationalize the medical system as a whole. Part 2 shifts the level of investigation from specialties and hospitals to hospital delivery systems. Bridging the first and last thirds of the century, it examines how the progressive reforms of the Committee on the Costs of Medical Care, national health planning, and perinatal regionalization tried to impose system-wide forms of corporate and industrial organization in the hope of controlling competition and rendering medical care more cost-efficient.

The privately funded 1927–1932 Committee on the Costs of Medical Care identified its high cost as the major problem in medical care and reform of its economic organization as the major solution. Chapter 4 describes how the committee tried to apply forms of financial management and other business strategies to medical care, seeking to organize hospital-based specialists in groups operated along business lines. Calling the proposed organizational forms and managerial methods a corporate practice of medicine, an American Medical Association–oriented minority dissented from the final report in favor of conserving individual entrepreneurial practice. Although commonly perceived as a failure, the CCMC's proposals for a national payment system and group organization of doctors and hospitals set the progressive reform agenda for the remainder of the century.

Illustrating how later reforms reiterated CCMC strategies, chapter 5 examines how national health planning starting in the mid-1960s encouraged business organization of medical delivery. Regional health planning and its regionalization strategy extended functional division of labor to the institutional level, differentiating hospitals by levels of specialization and technologic intensity. Harkening back to Britain's 1920 Dawson report, the levels system conferred competitive advantages on the larger, usually academic, medical centers at the apex of the organizational pyramid. Regionalization designated the geographic regions surrounding the highest-level providers as the market areas for organized delivery systems. Its institutional differentiation required managerial reintegration, and its system-wide planning and regulation endeavored to control capital investment and resource allocation.

Dominating the maternal and infant health care reform agenda in the time of planning, perinatal regionalization duplicated planning's strategies of regional organization. Chapter 6 examines how academic subspecialists in pediatrics as well as in obstetrics and gynecology sought to differentiate levels of care, consolidate services, allocate markets, and manage the resulting systems. In the context of growing academic practice plans, perinatal regionalization inflated tertiary care at the expense of primary care. Despite the fact that it missed its potential for developing perinatal systems based on population needs, by the end of the century regionalization became the worldwide vision of perinatal reform.

Perinatal regionalization built on and evolved alongside of developments in the economic organization of specialties and institutions. Moving the focus back to this level, part 3 examines the economic production of childbirth in the final third of the century. The three chapters in this part describe in turn the impact of specialty competition, intensive care, and managed care on perinatal therapeutics.

After summarizing specialty growth in the middle decades of the century, chapter 7 examines the effect of growing competition among obstetrics, family medicine, and midwifery on birth intervention. Obstetricians used their surgical and technologic procedures to compete with family physicians, midwives, and independent birth centers for the nation's finite number of births. This competition shaped physicians' and midwives' practice patterns as well as their birth paradigms. The great cesarean section boom of the 1970s and 1980s was linked to this professional and institutional competition, although it entailed a multiplicity of other factors, including the development of intensive care.

Chapter 8 describes how neonatal and obstetric intensive care units constituted the framework of perinatal regionalization. The new units built in new levels of professional and institutional division of labor and led to new levels of interventional intensity. Obstetric subspecialists reconstructed the labor and delivery unit as an intensive care modality by embedding electronic fetal monitoring and other technologies in its structure and function. Inflating capital as well as interventional intensity, these intensive care units served as strategic business units for their institutions and practice plans. Their competitive growth led to excessive use of intensive care technologies on birthing women and their babies.

Managed care strategies of the 1990s offered ways to reduce some of the excesses of the 1970s and 1980s, although not necessarily in consonance with measured health needs. Combining corporate organization with financial management, managed care epitomized a business model of medicine. Chapter 9 discusses how providers and insurance companies imposed industrial quality control methods to streamline clinical processes in birth and enhance its productivity and revenues. Obstetrics departments developed protocols that programmed the use of oxytocin to reduce cesarean section rates and the length of labor. Originating in Ireland, this strategy of active management of labor owed its growth to its close fit with hierarchic divisions of labor, department-based accounting, and industrial control methods under Britain's National Health Service and managed care in the United States.

Chapter 10 discusses implications of the book for health care reform. It raises ethical issues concerning the business model of medicine, describing how this approach warped ethical theory itself. It insists that it is necessary to re-form medical structures as well as reform itself to create a health care system that can use medical interventions appropriately. Such reform must continuously strive to restructure medicine according to the best available scientific evidence of efficacy. The discussion sketches possibilities for constructing a perinatal system based on meeting needs, emphasizing the necessity for developing new forms of democratic process in order to build it.

As we construct twenty-first-century health care, it is necessary to analyze twentieth-century structures and their (mal)functions. Well-intentioned planners and reformers often promoted medical care structures that could *not* meet their goals of equitable and appropriate care, but they hadn't analyzed them carefully enough to see this. Digging to the roots of the problems requires re-evaluating the organization and the work of medicine. It also requires scrutinizing the benefits and the beneficence of transferring organizational forms from the economy to medicine. As my contribution to these endeavors, I examine selected developments in the economic organization of medicine and how they shaped its content and theory. I hope the book contributes to a better understanding of how twentieth-century American medicine worked and didn't work.

Part I
Medical Specialism and Early-Twentieth-Century Economic Organization

Specialization in medicine, as in other domains, is an effective means by which the results of a given amount of work can be increased. By subdivision of tasks, operations that are easier in themselves result; by repetition of tasks, operations come to be performed with greater ease.
—Lewellys F. Barker, MD, 1922

Two

Academic Specialty Departments and Scientific Management

Hospital-based specialism, the pride and the foundation of twentieth-century American medicine, ironically became one of its major problems. Its development built in contemporary forms of economic organization, and these organizational forms had clinical impact. Scientific management and its pattern of specialization promoted efficiency and productivity in industry and equated both with scientific as well as economic progress.[1] They offered not only a new production method in the early decades of the century but also the ideology for a new economic order. To various degrees medical specialties professionalized on the basis of scientific management's division of labor and built hospital departments that provided the framework for it. Medical and business leaders consolidated medical schools, hospitals, and clinics, expanding them in size and complexity and thus creating a new kind of institution: the academic medical center. Specialization in these centers entailed a functional division of labor that fragmented medical work into a set of procedures performed by a range of personnel. This form of specialization and the management required to coordinate it transformed the work of doctors and nurses and led to a multiplicity of auxiliary hospital staff. Built in the name of efficiency, and perhaps making specialists more efficient, this division of labor did not make total health care more efficient. Developed only partially within medical care at this time, the business model profoundly shaped its structure and function for the remainder of the century.

Institution-Based Specialism

Medical leaders as well as historians conventionally identified specialism as scientific in nature, attributing it to an explosion in scientific and/or technical knowledge. Scientific knowledge was certainly expanding at the time, but much of it was generated by specialists practicing with their selected technologies.[2] The nascent specialty of radiology, for example, professionalized around the clinical use of X-ray machines and in so doing developed expertise in X-ray shadows of the body's internal structures. But other factors shaped specialization in addition to science and technology. In his classic study of ophthalmology George Rosen concluded that specialization resulted "at least as much" from social and economic factors as from scientific ones.[3] "Science and technology are not independent constructs that 'cause' scientific subdivision," Rosemary Stevens pointed out; "rather, they are embedded in a social process that may be driven by multiple personal, economic, and organizational agendas."[4]

Medical specialization entailed horizontal and vertical divisions of labor, both of which incorporated forms of economic organization. Horizontal division partitioned medicine by organs, diseases, technical procedures, and populations. This division was facilitated by anatomic concepts of disease specificity, but the cause and effect worked both ways; divvying up the body among specialists also reinforced anatomic concepts. "Instead of being an inevitable consequence of the human body's anatomy and physiology," physician-historian Joel Howell held, specialization was "forged by individuals and organizations to promote their specific interests, at particular times, in particular places, and in response to particular problems."[5]

Horizontal specialization is consistent with sociological views of professionalization as a competitive process in which service providers define their distinctive commodities and create markets for them.[6] This view of professionalism describes medicine's strategies to control entry, standardize production, produce distinctive products, eliminate competing products and producers, enhance demand, and engage in political activity to achieve and maintain these accomplishments.[7] In banning public identification of specialists as a form of advertising in the nineteenth century, the American Medical Association (AMA) acknowledged specialism's market potential.[8] With this restriction lifted in the twentieth century, specialties specifically engaged in market-oriented professional development, and the expanding urban middle-class population responded to their efforts. Pediatrics, for example, was both "status and market-driven," grounded in large part in providing well-child examinations to middle-class families.[9] Rehabilitation specialists also used monopoly over their knowledge and skills to organize their markets.[10] The specialty of obstetrics and gynecology (ob-gyn) developed different levels of care for different markets, as described in chapter 3.

Superimposed on the market-based horizontal specialization, which did not require an institutional base, a vertical division of labor fragmented hospital care into a sequence of discrete procedures assigned to a hierarchy of personnel. This division of labor was consistent with Frederick Winslow Taylor's scientific management. Based on features of "minute specialization," "rigid hierarchy," and "absolute control," scientific management controlled work and the worker.[11] Taylor's subdivision of production into component operations replicated the division of labor in Adam Smith's well-known pin factory. It analyzed elements of the work process, systematically subdivided it into standardized tasks, and assigned the separate tasks to separate workers.[12] Functional division of labor in medicine similarly divided clinical work into discrete procedures and portioned them out to different levels of personnel, primarily residents, interns, and medical students. This type of specialization was sometimes called "technical," and it often incorporated technology, but it neither required nor was determined by it. Pointedly referring to Adam Smith's pin makers, 1937 AMA president Charles Gordon Heyd credited increased productivity in medicine to specialist repetition of action and economy of labor.[13]

Scholars have varied in their (dis)agreement with Heyd's comparison of medical and industrial specialization. Rosen averred in the early 1940s that, although the view that equated division of labor with progress contributed to specialism's acceptance, functional subdivision did not apply to medicine, in which specialization occurred on a simpler level.[14] Twenty-five years later sociologist Eliot Freidson accepted functional division of labor in medical specialization as real as well as desirable. He named hierarchy and task differentiation as "essential attributes of formal organization…no less requisite for the production of health services by 'professionals' than for the production of material goods by 'workers.'"[15] Building on Freidson's work on professional autonomy but differing with him on division of labor, sociologist Paul Starr maintained that medicine's specialization was distinct from industry's because physicians themselves divided the labor and did not yield control of their work to management.[16] It is not that specialist division of labor was economic rather than professional in nature but that the concept of profession itself incorporated economic characteristics. Both horizontal and vertical divisions of labor in medicine were consistent with ongoing professionalization efforts, which contributed to their acceptance. Horizontal specialization allowed physicians to control their markets, and vertical specialization allowed them to control their work, their work organization, and their institutions.

The medical profession also held mixed opinions about specialization as a form of economic organization. Medical educator John Morgan wrote in 1765 that organization in the medical school and the division of medical practice "derived from the principle of division of function,"[17] although he was referring to the horizontal division of labor of his time. With the exception of Henry I. Bowditch of Harvard, members of the 1866 AMA Committee of Medical Ethics on Specialties repudiated the possibility of functional division of labor in medicine.[18] A Connecticut medical society speaker at the same time accepted its reality but rejected its desirability as a "perversion of the principle that justifies the subdivision of labor in the mechanical arts."[19] By the early twentieth century, however, growing numbers of academic leaders explicitly and favorably compared medical specialization with functional division of labor in industry. It was not that their business concepts overrode their scientific ones; many of them thought they were just superimposing order and efficiency on science-driven elements. Nor did the business view represent average medical thought at the time. Nevertheless, whether they perceived their organizational models in terms of business, science, or profession, they did apply elements of economic organization.

Former Johns Hopkins's dean William H. Welch saw subdivision of labor as necessary to both material and scientific advancement.[20] Recognizing that "the watchmaker no longer makes a complete watch or the shoemaker a complete shoe," a former Tufts medical school dean noted in 1906 that industrial subdivision manifested itself in the medical profession.[21] Even the more intellectual work of diagnosis could be compared with industrial production. As summarized by a 1915 Executive Committee report from the Massachusetts General Hospital, "modern scientific diagnosis is not so much *made* by one man as *assembled* like the parts of a machine, each part being made separately by a man specially skilled through practice in that one thing."[22] Although he assured the Sociological Section of the American Public Health Association that "shoemaking and doctoring are not seriously to be compared," Michael Davis, energetic reformer over the next several decades, did compare them.[23] Known for bringing scientific management and "modern principles of business efficiency" to the Boston Dispensary,[24] Davis described medical specialization in hospitals and clinics as a process of splitting work into pieces and separating them by function.[25]

As president of the American Urological Association in 1911, Hugh Cabot (of the Boston Cabots) also promoted functional specialization—although he bemoaned the amount of time the surgical assistant had to spend "with his eye glued to the butt of a cystoscope."[26] Cabot would call specialization a translation of the subdivision of labor from the industrial revolution.[27] Massachusetts General Hospital's Richard Cabot (Hugh's brother) also promoted "subdivisions of labor and specialization of function" in medicine, which he called characteristics of industry.[28] Both Cabots believed that medicine should be a "controlled monopoly" and that "salaried cooperative team work" provided a remedy for the competition of private practice.[29] Calling the dispensary an "economic and honest organization of medical industry," Richard Cabot advised that it represented a "powerful weapon against the evils and anachronisms of private [individualistic] practice."[30] With statements like this, the Cabots outraged many practicing physicians and came to be characterized as iconoclasts. The Cabots were indeed engaged in breaking down icons, but their initiatives were to become the major ideas for structural reform for the remainder of the century.

Lewellys Barker, hardly an iconoclast, was perhaps the clearest and most provocative advocate of an industrial model of specialism—although he saw specialism as scientific and technologic as well. In 1900 Barker, who would succeed William Osler as professor of medicine at Johns Hopkins University five years later, connected development in the specialties of ophthalmology, laryngology, and gynecology with their respective claims over the ophthalmoscope, the laryngoscope, and the speculum.[31] Barker attributed medical progress in internal medicine in part to scientific analyses that broke vital processes down into physical and chemical components, and he established research laboratories in his department to conduct such analyses.[32] These laboratories and their accumulation of data conferred on specialties a scientific identity.[33] Barker also advised that the complexity of medical work demanded a certain "division of labor," expanding the phrase in 1911 to "functional division of labor in the clinic."[34] To Barker specialization within internal medicine as well as other areas meant a systematic division of labor in diagnosis and treatment and its coordination in an institutional setting. This description was consistent with developments in academic medicine, and, like the Cabots, he called it "group medicine."

Barker explicitly recommended scientifically managing academic clinical departments, citing Frederick Winslow Taylor's 1911 book the year it came out.[35] He maintained that functional division of labor was necessary to increase medical productivity, as his description heading part 1 demonstrates. Medical task subdivisions, he held in 1922, "represent simpler units that in turn are further subdivisible into certain processes that can be finally resolved into still simpler constituent operations."[36] Such a specialty division of labor, Barker championed in the same article, increased "accuracy, speed and skill" and could be "almost as valuable for medicine and surgery as it has proved to be for commerce and industry." He described this form of medicine as "'large-scale production' of medical services." But organization and management were necessary to alleviate the "dangers" of specialization, which he named (among others) as "arrogance," "monotony of the 'piece worker,'" "objectionable aggressiveness," "stubborn opinionatedness," "boastful self-sufficiency," and "selfish materialism."[37] Echoing a principle of scientific management, Barker's paper described specialization as a "distribution of tasks in such a way that each physician may do the kind of work for which he is best fitted." Taylor himself affirmed that organized surgical practice provided an excellent example of the "modern subdivision of labor."[38] He told a U.S. congressional committee that the Mayo Clinic, with its coordinated teams of specialists, offered the "only complete and successful scientific management" that he knew.[39]

It was the teaching hospital more than the Mayo Clinic, however, that provided the model for specialization inherent in the hospital standardization program. Academic surgical leaders established the American College of Surgeons (ACS) and initiated its 1917 standardization efforts with financial support from the Carnegie Corporation.[40] They took on the role of defining requirements for hospital facilities, equipment, and their departmental organization.[41] Consistent with the economic organization and progressive reforms of the time, medical leaders accepted the standardization movement as a strategy designed to emulate "modern industrial organization."[42] An obstetrician participating in the standardization process approvingly compared it to methods of efficiency engineers in large industrial plants.[43] Concepts of scientific management were "imbedded in the background of hospital standardization," a health services administration professor later noted.[44]

Following the beginning of the standardization movement by a decade, the Committee on the Costs of Medical Care (CCMC), chaired by Ray Lyman Wilbur, assumed an industrial model of specialism in its studies of medical care payment and organization. With Lewellys Barker and Michael Davis among the instigators of the project, CCMC reports accepted specialty divisions of labor in an institutional context as desirable and inevitable both scientifically and economically. The committee's *The Costs of Medical Care* credited group medicine with coordinating specialty organization. *Costs* recognized a "horizontal" specialization in which physicians of equal training restricted their range of practice. As *The Incomes of Physicians* further noted, horizontal specialization was based on the "same economic principles and forces which give rise to trademarks and labels in commercial enterprises," creating what was "technically known as monopoly value in an otherwise competitive field."[45] *Costs* also recognized a "vertical" specialization in which physicians assigned routine tasks to subordinates. It identified this division of labor as characteristic of "large-scale production as exemplified in modern industry."[46] In vertical division, *Costs* observed, the physician performed the "special services which only he is equipped to render."[47]

Concepts of scientific management became conflated with those of science, in itself contributing to their legitimacy.[48] Industrial engineer and future CCMC member Morris Llewellyn Cooke, known for extending scientific management to a wide range of social institutions, called scientific management the "science of human labor."[49] He credited science in industrial process with providing a "measure of order, of definition, of standardization and of control."[50] Barker himself did not give up his views of specialism as consonant with science and technology; he superimposed on them a view of medical science as consonant with scientific management. He knew that scientific management subdivided work into measurable and manageable units, and he promoted an analytic method that subdivided the body into measurable (and presumably manageable) units as the basis of scientific diagnosis and treatment. Like his contemporaries, he held mechanistic concepts of the body consistent with his work organization.[51] In "The Unveiling of the Cell" he broke down vital processes into constituent parts and explained cell function as the "harmonious co-operation of certain ultimate units in the cell . . . [that] work together like the parts of a machine."[52] This concept of the cell continued a historical conjunction of division of labor in scientific process with mechanistic concepts of the body.[53]

Many physicians undoubtedly meant their positive and negative comparisons of medicine with industry as analogies or rhetorical devices. Progressive ideology and popular imagery of the time assimilated economic concepts of efficiency from industrial production and its scientific management.[54] But efficiency had material meaning; it entailed functional specialization and central coordination.[55] The concept of efficiency also had many meanings in medical care.[56] Michael Davis used it to challenge medicine's "fundamental structural and financial features."[57] Vertical division of labor was the structure of scientific management, efficiency its ideology. This division of labor required an institutional base; it coevolved with institution-based specialty departments.

Specialty-Based Institutions

Columbia-Presbyterian materialized its founders' visions of a great medical center in New York City by consolidating Presbyterian Hospital, the Vanderbilt Clinic, and the Sloane Maternity Hospital with Columbia University's medical school.[58] Abraham Flexner's well-known 1910 report to the Carnegie Foundation planned a nationwide network of such centers.[59] Reinforced by the example of industrial consolidation and financed by an outpouring of public and private funding following the Flexner report, medical schools integrated teaching units with hospitals and clinics. In the process they invented the specialty-based academic medical center. After building the grand St. Louis railroad station, lumber magnate Robert S. Brookings envisioned a grand regional medical center at Washington University.[60] At the end of the exuberant 1920s (and terminating with the Depression) hospital journals were brimming with photographs and blueprints of multimillion dollar "medical teaching plants," fully equipped with specialty technologies.[61] In parallel with the biomedical paradigm of disease specificity, the architecture of these hospitals expressed scientific management's "efficiency and functionalism."[62] Representing an elite among hospitals, these burgeoning academic medical centers were to have a far-ranging impact on medical care development. Teaching hospitals already dominated hospital care, accounting for 66 percent of the total bed supply and 60 percent of the total capital investment in hospitals by 1929.[63]

Specialty departments in the new academic centers were developing a form of group medicine.[64] Barker described institution-based specialism as consistent with the "general tendency toward association and co-operation in modern society."[65] He felt that such a group organization was necessary to synthesize clinical information into a "well-proportioned view of the patient's total physical, mental and social status." Arguably, such a vision never developed in any setting. Davis, the Cabots, and Barker accepted vertical specialization only on the condition that organizational structures and managerial processes exist to recombine the fragmented tasks and integrate the separated workers. Medical policy leaders frequently described such specialty group organization in industrial as well as educational terms. "In medicine, as in industry," Michael Davis wrote with Andrew Warner (who would become executive secretary of the American Hospital Association), specialists working in institutions offered the most efficient and profitable organization.[66] Harry H. Moore, economist and future lead staff for the Committee on the Costs of Medical Care, defined the necessary medical organization as a "systematic union of individuals, machinery, and techniques into a body or unit agency whose members work together for the economical production of goods or services."[67] Moore's description became the CCMC's vision of group medicine. Hugh Cabot similarly described the medical group as a "conglomeration of specialists" made up of departmental chiefs and their "necessary subordinates," and he advised that such a group organization could enhance specialist efficiency. Cabot attributed his preference for group medicine to his "abiding dread of state medicine in a democracy."[68] He was serving at the time as chief of the Massachusetts General Hospital's Genito-Urinary Department, which would have matched his description.

Mandated by hospital standardization, the departmental structure of clinical specialties provided the template for the vertical division of labor. Michael Davis affirmed that organization in the "business" of hospital care meant "specialization and its concomitant departmentalization in hospitals and clinics."[69] In a 1902 Johns Hopkins's alumni society address Barker issued a "plea for the better organization and endowment" required to elevate the level of clinical departments to the level of basic science departments.[70] A decade later he somewhat circularly credited the Flexner report—which had used Hopkins as its model when Barker was professor of medicine—for strengthening clinical departments. He advised that each internal medicine department, for example, should have salaried staff, with clinical, clerical, and technical assistants, as well as its own wards, laboratories, outpatient clinics, private rooms, and budgets.[71] Other specialty chiefs embarked on similar department-building campaigns and competed with one another to achieve the "dignity of full department status."[72] Department chiefs published papers with lists of equipment and personnel necessary for them to attain a respectable position in the medical center. Building such fully equipped specialty departments entailed a huge expansion in institutional capitalization. University of Pennsylvania obstetrics professor Barton Cooke Hirst enthused that, since the United States was the only country rich enough to equip its specialty departments fully, the "hegemony of the medical education of the world lies within our grasp."[73]

Barker's 1902 address was in part a fund appeal; he was seeking endowment for his proposal that specialty department professors become full-time, salaried employees of their institutions in order to reduce their dependence on practice income.[74] Writing to Barker in 1913 for more information about full-time, Ray Lyman Wilbur, dean of Stanford Medical School, accurately predicted an "endless amount of trouble."[75] Barker himself ironically rejected the full-time offer in the same year and resigned his Johns Hopkins chair in order to maintain his private practice. Barker seems not to have seen the full-time system as an important means of institutional revenue generation in 1902, but by the early 1920s he recognized that full-time plans could generate significant patient care revenues for clinical departments and their institutions.[76] Obstetrician John Whitridge Williams, the dean who accepted Barker's resignation and implemented the full-time plan at Hopkins, approved of medical schools' charging middle-class patients for their services and specifically advocated developing specialty department–based pay clinics.[77] Abraham Flexner also probably did not mean in 1910 that academic hospitals should develop revenue-generating services, but he condoned them in 1925 on the grounds that the original benefit of the full-time arrangement remained—the individual physician was "stripped of business or professional motive."[78] It seems reasonable to assume that Flexner or at least his employer, the Rockefeller-funded General

Education Board, recognized that the new academic centers they were capitalizing would require substantial operating revenues.

Providing clinical services to paying patients played a growing role in supporting the high overhead and operational costs of academic medical centers and their specialty departments. Flexnerian full-time evolved into revenue-generating faculty practice plans in some centers. Although an academic himself, George Dock called it "ominous" when the Universities of Virginia and Michigan expected their faculty members to cover their salaries and other departmental expenses by providing clinical services to wealthy patients.[79] Private physicians in the late 1920s clearly saw academic practice as a competitive threat. Former American Medical Association president William Allen Pusey, while calling group medicine the "chief positive contribution of physicians in the field of corporate medical practice," charged that some hospitals, usually academic ones with full-time staff, had "frankly gone into the practice of medicine for pay."[80] Private practitioners and smaller hospitals similarly complained that they could not "compete with the advertising power of a great university."[81]

The full-time salary system removed faculty members from the individual private practice market and made the institution the unit of competition. Many academicians, however, successfully resisted full-salaried status. Harvey Cushing and his Harvard colleagues applied the rather meaningless phrase *geographic full-time* to plans that allowed faculty to add private practice fees to their salaries. The difference between "strict" and "geographic" full-time was not whether the faculty member generated practice revenues but, rather, where the revenues flowed. Under strict full-time they flowed into university and departmental coffers; under geographic full-time they (or a portion thereof) flowed into faculty members' wallets.

Consistent with the evolving institutional practice, many economists and progressive reformers deemed the persistence of the individual medical entrepreneur problematic. Concerned with controlling capital investment and operational costs and assuming a natural development from entrepreneurial to corporate organization, they seemed to feel that medical authority, financial interest, or general obtuseness was obstructing this evolution. The final report of the Committee on the Costs of Medical Care assumed that most physicians would eventually work as salaried medical center staff. Its minority report condemned such a salaried status as corporate practice of medicine. AMA spokesman and CCMC dissident Nathan Van Etten called the "competitive practice of medicine by an incorporated medical school or clinic" a "corporate practice of medicine."[82] This tension between proprietary and corporate practice led to a variety of curious hybrids for the remainder of the century. In the late 1930s the National Bureau of Economic Research distinguished physicians from other professionals by the extent to which they were not yet salaried employees.[83] But the study did not distinguish specialists from general practitioners or recognize the extent to which the specialists were more likely to be salaried. Thirty-four percent of U.S. specialists in 1920 had full-time salaried employment, compared with 8 percent of general practitioners; more than half of all specialists at the time had full- or part-time salaries.[84] The organization deemed necessary to replace the individual entrepreneur was the academic medical center, whose specialty departments required a range of ancillary occupations to take over most of vertical specialization's fragmented tasks.

Managing Workers

Academic centers such as Johns Hopkins, Columbia, Harvard, Duke, and Washington led the way in developing a range of clinical jobs for different levels of medical and nonmedical staff. Osler initiated the clinical clerkship at Hopkins in 1896 primarily to enhance the quality of clinical work.[85] Hopkins's leaders found that medical student clerks could carry a significant workload, and they advised that using students in this way increased hospital efficiency.[86] Barker described how students became an "integral part of the working force of the clinic."[87] Comparing the organization of work in the clinic with that in a factory or business office, Barker credited Osler with contemporary managerial capabilities and an intuitive grasp of "the newer principles of association and of group organization."[88]

The system of "graded responsibility" in teaching hospitals classified medical tasks according to technical complexity and assigned them to a hierarchy of residents, interns, and clerks.[89] Interns and clerks took histories, performed physical examinations, did laboratory work, presented cases at rounds, and wrote reports.[90] The medical hierarchy was also a managerial hierarchy, with the different levels managing the work of the levels below them. As part of redefining residencies as training positions, department chiefs assigned the growing numbers of residents the tasks of performing more complex clinical tasks and supervising interns and clerks.[91] The senior resident had complete responsibility for the "ward," or nonprivate patients.[92] Interns and residents became hospital employees, and by the 1930s most residents were salaried.[93] The dual purpose of clerkships, internships, and residencies was training for the doctor and "cheap labor" for the hospital.[94] This cheap labor fed the growth of specialty departments and their residency programs. The number of hospitals approved for residencies by the AMA Council on Medical Education, already 270 by 1927, expanded to 410 by 1935 and to 610 by 1941.[95]

Michael Davis advised the Rockefeller Foundation that residents' roles should be predominantly managerial.[96] But residents were also expected to

perform (and learn) the highest-level procedures identified with their specialties. The role of the department chief was also becoming more managerial.
The American College of Surgeons's standardization program expected chiefs
to plan, coordinate, standardize, supervise, and control all the practice activities in their departments.[97] Their major purpose, according to the managerial
philosophy of one hospital superintendent, was to improve productivity and
ensure full utilization of the resources in their departments.[98] Barker later
explained his own work as departmental chief in terms of scientific management. Comparing himself to a business executive keeping a large organization
steadily functioning, he described how he had analyzed medical functions and
delegated portions according to the special aptitudes of the graded staff in his
department.[99]

Barker's leadership in internal medicine notwithstanding, surgical specialties took the lead in developing teams of medical and nonmedical personnel.
As a president of the American College of Surgeons later noted, "surgeons operated with trained assistants as a team. The classic picture of Agnew in his
clinic depicts an anesthetist, a surgical assistant, a nurse, and an orderly, all
performing specific functions."[100] The Mayo Clinic operationalized the type of
teamwork in which surgeons parceled out nonsurgical and routine surgical
tasks to assistants, retaining the complex surgical functions for themselves.[101]
Relationship with the patient often became one of the parceled-out tasks. "It is
not unusual," an academic obstetrician-gynecologist observed in 1918, "to hear
an operator say of the patient under the anesthetic, 'this is the first time I have
examined the patient.'"[102]

Harvey Cushing exemplified allocation of the most complex tasks to specialists. As Harvard's chief of neurosurgery at the Peter Bent Brigham Hospital, Cushing did not examine ward patients in his department prior to
performing surgery on them. He personally performed the most specialized
task, such as dissecting out a brain tumor, leaving the more routine tasks of
cutting patients open and stitching them back up to his residents and surgical
assistants. A visiting surgeon described how Cushing controlled the work of
his subordinates, who rounded with him in hierarchical order. Cushing's self-
proclaimed goal was to keep everyone, including himself, "working at their
greatest possible efficiency."[103]

Since the work assignments of the different medical levels were strongly
identified with education, vertical divisions of labor may perhaps be more obvious among the hospital occupations considered ancillary. Specialists and hospital administrators could not have divided up and divvied out medical care
without other institutional workers to take over many technical tasks as well
as caring. Richard Cabot initiated the social work unit at the Massachusetts

General Hospital to supplement, and counteract, the "necessarily brief" patient-physician encounter.[104] Michael Davis advised that trained assistants should perform "executive, social service, nursing, clerical and technical functions."[105] Efficient work in hospitals and dispensaries, according to Davis, required a range of registered nurses, practical nurses, nursing students, aides, orderlies, and technicians to perform most of the tasks involved in running machines and caring for patients.[106] Harry Moore attributed increased productivity to such a vertical division of labor. He observed that "nurses and social workers may do so much of the routine work that a physician may deal with many times the number of patients he would see under other conditions."[107] A Committee on the Costs of Medical Care report supporting further use of *Midwives, Chiropodists, and Optometrists* (particularly in the context of group practice) recapitulated the scientific management mantra that it was "uneconomic to employ a person whose time is more valuable when a person whose time is less valuable is available."[108]

As the CCMC suggested, a more economic use of health care personnel in maternity care would have employed (nurse) midwives. This suggestion countered the obstetric specialty's strenuous efforts to abolish midwifery, although a few of its leaders did go against the mainstream. Benjamin Watson, obstetric chief at Columbia, for example, advised that using midwives for the majority of births—along the lines of his native Scotland—would be of "economic advantage" to the physician.[109] But private obstetricians and the majority of academics rejected midwifery for many reasons: economic competition, professional and institutional needs to hospitalize birth, gender discrimination, practices incompatible with specialty therapeutics, and fear that midwife inclusion in the medical system would lead to more governmental regulation.[110] Although a few leaders trained midwives to provide maternity care for poor women in their areas, most viewed replacing the midwife with the "clinico-educational organization" to be a professional necessity.[111] Obstetric leaders opted instead to develop and control specialty nursing within the division of labor in their departments. In so doing, they built the class and gender hierarchies of the doctor-nurse relationship into those of scientific management.

Until the late 1920s nurses had three primary forms of employment open to them: private duty in the home or hospital, accounting for around 54 percent of employed nurses; public health nursing, accounting for 19 percent; and hospital staff nursing (where students had been performing most of the nursing), accounting for 23 percent.[112] Nursing as well as medical policy promoted a shift in nurse employment from independent practitioner potentially competing with physicians to that of hospital employee.[113] The Rockefeller Foundation–sponsored Committee for the Study of Nursing Education advised hospitals that they could attain higher nursing productivity by employing graduate nurses.[114] The Committee on the Grading of Nursing Schools also recommended hospital employment of graduate nurses. Referring to the grading committee's work, accountant C. Rufus Rorem calculated that institutional staff nursing was more efficient in terms of cost as well as in use of nursing knowledge and skills.[115] Rorem contributed to the National League of Nursing Education's similar conclusion that graduate nurses were more efficient and more productive than student labor in the hospital. In the name of efficiency the league recommended that hospitals replace student nurses with a range of graduate nurses, clerks, maids, porters, and orderlies.[116]

At the same time that hospital administrators and department chiefs were seeking to manage their expanding workforce, nursing was endeavoring to professionalize itself. One of its tactics applied Tayloristic methods of scientific management to its own labor process in the hospital.[117] A nursing manager later attributed such a functional nursing to "industrial engineering principles of the division of labor and mass production."[118] Its methods sought to "simplify production by reducing each task to its smallest components," which were "divided among a number of workers, each assigned to a few repetitive tasks."[119] But, cautioned nursing historian Barbara Melosh, "in nursing, as in other work, the actual application of scientific management was partial and incomplete . . . no simple functional definition can capture the intricacy of the medical division of labor." Over the subsequent decades nursing organization swung back and forth between such a functional organization and a less fragmented primary nursing organization.[120]

Consistent with the managerial approach, the grading committee identified desirable professional characteristics for nursing to be reasonable hours, adequate (salaried) income, hierarchical supervision (which it also called constructive leadership), development of new techniques, and close contact with medical men (which it called professional growth).[121] These characteristics obviously pertained more to the needs of institutional management than those of an autonomous profession. The grading committee's activity analysis found that hospital nurses spent less time than private nurses did in evaluating patients' health and more time assisting physicians and performing procedures.[122] Consistent with this finding, it recommended reconstructing undergraduate and postgraduate nursing curricula around medical specialty areas.

Medical specialties for their part were actively establishing their own special nursing branches. Barker held in 1900 that specialties, especially surgical ones, required a trained corps of assistants and nurses.[123] He advised the 1909 graduating class of the Johns Hopkins Hospital School for Nurses that they were at that point trained to be general practitioners of nursing but that many of them would go on to specialize in obstetrics, pediatrics, surgery, and other areas.[124] He advised them to continue developing the technical skills required to administer drugs and perform injections and catheterizations. Academic obstetrician Herbert Marion Stowe described at the following year's meeting of the Chicago Society of Superintendents of Training Schools for Nurses how the tasks of the specially trained obstetric nurse must complement those of the specialist. Nursing textbooks similarly detailed how the work of the specially trained nurse fit in with medical specialism.[125] There was a tension between Stowe's expectation that the nurse should be "fully prepared to manage a normal delivery, to recognize many complications, and to treat them properly" (called diagnosis and treatment when performed by doctors)[126] and the expectation that the nurse should prepare for the physician's every need, "to anticipate his wants, to carry out his orders accurately and intelligently."[127] A Massachusetts nurse told the grading committee that a doctor once ordered her: "If you see anyone dying, let him die unless I tell you what to do. If you know the medicine I have ordered is going to kill him in the next minute, give it!"[128] This was, one hopes, an extreme example of nurse (and patient) subordination to medical hierarchy. Nevertheless, the contradictory requirements of competence and subservience remained with nursing throughout the century.

Specialties and their clinical interventions coevolved with the new division of labor and the new academic centers, together creating a "new capital-intensive medicine."[129] Elements of large-scale production were not just applied to the organization of doctors and hospitals early in the century; they also reconstituted the structure of specialties, nursing, and academic medical centers. But characteristics of scientific management were not uniformly applied across the developing specialties. They better fit specialties based on surgical and/or technological procedures, such as obstetrics and gynecology. Reciprocally, they reinforced ob-gyn's use of procedures in childbirth.

Three

Dividing Labor,
Industrializing Birth

Business models shaped not only the organization of specialties in the early decades of the twentieth century but also their therapeutic content. Internal medicine chief Lewellys Barker credited uniformity in clinical technique to the functional division of labor at the department level as well as its scientific management.[1] The specialty of obstetrics and gynecology (ob-gyn) offers a particularly good perspective on the development of specialty departments in the new academic medical centers and their use of clinical procedures. Obstetrics departments established hierarchies of residents, interns, student clerks, and nurses, parceling out birthing tasks among them. They selected surgical and technological interventions that fit this division of labor and, as a consequence, reconstructed the process of birth as a surgical procedure. Birth intervention patterns also reflected hospital differentiation of services according to the market. Building institutions and using procedures shaped the specialty's diagnostic and therapeutic paradigms. Leaders at the time identified excessive medical intervention in birth to be a major problem, yet they rejected research findings that conflicted with their profession- and institution-building achievements.

Specialization and Scientific Management of Birth

Academic obstetrics and gynecology strove to expand its departments in number, size, and technologic capacity. Howard C. Taylor, an ob-gyn chief at Columbia University, later called the academic department the "materialization of the specialty—in bricks and mortar, in organization, in the development and nurturing of ideas."[2] Barton Cooke Hirst, the University of Pennsylvania chief who sought hegemony over world medical education, insisted that ob-gyn should have its own hospitals or units with at least one hundred beds in order to attain full department status in the medical school.[3] Drawing attention to what the profession called the "midwifery problem," Charles E. Ziegler of the University of Pittsburgh called on the recent 1910 Flexner report to support his proposal to construct thirty new fully equipped academic obstetrics departments like Columbia's Sloane Hospital.[4]

Like scientific management in industry—if not so highly fragmented—ob-gyn and other procedure-oriented specialties divided their clinical care into separate tasks assigned to different levels of hospital staff according to technical complexity. In the words of nursing scholar Barbara Melosh, "managerial innovations redesigned the hospital, changing its physical arrangement, the flow of work, the division of labor, even the performance of individual procedures."[5] The division of work labor in ob-gyn departments routinized birth procedures and divided the biological process of childbirth labor into "labor" and "delivery." Laboring women were wheeled from one workstation and function to another. In the prep room student nurses routinely administered enemas and shaved perineal areas (despite a 1922 report concluding that routine shaving was associated with slightly worse outcomes).[6] Graduate nurses administered analgesics and supervised fetal heart rates and labor progress in the labor room.[7] As birth became imminent, patients were dashed in their beds to the delivery/operating room—the workstation of the specialist. These professional and spatial divisions remained the dominant organization in maternity units throughout the century. The 1997 specialty-oriented *Guidelines for Perinatal Care* identified six separate functional units.[8] Alternatively, hospitals that had developed single-room maternity care criticized their competitors for moving laboring women from room to room at least six times.[9] For both configurations the incentive was to "maximize economy and flexibility of staff and space."[10]

Consistent with their functional division of labor, obstetrics departments trained special nurses to take over many tasks in prenatal, labor, and postpartum care yet not compete with doctors for the delivery. In a common, if bizarre, inversion of the goal of facilitating the birth of a healthy baby, the delivery nurse was expected to hold back the head of the emerging baby for an hour or more pending the late arrival of a doctor. Carolyn Conant Van Blarcom, whose textbook instructed nurses how to hold back the baby's head, was explicit about the nurse's role in supporting medical interventions: "In her relation to the doctors the nurse must be so convinced of the rightness of their procedures that she gives unquestioning loyalty and confidence . . . As to the patients, the nurse in her turn must win from them trust and confidence as she imparts the things it is decided they should be taught."[11]

In accord with such a division of labor, the obstetrics profession defined its own clinical role in terms of performing short-term technical and surgical procedures at the end of labor. Sloane Hospital chief Benjamin P. Watson—who had appreciated the midwives in Scotland—maintained that the obstetrician's attendance was primarily required to apply procedures "at the actual time of delivery."[12] Watson appreciated that this division of labor enhanced obstetricians' job satisfaction. The intern and resident systems "infinitely lessened the drudgery of obstetrics," extolled another academic.[13] As University of Iowa ob-gyn chief E. D. Plass later explained, obstetricians favored the hierarchic division of labor because they need "spend less time with each patient who is always under competent supervision by the nursing and resident staff."[14] One teaching hospital ob-gyn chief advised that his new resident system considerably augmented his department's productivity.[15] Using student clerks and interns to perform most of the clinical tasks also enhanced specialty department productivity. Interns at Washington University took responsibility for all histories, physical examinations, laboratory tests, and records. They prepared patients for delivery or operation, assisted in major operations, and performed minor ones.[16] Since Washington's Barnes Hospital was at the time a full-time institution with capacity for four paying patients for every one charity patient, the house staff also took over many of the responsibilities in caring for faculty members' patients. Leaders in the hospital standardization movement came to recommend that all hospitals providing maternity care should have residents and interns.[17] An obvious corollary of this policy would be that only teaching hospitals should provide obstetrics services.

The standardization programs initiated by the American Hospital Association and the American College of Surgeons solidified the organization of specialty departments and scientific management. In obstetric departments standardization reinforced the development of separate function rooms for separate staff, contributing to procedural routinization and control of workers as well as childbirth.[18] Obstetric chiefs standardized the instruments and operative techniques for each of the rooms.[19] They required that nurses, house staff, and often even attending obstetricians follow the standardized procedures. The Philadelphia maternal mortality study similarly recommended that all of its city's hospitals establish standard techniques for all physicians delivering in their obstetrics units.[20]

Functional division of labor and procedural standardization augmented the development and routine use of surgical and technological interventions in birth. Like many specialists, ob-gyns attributed their organizational and therapeutic developments to scientific and technologic expansion. Also like other specialists, they conflated scientific management with science. Academic specialty departments organized their procedure rooms to enhance productivity and speed of clinical process. Managing the flow of patients through the labor and delivery unit became an objective of obstetric therapeutics as well as delivery unit design.

Long Island College Hospital ob-gyn professor Robert Latou Dickinson became infamous in some circles for applying scientific management to clinical process and advocating the adoption of clinical process management in hospital standardization. Criticizing the "old one-doctor-one-patient scheme," Dickinson maintained that hospital standardization—like scientific management—required a rigorous analysis of all patient care tasks and their assignment to teams of workers.[21] He advised that medical school hospitals, dispensaries, and group practices were the best suited organization for this kind of management.[22] Joining the burgeoning enthusiasm for Taylorism in medicine, a Cornell professor commended Dickinson for seeking the "one best way" to give an enema during labor.[23] Whether or not Dickinson's colleagues agreed with him philosophically about applying scientific management to surgical process (and many did not), they increasingly adopted its organization. Birth historians later noted that hospital birth at this time became "streamlined" and "a kind of industrial production."[24]

A dominant metaphor over the next several decades, the assembly line, pervaded obstetric unit design as well as its imagery as patients were conveyed from one workstation to the next. The editors of *Obstetrical and Gynecological Survey* referred to their "assembly-line methods for practicing obstetrics" in the 1940s.[25] A few years later the U.S. Public Health Service (PHS) published a report that brought teaching department organization to community hospitals that were building or rebuilding under the 1946 Hospital Survey and Construction Act (the Hill-Burton program). Noting how hospital architectural textbooks of the time incorporated principles of industrial production into obstetric unit design, architect Roslyn Lindheim also attributed the spread of academic birth practices to community hospitals to the PHS report.[26] Illustrating how hospital architecture could routinize obstetric intervention, a subsequent PHS report advised community hospitals that principles of standardization required "proper sequential arrangement" of delivery unit functions.[27] By the mid-1960s the American Hospital Association's journal championed a "maternity center designed for 'assembly-line' efficiency," advising that the purpose of such a center was to achieve a "continuous operational flow" of patients.[28] Not quite so enthusiastically, patients also compared hospital delivery to assembly lines in manufacturing or meatpacking industries. Resonating with a 1958 *Ladies' Home Journal* article on "Cruelty in Maternity Wards," readers complained that they had been "herded like sheep through an obstetrical assembly-line."[29] Obstetric production did not, of course, became as standardized or as mechanized in labor and delivery units as it did in Ford plants. For one thing, nurse power rather than electric power propelled the beds carrying patients from station to station.

The ob-gyn specialty constructed labor and delivery units along the lines of industrial production, interventions to fit this design, and congruent mechanistic paradigms of birth. Although their modalities were primarily surgical and instrumental, obstetricians were not averse to using pharmacological agents. They administered drugs for pain control and to initiate and/or to speed labor. Many obstetricians at the turn of the century were still using ergot—a product of bread mold—to stimulate uterine contractions. But ergot's therapeutic effects ranged from nil to catastrophic. The profession subsequently substituted posterior pituitary gland extract, which owed its commercial availability to the centralization of the meatpacking industry. One pound of dried extract became the profitable by-product of pituitary glands from twelve thousand young cattle.[30] The assembly line in slaughterhouses thus contributed to assembly line obstetrics.

Pituitary extract for accelerating labor enjoyed a burst of popularity in the 1910s.[31] By standardizing the length of labor, obstetricians reduced the risk that they would arrive too late—or too early. One obstetrician boasted that he used the extract on three-quarters of his patients and that, consequently, he never had to spend more than two hours waiting on the labor of his multiparous patients (women who had previously given birth).[32] Another obstetrician—with a caseload of up to two or three deliveries a day—claimed that faster labors entailed less risk.[33] The diagnostic incidence of uterine inertia and slow labor expanded along with the use of pituitary extract to accelerate it.[34] Yet a professor at the Philadelphia Lying-in Hospital called uterine inertia a nonspecific concept covering many factors that prolonged labor. He criticized the common obstetric assumption that the diagnosis itself called for immediate delivery with pituitary extract or "instrumental interference."[35] Another professor accused obstetricians of using pituitary extract acceleration too often and for their own expedience.[36]

Induction, which standardized when labor began, developed alongside of acceleration, which tried to standardize when it would end. Benjamin Watson was already using a variety of chemicals such as castor oil and quinine to induce labor when he added pituitary extract to the brew.[37] Charles Reed routinely inserted Vorhee's bags into the uterus to induce labor, describing his purpose as "scientific control of the labor from the very beginning."[38] Reed developed ideas about dangers of fetal postmaturity that reflected his policy of routine induction at term.[39] The first wave of pituitary extract enthusiasm subsided, however, as obstetricians found that (like ergot) commercially available preparations did not have a consistent physiologic effect. They found that its use during labor could lead to severe consequences, including uterine rupture.[40] As routine use of pituitary extract waned, routine use of technical and surgical procedures expanded.

Obstetrics emulated surgery and actively sought to merge its departments with those of gynecology to enhance its identity as a surgical specialty.[41] The "tight connection between therapeutic intervention and professional identity," which historian John Harley Warner described for the nineteenth century, applied to the development of the obstetrics specialty and its therapeutics in the twentieth century.[42] Obstetrics' use of surgical and technological procedures delineated its domain in the medical school and hospital. John Polak of Long Island College Hospital articulated a 1922 obstetric credo: "We believe that labor is a surgical procedure, [and] that the delivery of the primipara is just as important as the opening of the abdomen."[43] Such a conviction rationalized obstetricians' lobbying medical school deans for more departmental funding as well as conducting birth as surgery. Leaders at Herbert Hoover's 1930 White House Conference on Child Health and Protection recognized that the acceptance of obstetrics as a major academic specialty owed a great deal to its surgical identity.[44]

Ironically, despite the continuing growth in scientific knowledge and surgical technique, the new obstetrics departments did not have much new to offer their patients. Other than pituitary extract, academic obstetricians did not owe their treatment innovations to contemporary developments in medical science. Instead, they promoted routine use of procedures previously devised to treat complications. Teaching hospitals led the way in routinizing technological and surgical interventions in birth—although there was considerable variation among them. The Boston Lying-in Hospital, for example, used forceps, cesarean section, version (turning the baby around in the uterus), and/or instrumental induction (rupture of the amniotic membranes) in 29 percent of all its deliveries in 1910, increasing this rate to 45 percent by 1921.[45] Sixty-three percent of deliveries at the Philadelphia Lying-in in the 1930s were operative.[46] Consistent with these rates, an obstetrics professor asserted that only the "competent gynecological surgeon" should practice routine intervention and then only with the availability of "full operating-room equipment, proper assistants, and an expert anesthetist."[47] Outside of academe only a very few well-endowed hospitals could have met these criteria.

Obstetric critics at the time and for the remainder of the century accused the specialty of intervening excessively and blamed the situation on obstetricians' (patriarchal) perceptions of birth as pathologic.[48] Indeed, delivery was more dangerous in the days before antibiotics, blood transfusions, and an understanding of how doctors and hospitals themselves contributed to infection and hemorrhage. Historian Irvine Loudon showed how obstetricians' high intervention rates both in Britain and in the United States in the early decades of the century actually increased maternal mortality and morbidity, which in turn supported professional views of birth as pathologic.[49] Critics pointed their fingers at Joseph B. DeLee, founder of the Chicago Lying-in Hospital, as a key innovator and a key villain: the "architect of obstetrical intervention" and the "principal protagonist of the 'birth as pathology' school."[50] DeLee did in fact provide considerable ammunition for these labels. He owed much of his fame to his use of routine outlet forceps just as the baby's head was about to emerge from the birth canal. In what would become a frequently quoted paper on this procedure, he dramatically compared potential damage during the final moments of delivery to falling on a pitchfork for the woman and catching its head in a closing door for the baby.[51] DeLee's legacy continued at the Chicago Lying-in, where the forceps rate expanded to 28 percent of its births in the 1930s, 44 percent in the early 1940s, and 68 percent in the late 1940s.[52] These rates compared to statewide forceps use rates averaging 26–27 percent from the mid-1940s to the mid-1960s.[53]

Birth intervention critics tended to portray Johns Hopkins's John Whitridge Williams as DeLee's interventional and philosophical antithesis. Williams did in fact criticize DeLee's routine forceps, and he did contrast a pathological model of birth with a more physiological one, yet his own textbook also cast birth in a pathological framework.[54] The key divergences between DeLee and Williams were not conceptual but institutional and situational. Williams's institutional base was the medical school where he served as dean as well as department chairman, and he wrote clinical policies for his residents to manage interns and students delivering indigent patients. Although he was an academic chairman himself, DeLee was primarily a hospital builder; he developed routine intervention for obstetricians delivering private patients in his Lying-in Hospital. DeLee may have used feistier language than his peers, but many of them were already using forceps routinely by the time of his famous paper. Arthur Bill, professor at Western Reserve School of Medicine, reported that he had used forceps on 72 percent of his most recent five hundred deliveries.[55]

Ralph Pomeroy, the professor insisting on full operating-room equipment, made a name for himself by hastening delivery with routine episiotomy.[56] Bertha Van Hoosen, obstetric chief at Loyola University Medical School, later accepted that episiotomy had relegated fifteen to twenty minutes of perineal massage to obscurity as obstetricians used the knife or scissors with a quick snip: "The most widespread innovation in modern obstetrics is the cutting of the muscles at the vaginal outlet. This goes under the name of 'episiotomy' and is taught, advocated, and applied universally. The older midwives and obstetricians made an art of the slow and careful delivery of the baby's head without inflicting any injury to the muscles of the perineum at the outlet of the birth canal. Now . . . the obstetrician assumes the responsibility for the time when the baby shall come, and the depth to which the mother shall be laid open to hurry the birth."[57] Known for her technical and surgical skill, Van Hoosen participated in the process that diverted birth from a "delicate natural process, consuming hours," as she described it, to a "short surgical procedure directly under the control of the operator."

Episiotomy became the most frequently used obstetric procedure by midcentury. Some U.S. hospitals reported episiotomy rates of 85 percent in 1950; nearly all in the 1960s and 1970s reported rates exceeding 70 percent.[58] Yet a 1979 report from the Congressional Office of Technology Assessment belatedly concluded that there was no scientific evidence supporting routine episiotomy and that there never had been.[59] Joint guidelines of the American Academy of Pediatrics and American College of Obstetricians and Gynecologists shortly thereafter advised against routine episiotomy.[60] Rates declined after that to 64 episiotomies per one hundred vaginal deliveries in 1980, 56 in 1990, and 33 in 2000.[61] Episiotomy remained the number one inpatient operative procedure in the country in the 1990s, although a number of random controlled trials had found no evidence that routine performance of the procedure benefited either the mother or the baby.[62] Instead, technology assessors would ironically conclude that routine episiotomy inflicted more perineal trauma than birth did.[63] It appeared that DeLee's metaphoric pitchfork was the episiotomy more than the birth.

Bertha Van Hoosen's practices seem to have been as interventionist as those of male physicians. This observation calls into question later feminist accusations that DeLee and other male obstetricians used birth procedures as a means of patriarchal dominance. Van Hoosen promoted "twilight sleep" drugs because they moved birth into the hospital. Like her male colleagues, she promoted hospitalization of birth because it decreased the "time and inconvenience of the physician by seventy-five per cent," in part by relieving the doctor of the "job of morale-keeper."[64] Consistent with Van Hoosen's practices, historian Regina Morantz-Sanchez found that obstetricians at Boston's woman physician-controlled New England Hospital did not intervene in birth any less than their colleagues in male physician-controlled institutions and that their thinking on the pathology of birth also mirrored that of male obstetricians at the time.[65] Historian Ornella Moscucci also disputed the identification of patriarchy as the major driver of medical intervention in obstetrics and gynecology. Moscucci found that explaining its intervention practices required integrating gender dynamics with technologic, scientific, and institutional developments; professional competition; public policy; and social class.[66] Although Moscucci's context was nineteenth-century Britain, all of these elements pertained to the development of U.S. ob-gyn in the twentieth century.

Some obstetricians at the time themselves attributed excessive birth intervention to concepts of birth as pathologic and tried to counteract it with concepts of birth normality. Rush Medical College professor Rudolph W. Holmes disparaged the view of pregnancy and labor as "pathologic entities" that "must be terminated by some spectacular procedure."[67] A White House conference report similarly contended that "while progress has been impeded by the attitude assumed by some of the medical profession and laity alike in regarding childbirth as a consistently physiological process, we have even more grievously erred in the assumption that childbirth is a pathologic process. The latter view has led to unwarranted and meddlesome interference and is responsible in no small degree for our deplorable results."[68]

But obstetricians' views of birth as normal did not necessarily curb their interventions, either. Advising that "nothing should be done to interfere with the natural mechanism" of birth, one academic reported that even in labors he called normal he usually administered anesthesia, ruptured amniotic membranes, and performed episiotomies.[69] Some obstetricians tended to invoke nature to support whatever their practices were. Some saw themselves as controlling nature, others as "aiding Nature's efforts" in their routine use of birth interventions.[70] Some recognized that it was the very normality of childbirth, ironically, that permitted procedural routinization. In addition to using concepts of normality for their own purposes, obstetricians also did not use concepts of pathology consistently. DeLee used the language of abnormality to justify his preferred interventions when performed by trained obstetricians and the language of normality to criticize competing interventions and competing birth attendants.[71] Graphic and rhetorical, his analogy with falling on pitchforks was obviously meant to advance the profession of obstetrics more than the science of pathophysiology.

As the White House conference committee recognized, treating birth as pathologic was an important strategy in obstetrics' effort to professionalize as a specialty[72] and to achieve the dignity of full departmental status in the medical school. Pittsburgh's Ziegler blamed obstetrics' low professional and low economic status on the perception that birth was a normal process.[73] A

Georgetown University professor correspondingly called for "national propaganda" challenging the "long-cherished fallacy that pregnancy and labor are normal physiologic conditions and therefore require no special care."[74] Pathology provided a scientific basis for Flexnerian reform and the development of specialty institutions, and it loaned a scientific legitimacy to obstetrics.[75] Academic obstetricians crusaded to upgrade the status of their departments and their interventions to the level of surgery, and they used the concept of birth as pathologic to justify these upgrades.

Actions and ideas coevolved in the ob-gyn specialty. Obstetricians developed the paradigm of birth as pathologic intrinsic to their activities of building institutions and intervening in birth. Obstetric diagnostics and therapeutics were not just translations of scientific knowledge into clinical practice; they were also translations of clinical practice into scientific knowledge. Williams himself suggested that the operative approach molded obstetricians' concepts of labor as pathologic.[76] Specialty divisions of labor and the separation of clinical functions in different rooms in the labor and delivery unit reinforced (although they did not invent) an analysis of labor as "arbitrarily, and for matter of convenience, divided into three stages."[77] Dividing labor into stages permitted assigning the long first stage, the dilatation of the opening of the uterus (the cervix), to nurses.[78] It also justified the arrival of the obstetrician near the end of the second stage—between full dilation and expulsion of the baby—to perform exit procedures. According to this work definition, obstetricians identified themselves as doctors who shortened the second stage by "timely intervention."[79] The "two-hour rule" rationalized the maximum amount of time they had to wait on the second stage before intervening.[80]

This discussion (and those to follow) on the mutual construction of obstetric institutions, interventions, and ideas builds on the work of historians who found similar relationships in other medical areas. Charles Rosenberg noted the "interdependence of ideas and the institutional contexts in which they are elaborated."[81] Elizabeth Fee held that institutional developments at the turn of the twentieth century provided an "infrastructure for the development of new forms of medical theory and practice."[82] As Keith Wailoo put it, specialties were competing to identify the "true location (both institutionally and corporeally)" of diseases.[83] Obstetricians developed diagnostic concepts consistent with their specialty interventions and their departmental infrastructures. The concepts, the interventions, and the infrastructures were also oriented to the market.

Market Stratification and Birth Intervention

The growing industrial wealth in urban America at the turn of the twentieth century substantially extended the number of people able to pay for higher-priced goods and services. This growth led to a widening gap between rich and poor and increasingly distinct levels of purchasing power. Academic obstetrics departments divided labor by patient class as well as staff training levels. They initially assigned home delivery of low-income women with normal pregnancies to medical students (sometimes supervised by interns). Students, interns, and residents delivered low-income women with complications in academic hospital units. Full-fledged specialists delivered their private patients in the hospital, complicated or not. Charles Ziegler's ideal was Boston, where medical students attended nearly 20 percent of the city's births.[84] In New York City hospital staff conducted 30 percent of the city's deliveries in the mid-1910s, private physicians conducted about 40 percent, and midwives the remaining 30 percent.[85] Wealthier women traditionally comprised obstetricians' private practice, and the specialty flourished in the new century by adding the growing middle class to its clientele. Obstetric specialists in Michigan's urban areas attended 21 percent of women in "comfortable circumstances" in the mid-1930s, 12 percent of the deliveries of women of moderate means, 5 percent of those of poor women, and 1 percent of women on relief.[86] Birth became an important way to fill hospital beds with paying patients and contributed substantially to their growth and financial viability (second to tonsillectomy).[87] The building programs of the 1920s added many private obstetric beds to teaching and other hospitals. By the early 1930s 77 percent of the women in the nation's highest income group delivered their babies in a hospital, compared with 26 percent in the lowest income group, with incremental intermediate values.[88]

Expanding the hospitalization of birth supported obstetrics services both financially and professionally, and it supported elevation of the specialty to departmental status.[89] The new departments required more and more patients to fill their growing numbers of beds; to keep their students, interns, and residents working efficiently; and to bring in patient revenues. Prenatal care aided the necessary patient recruitment efforts. Fred Lyman Adair, who would succeed DeLee at the University of Chicago, told Sheppard-Towner program administrators at their 1926 conference that the purpose of prenatal care was to get pregnant women away from midwives and into the medical system.[90] Obstetric leaders established a Committee on Maternal Welfare and other organizations to promote public and professional acceptance of their specialty and to move childbirth into the hospital, preferably the teaching hospital.[91]

As they expanded, teaching and other larger hospitals internally segregated their services according to patient ability to pay (as well as by race), further reinforcing the socioeconomic stratification of patients and practitioners. Obstetrics departments built separate services for different class populations, with a high-cost, high-intervention level for patients who could pay for them. The Massachusetts General Hospital, for example, first established an obstetrics service for wealthy patients in its upscale Phillips House; two decades later it created an obstetrics service for middle-class women in its newly constructed Baker Memorial middle-rate hospital;[92] another decade elapsed before it provided obstetrics services for its charity patients. The White House conference classified birthing women into "three distinct groups of patients" to be served by three distinct groups of birth attendants. Interns, students, and residents delivered clinic patients' babies, general practitioners attended the "great mass of women," and wealthy women were "in a position to have the best available care" in teaching hospitals.[93] The Committee on the Costs of Medical Care similarly recognized—and apparently condoned—market differentiation of hospital services, clarifying that it also meant a treatment differential: "Differences in the prices of hospital service represent actual differences in the type or amount of service rendered, as evidenced by such features as privacy, complexity of equipment, number of diagnostic or treatment procedures, convenience of location, and number and classes of personnel involved."[94]

Like other medical specialties, obstetrics professionalized partly on the basis of providing special care to special people. Academic obstetrics consciously competed with general practice for the nation's births, using its technological and surgical procedures to gain a competitive advantage. Leaders warned that there was a "class of operations which should not be attempted by anyone who is not especially trained and skilled in their performance."[95] "We are specialists," proclaimed Polak at a 1921 symposium; "we can give these women something that the general practitioner cannot give them."[96] By "these women" he meant primarily middle- and upper-class women. "The time has come," DeLee announced at the same symposium, "for a division in the methods of treatment of natural delivery" performed by specialists and those performed by general practitioners. DeLee decreed watchful expectancy for general practitioners' normal births and routine intervention for obstetricians' normal births. Academic obstetricians held it as a point of pride that their private patients experienced considerably higher operative rates than patients in their clinics. But the specialty was only partly successful in monopolizing birth interventions. When Michigan's obstetricians were using forceps on 19 percent of their hospital births, general practitioners were using them on 12 percent of theirs; comparable episiotomy rates were 37 percent and 22 percent, respectively, and comparable cesarean section rates 4 percent and 1 percent.[97] On the demand side of the equation many middle- and upper-class women willingly chose obstetric specialists for their scientific and technologic methods, as historian Judith Walzer Leavitt demonstrated.[98]

Population-wide birth intervention patterns reflected the socioeconomic differentiation of patients, practitioners, and hospitals. In Baltimore in 1915 citywide use of instruments rose incrementally by patient income from 4 percent of deliveries in the two lowest income groups to 14 percent in the highest income group.[99] The socioeconomic gap persisted as obstetric intervention expanded. Nationally in the mid-1930s, around 12 percent of deliveries among women in the lowest income group were conducted by forceps, increasing to 27 percent in the highest group. National episiotomy rates similarly ranged by income from approximately 17 to 44 percent and cesarean section rates from 1 to 4 percent.[100] Separate maternity services in the same hospital also treated different classes of patients differently. One Philadelphia hospital had a total operative incidence of 50 percent for its private obstetric patients and 4 percent for its ward patients.[101] When it delivered 10 percent of its private patients by cesarean, the Philadelphia Lying-in Hospital performed cesarean section on 4 percent of its public patients.[102]

Diagnostic concepts of birth were congruent with the specialty's stratified institutions and practices, just as they were congruent with its functional division of labor. One obstetrician rationalized that the twilight sleep drug scopolamin particularly benefited the high-class woman due to her "highly organized nervous system."[103] Obstetricians identified pathologic entities such as "debility" and "neurasthenia" as indications for intervention in birth, attributing them almost exclusively to wealthier women.[104] Harvard's Franklin S. Newell maintained that affluent women with these conditions required obstetric intervention.[105] But it didn't take long for the specialty to recognize that the heavier use of anesthetics and analgesics on higher-class women often slowed their labors, necessitating further intervention.[106]

Like his contemporaries in Baltimore, Philadelphia, and Boston, Joseph DeLee instituted different intervention practices in his different obstetric services. He initiated the Chicago Maternity Center to provide medical (rather than midwifery) care for indigent women at home, and he built the Chicago Lying-in Hospital to provide full specialty (rather than general practitioner) care for complicated births and for all births of women who could pay specialist fees. DeLee authorized clinical policies of minimal intervention in the Maternity Center and routine intervention in the Lying-in Hospital. To explain this practice discrepancy, Leavitt held that DeLee maintained a conceptual consistency. He was committed to treating all women preventatively, she proposed, but (like Newell) he perceived women of different socioeconomic levels to be threatened with different dangers.[107] Leavitt recognized, however, that DeLee's concepts of prophylaxis were linked to his campaign to enhance the status of obstetrics. Categorizing birth pathology by class, DeLee's assertions were also marketing strategies. He wrote popular articles raising the specter of pathology and advising middle-class readers to engage obstetricians for their deliveries. He similarly counseled his colleagues that the "only way to get the public to appreciate" obstetricians' skills was to "let them know that we doctors consider a normal obstetric case of the highest pathological dignity."[108] DeLee built different types of maternity services employing different birth attendants for different classes of women. The services provided different levels of care and supported different concepts of risk. DeLee clearly linked a greater clinical intensity with a higher patient class. Obstetricians' patients got reduction of pain and length of labor, he affirmed, and they were "willing to pay for them. They should not be given a midwife's services and be asked to pay an obstetrician's fee."[109] DeLee clearly equated monetary gain with professional gain, like many professionals of his time.

For most of the twentieth century scholars as well as policy makers rejected the idea that financial incentives drove medical practices, but the tables turned in the last two decades, and the idea became an affirmation of economic faith. Yet both the idea's earlier rejection and its later wholesale acceptance were too simplistic. DeLee did take an entrepreneurial approach to his work. He charged wealthier clients up to five thousand dollars for delivery and recorded in his diary in 1926 that he had already amassed a personal fortune of a half million dollars.[110] Yet he was abstemious in his personal life, and he recirculated some of his wealth back into his institutions. John Whitridge Williams's entrepreneurship, on the other hand, was institutional. As dean of Johns Hopkins's medical school in the crucial decade following the Flexner report, Williams strongly supported the type of academic full-time system in which any financial surplus from patient care accrued to the institution rather than the individual physician.[111] Pittsburgh's Charles Ziegler also championed such a full-time system, advising that it maximized teaching as well as clinical efficiency.[112] Fully salaried himself, proceeds from his private practice added to his hospital's bursary. Ziegler's local medical society consequently suspended him on grounds of "dispensary abuse," the indictment community physicians used when patients with the ability to pay went to institutional services rather than private practitioners.[113] In contrast to Williams and Ziegler, DeLee strenuously opposed the full-time system and became the only member of his department allowed to hospitalize private patients in the Lying-in Hospital when the University of Chicago took it over. Chicago dedicated one of the three patient floors in its newly built lying-in facility to well-to-do women in order to bring in higher revenues from faculty practice.[114] Both DeLee and Williams sought to improve the childbirth situation for all women but, consistent with the ethos of their times, not necessarily to equal levels. Both men also raised the issue of excessive intervention in birth, and they both believed that further professional and institutional development would resolve it.

Professional Concerns about Routine Birth Intervention

Specialty medicine defined itself as scientific and assumed that its clinical activities enacted the march of scientific progress. DeLee and Adair identified a "highly refined obstetric technic" as scientific in itself.[115] Yet, even as they were instigating routine practices, many obstetric leaders, including DeLee, called excessive intervention in birth a problem. They were in part inveighing against general practitioners' competitive use of obstetric procedures. Noting the appeal of procedures in their "surgical age," an obstetrician/abdominal surgeon rebuked younger practitioners for rushing to perform procedures "as young chicks scramble for their corn . . . *They dislike obstetrics but love to operate.*"[116] But obstetricians also recognized to a certain extent that their clinical experimentation with technique had not been scientifically justified. Asking "to what extent should delivery be hastened or assisted by operative interference?" a 1921 American Gynecological Society symposium identified a burning question of its time. Rudolph Holmes accused obstetrics of being "pseudoscientific" in its "indiscriminate employment of operative intervention," claiming that the profession had "accomplished little in the way of conservation of life of the mother and child."[117] During the animated discussion DeLee rejoined that Holmes was "charging windmills."[118]

It was not a simple matter of radical interventionists versus conservatives. Obstetric leaders would champion one procedure and deprecate competing interventions. Although he regularly dilated the cervix manually, stuck his arm into the uterus, grabbed the baby by the ankles, and pulled it out feet first, turning it around if necessary, Irving W. Potter bragged that he had never done an episiotomy in his life.[119] Some obstetricians lauded routine forceps, others routine episiotomy; some promised elective, if not routine, cesarean section. Yet others ridiculed routine intervention and its perpetrators, accusing that "obstetricians are busy inventing operative procedures, looking to shorten or to eliminate the second stage of labor. One induces all women at term, another cuts the perineum of every primipara, while still another sections every eleventh woman and does version on the other nine or ten and, most remarkable of all, another calls all labor pathologic and advocates rapid delivery through a cut pelvic floor as soon as the head is through the cervix."[120] The 1930 White House conference incriminated cesarean section as "perhaps the most striking evidence of the present operative furor in obstetrics."[121] Such an accusation did not go unsubstantiated. A statewide study in Massachusetts identified cesarean section as a major cause of the state's continuingly high maternal mortality rates.[122]

Professional and policy organizations conducted a number of inquiries on birth intervention rates and outcomes besides the Massachusetts study. Their studies found wide practice variations and the profession used the variation itself as evidence of inappropriate intervention (as it would six decades later). A White House conference committee found forceps rates ranging from 1 to 81 percent of hospital births and cesarean section rates ranging from 0 to 15 percent.[123] The New York Academy of Medicine's study of maternal mortality around the same time also reported wide practice variations. Addressing a four-fold difference in cesarean section rates between private and ward patients in one New York City hospital, George Kosmak, a major instigator of the study, deemed it "doubtful" that the private service had an equivalently higher proportion of abnormal labors requiring intervention.[124] The White House conference committee disparaged DeLee's "convenience" prophylactic forceps operations, for which there was "no good evidence that they prevent anything but loss of time on the part of the operator."[125] Doubting the whole concept of preventative intervention, a Harvard Medical School professor questioned prophylactic forceps, prophylactic version, and prophylactic rupture of the amniotic membranes, sarcastically suggesting that such prophylaxis must be directed against normal childbirth.[126]

Policy studies raised the question of whether the profession and/or government should use regulatory means to restrict the performance of certain procedures to medical specialists.[127] The American College of Surgeons's standardization program initially sought to control the performance of surgical procedures, but it did not continue this approach. Specialty boards joined the effort, seeking to "establish monopolies based on specialist techniques."[128] The ob-gyn specialty used not only its clinical interventions but also its studies about them as competitive weapons. Williams's cesarean section analysis sought to reduce the "indiscriminate employment" of the procedure by nonspecialists.[129] Like the professor who wanted to restrict birth intervention to settings with full operating-room equipment, leaders hoped that the White House conference would be able to restrict use of obstetric procedures to physicians in "suitable surroundings."[130] The only surroundings that were suitable to most of them were their own academic departments—or at least their departments would be suitable if they were fully equipped. An Indiana University obstetrics professor blamed the high maternal mortality rates on medical school deans' recalcitrance to grant departmental status to his specialty.[131] Yet many also recognized that the field's successes had not reduced mortality.

The obstetrics profession had a dilemma: its own studies found that its professional, institutional, and therapeutic developments had not improved birth outcomes. City maternal mortality rates remained high in Manhattan, although (and in part because) birth hospitalization had risen to nearly 66 percent by 1927 and physician attendance to 84 percent.[132] Professional studies suggested that obstetricians were using their procedures on women who needed them the least and that a number of women and babies were being harmed in the process. One nonacademic taunted that it was "paradoxical to find that where obstetricians are highly trained, *elective operative interference has increased sufficiently to neutralize an otherwise descending maternal and infantile death rate.*"[133] Drawing attention to a comparable paradox, public health leader Julius Levy compared favorable birth outcomes in cities with high midwife delivery rates to the relatively poor maternal outcomes in Boston, "with its highly organized hospitals, medical colleges, prominent obstetricians, organized official and non-official health work, intensive prenatal work and a well educated general public."[134] The New York Academy of Medicine (NYAM) estimated that the proportion of "preventable" maternal deaths was lower in municipal hospitals than in specialty hospitals due to their excessive operative interference.[135] Yet it recommended more training and more upgrading of obstetrics departments and facilities. The specialty continued to use its research and policy studies not to reconsider its profession- and institution-building efforts but, rather, to reinforce them. The NYAM maternal mortality study model spread to other geographic areas, where obstetricians conducted similar studies and came to similar conclusions.

The ob-gyn specialty used maternal mortality studies such as that of the NYAM as well as policy initiatives such as the White House conference to establish its institutions, restrict competition, and monopolize procedures. On the grounds of keeping negative information from "people who belong to the extremely radical elements of socialism," one specialist proposed that the profession suppress studies showing better outcomes in areas where midwives were active.[136] Even Williams, one of the more scientifically oriented obstetricians, could not accept research findings that conflicted with professional and institutional development. He rejected the better midwife outcomes as "contrary to reason," maintaining that acceptance of such reports might lead to the abolition of the physician's role in birth, which, he affirmed, would be a "manifest absurdity."[137]

The development of specialty departments, routine procedures, and diagnostic concepts in obstetrics reinforced one another. The structural configuration of (academic) hospital maternity units and their work differentiation established production line–like processes in birth. This organization augmented labor induction and acceleration as well as routine use of surgical and instrumental procedures on patients of private obstetricians. Ward patients under the resident system underwent the assembly line without the special attention at the end. Obstetricians appreciated that this organization would enhance their control over their work, their subordinates, and their patients. They perceived such a scientific management of labor as scientific, despite the lack of scientific evidence to justify it. The specialty identified inappropriate intervention in birth to be a problem, but it used the issue as a strategy to further strengthen its specialty and its institutions, thus tending to exacerbate the situation. Even professional self-critique was not strong enough to resist the ways in which birth intervention was built into the very structure of labor and delivery.

As the massive construction of academic institutions and their specialty departments grew in the 1920s, it became increasingly obvious that they required large revenue infusions from full-time practice or other fee services to keep operational. Academic, social service, and business leaders organized the Committee on the Costs of Medical Care to propose ways of paying for institution-based specialty medicine as well as organizing it more cost-efficiently. The committee was the first of several important nationwide attempts to appraise and organize medical delivery as a system.

Part II
Designing Delivery Systems

The provision of medical care has become one of the largest industries of the country.
—Ray Lyman Wilbur, MD, 1933

Four

The Committee on the Costs of Medical Care and Corporate Organization of Medicine

The 1927–1932 blue-ribbon Committee on the Costs of Medical Care (CCMC) was the first of several reform initiatives that attempted to build medical delivery systems. Like the other two nationwide systemic efforts discussed in part 1, health planning and perinatal regionalization, the committee sought to reorganize medical providers collectively in ways consistent with contemporary economic organization. It looked to industry to organize and manage its growing institutions and specialties more cost-efficiently. One of its principal goals was full utilization of the institutions' productive capacities and the capital invested in them. Although the committee attributed its preferred organization to scientific and professional as well as business models, it sought to restructure medicine along corporate lines.[1]

The Committee's Origins

The CCMC project seems to have had multiple conceptions. In 1924 public health leader Haven Emerson and Paul Kellogg of *The Survey* magazine proposed a large study on the economic burden of sickness, sickness prevention, health insurance, health care administration, and the development of pay clinics and regional hospitals. They sent out a large batch of letters seeking to enlist the support of medical care leaders, many of whom ultimately did become CCMC members.[2] Emerson and Kellogg were not the only ones to envision a system-wide study of medical care. In his 1926 presidential address to the American Public Health Association, Charles-Edward A. Winslow suggested that the association "undertake a systematic study" of medical care organization.[3] U.S. Public Health Service economist Harry Moore subsequently credited economist Walton Hamilton for proposing the collection of material that served as the basis for Moore's 1927 book *American Medicine and the People's Health,* which provided the foundation for CCMC investigations.[4] Associate Director of Study I. S. Falk in turn identified Moore as the catalyst for the committee's creation.[5]

To summarize the committee's birth briefly, on April 1, 1926, fourteen leaders representing academic medical centers, foundations, policy organizations, and public health agencies met to discuss medical reform possibilities.[6] They appointed its instigators to a Committee of Five to develop a proposal for a large-scale study. Chaired by Winford H. Smith, director of the Johns Hopkins Hospital, the Committee of Five also comprised Lewellys F. Barker, then clinical professor of medicine at Johns Hopkins; Michael M. Davis, sociologist and administrator soon to be with the Julius Rosenwald Fund; Charles-Edward A. Winslow, of the New York State Department of Health and Yale; and Walton H. Hamilton, professor of economics at the Robert Brookings Graduate School of Economics and Government. Harry Moore staffed the committee.[7]

The Committee of Five presented an ambitious research proposal a year later at its May 17, 1927, invitational Conference on the Economic Factors Affecting the Organization of Medicine.[8] This conference formally established the proposed committee and appointed several conference participants to it. The new committee met briefly on the following day, named itself the Committee on the Cost of Medical Care, and elected academic physician Ray Lyman Wilbur (who had previously been contacted about the position) as chairman.[9] Wilbur was president of Stanford University, a member of the Rockefeller Foundation (which would be one of the major CCMC funding foundations), and former president of the American Medical Association (AMA), among his many positions. He would also simultaneously serve as President Herbert Hoover's secretary of the interior. Bridging the spheres of academia, medicine, philanthropy, and government, Wilbur was chosen, in the words of historian and foundation director Daniel Fox, as a "man for all factions."[10] The committee expanded to more than fifty members under Wilbur's direction. Its participants were by no means strangers to one another; they came from medical, educational, and philanthropic elites, and they had many institutional interconnections. They had worked together for the American Medical Association, the American Public Health Association, the American Association for Study and Prevention of Infant Mortality, the Committee on the Grading of Nursing Schools, the Cleveland Hospital and Health Survey, and the 1931 White House Conference on Child Health and Protection, to name just a few examples. They had served progressive reform efforts, including the campaign for national health insurance during the 1910s.

Progressive Reform Context

The CCMC's model for health care reform reflected the second industrial revolution as well as the Progressive Era reforms seeking to temper that revolution. Although conventional views of progressive reforms saw them as a reaction against industrial and corporate development, revisionist scholars have shown that they fundamentally accepted big business and its new economic order.[11] Progressive reformers assumed a natural evolution of capitalism from individual entrepreneurial to corporate organization, and they applied corporate models to a broad range of institutions.[12] Progress, defined Adam Smith's *Wealth of Nations* in the first industrial revolution, was continuous economic expansion.[13] Alfred P. Sloan similarly told his General Motors's stockholders in 1938 that economic evolution and progress meant growth in size and capitalization: " . . . for there is no resting place for an enterprise in a competitive economy."[14] Industrial growth owed a great deal to scientific and technologic developments, and it became identified *as* scientific and technologic development. From the dawn of (Western) science, historian Carolyn Merchant held, concepts of scientific progress were conflated with technologic and industrial development in capitalist economies.[15] Economic evolution married science and industrialism, and they were blessed by the doctrine of progress.

In the New Economic Era of the 1920s progressive reformers fused business management with social science.[16] Many social scientists thought that, by using surveys and other means of accumulating large amounts of empirical data, they could mitigate the inequities and injustices of industrialism and its twentieth-century organization. *Survey* magazine, for example, promoted planning as a means of protecting the weak from "economic exploitation" and providing public health, unemployment, and housing services for those who needed them.[17] Progressive reformers assumed that development and progress in medicine as well as in other economic endeavors required an industrial infrastructure, corporate organization, and a controlled market economy.[18]

The CCMC did not just follow progressive social reforms and theories of the New Economic Era; its membership included influential social scientists who were developing them. Its institutional economists Wesley C. Mitchell and Walton Hamilton regarded economic planning and regulation as mechanisms meant not to replace corporate capitalism but to enhance its productive capacities.[19] Mitchell's work formed the theoretical base for Herbert Hoover's efforts as secretary of commerce and as president to rationalize industry and to ameliorate recessional phases of what Mitchell called "business cycles."

Later histories revised conventional views of Hoover in terms of liberal versus conservative, describing him as a key leader in New Economic Era efforts to re-form industrial and social organization.[20] Historian Ellis Hawley, in particular, maintained that Hoover "preached the gospel of efficient production and scientific management" while simultaneously proclaiming his faith in "competitive individualism."[21] Hoover expressed his own purpose in initiating the "Waste in Industry" and "Recent Social Trends" compendia as increasing productivity by means of reshaping industry's economic organization.[22] Teamed with his secretary of the interior, Ray Lyman Wilbur, Hoover actively strove to consolidate production units, reduce excess capacity, and coordinate regional alliances (in other words, oligopolies) in the oil, power, coal, and grain industries.[23] It may be that, as CCMC chairman, Wilbur had similar reform goals for what he called at the time the "medical industry." Hoover was familiar with the CCMC's work, which was consistent with his activities to reorganize industry. Hoover was not invited, however, to the CCMC's final conference assembling a "battery of heavyweights" at the New York Academy of Medicine in November 1932, because "he might accept."[24] Funded by eight private business-endowed foundations, the CCMC project fit Hoover's (and Abraham Flexner's) premise that such foundations should play a key role in "democratic" social planning.[25]

CCMC reforms were consistent with the progressive evolutionary perspectives on economic development. A number of its studies applied sociologist and committee member William F. Ogburn's theory of cultural lag to the diagnosis of problems in medical care. Cultural lag was a "convenient metaphor" for reorganizing medical care,[26] but it was more than a metaphor; CCMC reports related it directly to their preferred organizational forms. Harry Moore cited Ogburn's cultural lag theory when he criticized medical care's inadequate organization in 1927. Quoting Barker's 1922 paper on functional division of labor (discussed in chapter 2), Moore affirmed that evolutionary progress in science, medicine, and industry meant specialization and its organization.[27] To the economists on the committee, cultural lag meant failure to conform to prevailing developments in economic organization as well as failure to adjust to them. Observing a "lag of economic organization behind technical development" in the coal industry, Walton Hamilton proposed to reorganize the industry's market structure, reduce the number of competitors, and create an oligopoly.[28] In his dissent from the CCMC's final report, Hamilton may have hoped for a similar design for medicine. As chairman of Hoover's Research Committee on Social Trends, Wesley Mitchell identified one of the trends as the "conscious drive to make our economic organization meet the need of the time." And, he charged, there had been a "lag in this process."[29] Mitchell compared medical development at the time with early stages of mechanization in industry.[30] "Most all doctors are economic Rip Van Winkles," Wilbur once commented more familiarly; "we have been asleep during the period of the world's greatest social and economic advances. We are economic misfits."[31]

The CCMC's Economic Purpose

Many of the CCMC's studies over the next five years assimilated forms and ideas of economic organization of the times. As its May 1927 conference title demonstrated, the committee was explicit about its economic purpose. It defined the key problem as the cost of medical care. One of its major concerns in this arena was that many middle-class people could not afford higher-priced specialty services. The first item on the May agenda was "the inability of the people to pay the cost of modern scientific medicine."[32] The supply side of this concern, as committee studies put it, was the "crisis in hospital finance."[33] The CCMC's proposed solution to supply and demand problems was to reform the "deficiencies of the present economic organization of medicine," as a confidential report to the executive committee phrased it.[34] Inefficiency was a key deficiency; the *Five-Year Program* identified the "ultimate question" to be what organization offered the "most efficient production of service."[35] The committee's summary volume defined its purpose to be diagnosis of the "economic organization of medical care," which, as mentioned earlier, it defined as "methods of producing and financing medical services."[36]

Most historical investigation on the CCMC has emphasized its broad spectrum of features and motives over its economic elements. Paul Starr, for example, associated its recommendations with expanded access and increased professional power as well as with bureaucratic organization.[37] Rosemary Stevens credited the committee with valuing entitlement to scientific medicine for the whole population.[38] Many of its leaders were indeed "partisans of universal access."[39] Calling CCMC reformers "altruistic," Forrest Walker contended that they had not sought to change existing medical institutions radically.[40] Differing with Walker on the extent of desired change, foundation director Steven Schroeder distinguished CCMC encouragement of group medicine on the basis of quality of care (as he saw their activities) from financial strategies of managed care's group medicine in the 1970s.[41]

I do not dispute the committee's intentions to expand access and spread the benefits of modern medicine across the population. CCMC leaders believed in the scientific nature and therapeutic power of twentieth-century medicine, as Fox attested. Fox indicated that CCMC leaders saw changes in society as "subordinate to changes in medical science as determinants of economic relations between physicians and patients."[42] I find that the report *The Crisis in*

Hospital Finance attributed the need for change equally to science and economics. It held that "the advance of the science and art of medicine, on the one side, and the economic development of 20th-century America, on the other, compel changes in the forms of medical practice."[43] The subject of the present discussion, however, is not determinants of change but, rather, the nature of the chosen forms. Although CCMC leaders attributed the need for change equally to science and economics, they generally identified the necessary structures as forms of economic organization. CCMC reformers assumed that they could superimpose the new economic order on medical care without affecting its science. They did not develop a mode of organization specific to medical science, nor did they claim to do so; they looked to the economy for their models to increase productivity and achieve a more efficient use of capital.

CCMC reports associated their recommended organizational forms with popular images of efficiency and mass production. Comparing medical delivery with "production in any industry," *The Fundamentals of Good Medical Care* defined its reorganization goals as producing the "maximum amount and the highest quality of service with the minimum of wasted effort."[44] It was not that such a concept of efficiency drove CCMC reforms but that CCMC reports attributed enhanced efficiency to each of their recommended organizational forms to strengthen their argument. CCMC leaders promulgated models of economic organization, and they honestly believed that their preferred models would provide the best that medicine could offer by joining scientific medicine with scientific management. They did not see an either-or issue of access and quality versus economy. Consistent with and contributing to the progressive tenor of the time, they assumed that matching medicine's economic organization with contemporary financial, institutional, and managerial modes would contribute equally to medical progress, access, and cost-efficiency.

Business Organization

To accomplish its multilevel goals, the CCMC applied business models to medical care organization. Its 1930 report *Capital Investment in Hospitals* explained that the hospital had become a "place of business, and its business is medical care."[45] The report did not see the hospital as all business, however. It went on to say that it was "at once a hotel, an industrial plant, a repair and rehabilitation shop, a haven of refuge . . . and an educational institution." This dual perspective of business and service pervaded CCMC publications. Hospitals were in many respects "typical of all business enterprise," another report held, yet even when organized as business, it continued, they maintained a spirit of public interest.[46] CCMC reformers held a strong public interest ethic, but, like their progressive contemporaries, they thought it could best be dispensed by experts—that is to say, themselves.[47] Feminist public administration scholar Camilla Stivers held that progressives used the term *the public* not to refer to the citizenry at large but to professional experts: they were "the public," and their opinions represented "the public interest."[48] Staff member C. Rufus Rorem used the phrase "the public's investment" to suggest a service-oriented management of capital as well as to emphasize that approximately half of the three billion dollars invested in hospitals was tax-originated funding.[49] Combining business structures with service motives, the CCMC majority and staff seemed to assume that medical care could be structured as business and function as service. Chairman of the Executive Committee C.-E. A. Winslow answered yes to his question: "can the business analogy, however faulty and incomplete, help us towards methods of realizing the nobler functions of medicine as an art and a science and a profession?"[50]

Historian Douglas Parks made the case that CCMC leaders had chosen their desired forms of organization long before completing their studies.[51] Many of them had worked toward their preferred organization for a decade or more. As director of the 1920 Cleveland Hospital and Health Survey, Haven Emerson had advised applying to hospitals the same "principles of organization and efficiency" as "up-to-date business enterprises."[52] Before the CCMC's research was finished, the executive committee's confidential report identified group medicine, pay clinics, and middle-rate services as the top three organizational priorities.[53] The following discussion examines in more detail the business elements of the CCMC's recommended reforms in medical delivery.

Financial Management

The erection of large, complex (academic) medical centers described in chapter 2 signified a quantum leap in hospitals' capital intensity. To many reformers of the time, such a capital expansion itself mandated business management. As Michael Davis advised the Rockefeller Foundation's 1929 hospital administration training efforts, "a billion dollar business needs the kind of management appropriate to large enterprises."[54] CCMC economists and accountants similarly held that the hospital's large capital investment made its service a business requiring accounting and other managerial "techniques borrowed from industry."[55]

Business executive Julius Rosenwald, whose foundation contributed to the CCMC and employed Michael Davis, advised hospital administrators attending the 1930 meeting of the American Hospital Association that private sources of capital were requiring more control over it and more accountability with regard to its use.[56] The CCMC's final report described a partnership between medical professionals and the owners of capital, delegating financial responsibility to the owners.[57] The committee's financial proposals would have (and similar endeavors eventually did) reduced the power of organized medicine and increased that of the owners of capital.

In a campaign against institutional medicine and its shifting control, the American Medical Association's Bureau of Medical Economics ironically charged the CCMC with making a "false analogy with industrial capital."[58] Declaring a need to develop an alternative economics, the bureau held that, along with other professions, medicine did not fit into the system of economics based on analysis of the "existing stage of industrial production." The bureau challenged the committee's three billion dollar appraisal of the hospital system in terms of exchange value. In contrast, the bureau director maintained, accumulation of scientific knowledge was the chief capital investment in medicine.[59] This kind of capital, the bureau report asserted, did not encourage growth of productive units, it did not usually return a profit, and, most important, it did not "confer on the owners the power to control the employment and the actions of the physicians."[60]

In contrast to the bureau's denial of profit making, Walton Hamilton advocated supplanting the private practice profit-making dynamic in medicine with nonprofit institutions.[61] Like Hamilton, CCMC leaders' interests in financial management and the bottom line were not for the purpose of establishing profit-making institutions that would generate a return on investment for owners or stockholders. Davis and Rorem emphasized that most of the capital invested in hospitals was "social capital," by which they meant it was invested for nonprofit purposes.[62] The committee's endorsement of nonprofit status was consistent with Hamilton and Mitchell's belief as institutional economists that the profit motive should (and could) be separated from other economic activities of enterprise.[63] Nonprofit hospitals would be structured and managed like businesses in terms of managing capital and developing self-supporting units, but they would reinvest any surplus in further institutional growth.

CCMC leaders supported managerial strategies designed to maximize institutional growth and productivity, and, like market economists, they assumed that these strategies would also maximize utility. A CCMC credo was that increased use of scientific (by which they generally meant specialty) services and equipment would increase benefits to the population.[64] Yet promoting utilization had a strong element of finance as well as beneficence. Using specialty departments at capacity would not only spread their benefits; it would also enhance their economic status. CCMC reports promoted higher hospital occupancy rates to enhance productivity of the capital invested in them.[65] *The Crisis in Hospital Finance,* a collaborative publication with the Julius Rosenwald Fund, reflected the concerns that Rosenwald had expressed at the American Hospital Association meeting. It criticized inefficient use of large amounts of capital that had been "diverted" from business or other public services.[66] *Capital Investment in Hospitals* correspondingly advised hospital administrators that their large capital investments could be justified only if their facilities were used at "maximum capacity."[67] As the CCMC was winding down, Rorem told the Taylor Society for the Advancement of Management that efficient use of fixed capital required maximum use of the hospital plant and its scientific apparatus.[68] The committee recommended group medicine as the form of organization that could best maximize capital and specialist productivity.

Institution-Based Group Medicine

CCMC leaders had already promoted group medicine to coordinate specialists and provide an efficient form of organization. In 1919 Michael Davis had praised group medicine for its principles of business organization.[69] Lewellys Barker around the same time had seen the association of academic specialty departments as a key form of group practice. Endorsing the "commercial spirit" it brought to medicine,[70] Barker described group medicine as "large-scale production" of medical care.[71] Reflecting its authors' apparent preference for group medicine, the Executive Committee confidential report called individualistic practice "defective," "inefficient," and an anomaly in a "world dominated by the methods of large scale enterprise." The report offered the hospital as a "highly organized unit for the large scale production of medical services."[72] Executive Committee member (and coauthor of the confidential report) Haven Emerson favorably viewed hospital-based group medicine as exemplifying "mass production methods in diagnosis and treatment."[73] Leaders, including Barker, touted group practice as a way to ensure professional control and avoid any "premature state control of medicine."[74]

CCMC reports examined a variety of organizations that held in common an institution-based organized group of physicians. *Private Group Clinics* identified the characteristics of such groups as shared use of facilities and equipment, full-time salaried specialists, and fee services.[75] It described the "dual character" of the groups it examined; on the one hand, they were "cooperative ventures"; on the other, they were highly capitalized "business organizations."[76] Although medical leaders on the CCMC expressed concern about maintaining general practice, and *The Fundamentals of Good Medical Care* estimated that specialists were needed to provide only 18 percent of medical care, group clinics—especially academic ones—generally emphasized specialty care over general practice.[77] Authors of *The Costs of Medical Care* appreciated that organizing specialists into groups represented the next step usually followed in making production more efficient. But, applying an evolutionary argument, it charged that "modern medicine has not, generally speaking, taken the next step ordinarily followed in attempts to make production more efficient—namely, to develop a plan to coordinate the services of specialists with each other and with the available capital investment in plant and equipment."[78]

Many of the private group clinics that the CCMC surveyed had forms of group payment as well as group delivery. The CCMC-supporting Twentieth Century Fund promoted prepaid group medicine, which its founder, retailer Edward Filene, favorably compared to "modern business practice."[79] A letter from the director of the fund to Executive Committee chairman Winslow commended Winslow's encouragement of group practice combined with group payment. But the director chided Winslow for condoning management of insurance funds by "outside" organizations instead of by medical centers themselves.[80] Sidestepping the issue of prepaid group practice, recommendation number three of the CCMC final report supported group payment via insurance, taxation, or both.[81]

Separating delivery from payment, recommendation number one of the CCMC's final report held that medical care should be delivered by groups, preferably those organized around hospitals. An April 1931 internal discussion paper prepared for the executive committee apparently attempted to prod it into defining its desired organization in greater detail. Framing the question in terms of which form of organization offered both the highest quality of care and the most economic use of capital, it offered two alternative answers. The first succinctly stated that the current organization was sufficient and "probably not far behind the mercantile industries in efficiency of organization." The second choice was considerably more detailed, proposing that "economies through mass production" could be achieved by building highly equipped group facilities operated by professional managers and salaried personnel.[82] It appears that CCMC leaders preferred the second choice but that it was not spelled out in the final report in an attempt to avoid dissent.

The opposition to the CCMC final report's endorsement of group medicine did not have to be paranoid to see the threat to private entrepreneurial general practice. Harry Moore concurrently wrote for *Recent Social Trends in the United States* that medicine remained individualistic in the "midst of a highly organized economic world."[83] Reminiscent of Richard Cabot's "evils and anachronisms of private practice" (if not so strident), other CCMC researchers wrote for the *Encyclopaedia of the Social Sciences* that medicine was a "major industry" within which the private practitioner was an "unnecessarily wasteful economic unit."[84] Group practice, especially in academic settings, provided a means for specialists to dominate managerially and medically. Regionalization proponent Kerr White later held that the CCMC identified problems from the "viewpoint of the academic community."[85] Not surprisingly, many private and general practitioners did not accept the diagnosis that identified them as wasteful units or the prescription of group medicine. The final report did not call private practitioners wasteful, and it soft-pedaled the leaders' apparent goals to such an extent that Edgar Sydenstricker, of the U.S. Public Health Service and the Milbank Memorial Fund (the leading CCMC-supporting foundation), and Walton Hamilton each dissented from it.

But weakening the final report was not enough to prevent an AMA-oriented secession. A minority report signed by eight of the twenty-six physicians on the committee, along with Alphonse M. Schwitalla, dean of the St. Louis University School of Medicine, countered with a recommendation to "restore the general practitioner to the central place in medical practice."[86] Schwitalla enjoyed the irony of the CCMC's advocacy of "methods of big business" in 1932, a time of massive business failure.[87] Although the notion was widely ridiculed in the decades to come, the minority report rather accurately portrayed the majority's recommendations as a "corporate practice of medicine."[88] But both sides supported business models: the minority held a conservative view of retaining the individual entrepreneur; the majority preferred a form of corporate institutional medicine. This entrepreneurial-corporate continuum framed structural reform strategies in medicine for the remainder of the century and restricted serious search for alternative forms of medical care organization.

The final CCMC report envisioned that hospitals would develop into comprehensive groups organized as corporations, which it called "community medical centers." Where this organization could not be achieved, leaders advocated more limited forms of group organization that linked hospitals with networks of affiliated physicians. Rorem subsequently described such affiliated physician use of hospital services as "group practice a la carte."[89] It also became known as the physician workshop model, which economists later described as a system in which "physicians structure their relationship to the nonprofit hospital in a manner that allows them to maximize their personal revenues, socializing the costs of production while privatizing the net revenues."[90] Group organization in this sense became a prevalent form of organization. As another way of achieving limited forms of group medicine, the final report promoted specialty-based pay clinics and middle-rate hospitals.[91]

Revenue-Generating Services

Hospitals, specialty clinics, and academic centers were becoming increasingly dependent on revenue-generating services.[92] Specialism was particularly conducive to charging fees for its technical and surgical procedures, which, in turn, reinforced procedural development. Radiology departments led the way in revenue generation in many hospitals.[93] CCMC leaders such as Lewellys Barker had supported further development of specialty-based pay clinics.[94] Michael Davis organized the ophthalmology clinic of the Boston Dispensary as a fee service in 1913. The clinic was held in the evening for working people able to pay its costs.[95] Its price structure covered all the dispensary's expenses and paid a flat fee to the specialists.[96] Its economic goal was to cover its expenses with revenues generated by the services provided. Davis also helped Cornell University and the University of Chicago design pay clinics for their faculty and staff practices. Chicago's exemplary practice plan was known as a "strict" full-time system—although exceptions such as Joseph DeLee remained. Chicago compensated its full-time faculty group practice by salary, and surplus revenues flowed to the institution.[97] Pay clinics at both Chicago and Cornell shifted some of the costs of clinical training from the institution to the patient (and shifted some of the indigent patients out of the academic institution).[98] In his 1920 work for the Cleveland Hospital and Health Survey, Davis classified pay clinics as "public services" because they were open to paying clientele as well as the poor.[99] Davis described pay clinics as a "co-operative practice of medicine on a business basis."[100] By *business basis* Davis specifically meant employment of salaried specialists and patient fees.[101]

After an earlier growth in private pavilions for the wealthy, much of the 1920s hospital construction boom built semiprivate rooms and middle-rate units for middle-class patients.[102] By the middle of the decade paying patients provided urban voluntary hospitals with one-half to two-thirds of their operating revenues.[103] At the same time, state welfare departments were investigating the extent to which public hospitals also could establish rates that covered their costs.[104] Reform leaders continued to press for more fee services. Julius Rosenwald told American Hospital Association members in the early months of the Depression that "to meet the new economic order" they had to reduce their charity services and further expand their fee services.[105]

The CCMC promoted continued growth in fee clinics and middle-rate hospitals. A physician who would sign the majority report identified the middle-income patient as a "business proposition" for hospitals.[106] Maintaining that the wealthy could pay for specialty services and that the poor (some of them, anyway) received specialty services in teaching units, the CCMC's access concerns focused on its estimated 75 percent to 90 percent of the population who were people of "moderate means."[107] It was this middle-class population that provided a large market for fee services and offered a solution to the crisis in hospital finance. The published report *Hospital Service for Patients of Moderate Means* praised the newly constructed Baker Memorial at the Massachusetts General Hospital and the high proportion of pay beds in New York's new

Columbia-Presbyterian Medical Center. It specifically stipulated that middle-class services should be "economically self-supporting."[108] *Self-supporting* meant covering all operational costs with fees for services, but it did not yet mean covering capital costs with patient fees.

The Crisis in Hospital Finance advised administrators to use standardized accounting methods to identify their "revenue-producing departments."[109] To Rufus Rorem, certified public accountant and coauthor of the report, accounting assumed the "prevailing economic order" and enabled administrators to set the price of each service at full cost, including fixed costs.[110] By embedding such economic rules, accounting methods took the place of economic incentives. Other CCMC leaders deemed pricing at full cost "no less desirable in medicine than in industry."[111] Once the actual cost was determined, it would be a managerial decision whether or not to charge the full amount in individual cases. Davis and Rorem noted, however, that hospital administrators were beginning to define the practice of setting prices lower than full cost as unfair competition.[112] The principle of self-support itself thrust hospital services and group medicine into the market. It compelled them to compete for paying patients, manage their institutions according to the bottom line, and design their services for the market in ways not necessarily consistent with the population's need.

CCMC leaders valued efficiency, accountability, and control, economic concepts congruent with the components of economic organization they recommended. Did they use the imagery and language of business as analogy and rhetoric in their arguments? Of course they did, as did their opponents. Both sides also used the rhetoric of science, service, and the doctor-patient relationship. But the CCMC's reform model was not just analogous to business. It materially built business components into the structure of medical care. These components carried inherent economic dynamics, whatever their promoters' intentions were. The committee did not initiate the application of financial management, institution-based group organization, and revenue-generating services, nor was it actually effective in implementing the business components. Nevertheless, it strengthened the position of these business strategies on the twentieth-century health care reform agenda. In the process it also invented the social and economic aspects of what came to be known as "health services research."[113]

It was not such a leap as commonly thought from health reform in the 1920s New Economic Era to national health planning in the 1970s and 1980s and to competitive managed care in the "economic era of health care" of the 1990s.[114] The CCMC tried to integrate doctors and hospitals (and sometimes payments) into corporate organizations; organizational strategies of managed competition and competitive managed care would recapitulate this integration. In his 1924 AMA presidential address Wilbur had challenged medicine to choose between emulating the nineteenth-century railroad industry or the up-to-date telephone industry.[115] Emphasizing the latter, CCMC proposals for regional coordinating agencies to control capital expenditures and integrate medical providers by geographic areas—thus creating regional oligopolies—would provide the basis for the regional health planning programs.

Five

Regional Health Planning and Economic Organization of the Medical Industry

Future U.S. Supreme Court Justice Louis Brandeis proposed in 1912 that regulated monopoly and regulated competition were the two systemic strategies for establishing industrial order.[1] The two terms fit two key system-wide medical delivery reform efforts: regional health planning and managed competition. With the idea of regulated competition Brandeis was attempting to distinguish an approach to progressive regulation for Woodrow Wilson's successful presidential campaign against Theodore Roosevelt. Brandeis was against big business—although he was for scientific management. Most progressives of the time, however, saw the trend to "corporate giantism" as "natural and inevitable."[2] Roosevelt articulated the progressive view that industrial combination was necessary because it stimulated economic growth, and he believed that government planning and regulation could prevent destructive competition and monopolization.[3]

Progressive Era reformers saw planning as an appropriate tool for managing the country's economic order. Not content with leaving supply and demand to the market, planners aspired to allocate resources efficiently and maximize productivity. The mobilization of World War I called this planning into service, and the New Economic Era of the 1920s as well as the New Deal of the 1930s continued to develop planning mechanisms.[4] Herbert Hoover and the social scientists he recruited developed planning as a form of scientific management of the economy.[5] Many progressive reformers and business leaders in the New Economic Era endorsed government working with business to stimulate national economic growth and secure the economic order. After Hoover's more corporative measures failed to lift the country out of the Depression, progressives turned to the government itself to establish regulatory and planning agencies to manage industrial systems.

Planning sought to stabilize industry by transferring productive as well as political decisions to a professional elite.[6] Experts in management and economics, planners came from "corporate management with its allies in philanthropic organizations and premier private universities."[7] They worked for groups such as the American Economic Association, the Taylor Society, the Brookings Institutions, and the National Bureau of Economic Research (NBER). As NBER director, chairman of the New Deal's National Planning Board—and presumably as member of the Committee on the Costs of Medical Care (CCMC)—economist Wesley Mitchell envisioned that national planning would guide the economic evolution and market structure of industry. Assimilating the "existing economic order," planning would maximize industrial output for the "highest economic and social purposes."[8] National economic planning strove to create a "system of economic organization in which all individual and separate plants, enterprises, and industries are treated as co-ordinated units of a single whole."[9] This model of systemic organization was based on regional industrial organization, which served as the model for health systems planning.

Developing the Health Systems Model

Regional health care organization under the 1966 Comprehensive Health Planning law and the 1974 National Health Planning and Resources Development Act built on principles of progressive reform and national economic planning. The deregulation bandwagon of the 1980s—the health planning system was allowed to expire in 1986—obscured the fact that medical, hospital, insurance, and other corporate leaders had long encouraged health systems planning and management. Models of regional organization informed a wide range of twentieth-century health care reforms.[10] Proposing a nationwide consolidation of medical schools, the 1910 Flexner report mapped one per metropolitan area.[11] Three years later the Philadelphia Medical Society's Committee on Hospital Efficiency, chaired by Edward Martin, a leader in the American College of Surgeons's standardization program, presaged the Certificate of Need programs. Seeking to prevent any "unnecessary duplication" of equipment and facilities, the committee viewed Philadelphia's hospitals like an industry that required central management.[12] Great Britain's 1920 Dawson report provided a guide for American academic leaders' efforts to organize regional, three-level systems centered on teaching facilities.[13] In his presidential address to the American Public Health Association a few years later, Yale's Charles-

Edward A. Winslow identified Dawson's voluntary hospital system as a viable alternative to individualistic medical practice as well as to state medicine.[14]

The Cleveland Hospital and Health Survey incorporated features of regional organization and planning in the same year as the Dawson report. The survey recommended controlling capital expenditures in its area's hospitals and managing them according to business principles. Like Dawson, contributor Michael Davis proposed a three-level system comprising large, fully equipped hospitals and dispensaries serving the whole city; smaller and less technologically equipped district hospitals; and minimally equipped health centers serving local areas.[15] Survey director Haven Emerson—like both Davis and Winslow, a CCMC leader-to-be—held what would become by the end of the century a popular concept of accountability in medical care: he viewed the public as "investors" in the Community Fund and as "stockholders" of the institutions supported by it.[16] Emerson identified "duplication of function" in hospitals as a problem that could be solved by assigned geographic areas for each institution. As a favorite tool of progressive reformers, health care surveys effectively served as market surveys of supply and demand. The Cleveland Survey supported the plans of three downtown hospitals to upgrade their levels and their markets by moving to "more salubrious quarters" in suburban areas.[17] Several of the hospitals were moving to form the University Hospital Group of the Western Reserve University School of Medicine. Yet Davis warned that their move would render the central (and poorer) sections of the city bereft of medical facilities.

The Committee on the Costs of Medical Care further encouraged development of regional planning to allocate capital investment and supervise growth of technology-intensive medical services.[18] The Bingham Plans, also starting in the 1930s, provided a model for regional organization—as well as for group practice. The plans linked community hospitals in Massachusetts and Maine to specialty departments at Tufts University medical school's newly consolidated (and newly named) New England Medical Center in Boston.[19] Specifically commending the Bingham Plans, Surgeon General Thomas Parran promoted their stratified hospital system as a national model. Parran told the U.S. Senate in 1944 that such systems would allow hospitals to operate in a "more business-like manner," by which he meant receive "full cash value of services rendered" and use their large capital investment to "full capacity."[20] He emphasized designing area wide hospital service plans before building new hospitals. The subsequent Hill-Burton hospital construction program did require regional planning, but it did not implement Parran's systemic vision. Although none could be called a complete realization, regional organization also shaped the 1965 regional medical programs (RMPs), the 1971 Area Health

Education Centers (AHECs), the 1966 and 1974 health planning programs, the 1993 managed competition bill, and the integrated hospital systems of the 1990s.

Recapitulating the Committee on the Costs of Medical Care's theme that medical care lagged in its economic evolution, health planning projected a progression of economic development onto medical care. As advisor to the Health and Hospital Planning Council of Southern New York just prior to national health planning, former CCMC staff C. Rufus Rorem saw regional planning as a means of controlling the "economic development and administration" of medical services.[21] Johns Hopkins's regionalization enthusiast Kerr White similarly held that health systems remained in a "rudimentary stage of evolution compared with systems for the mass production of manufactured goods."[22]

Health planning leaders explicitly linked regional health planning theory and practice to regional economic planning.[23] Promoters of the Public Health Service model consciously applied precepts of regional planning as well as regional economics in designing comprehensive, hierarchic, self-sufficient medical delivery systems.[24] Health planners in the United States and Britain called on the fields of regional economics and economic geography to map centralized specialty services in a three-level hierarchy of facilities serving a geographic area.[25] Economic geography defined its purview as the spatial differentiation of economic activities and the growth of economic systems, and it identified integration, hierarchy, and growth as "fundamental system principles."[26] Planning professor John Friedmann held that regional planners were particularly concerned with economic growth, or "more precisely . . . the *spatial incidence of economic growth.*"[27] He and other planners maintained that regional industrial organization promoted productivity, expanded scale, differentiated functions, concentrated specialists, and integrated production units.[28] These regional strategies were precisely those sought by regional health planning (as well as by managed competition),[29] and they were sought for the same purposes as in industry—to promote system-wide economic growth and productivity.

Many professionals advising or working in the national health planning programs trained in the disciplines of regional economics, urban planning, and business management, and they brought the precepts of these fields to their health planning. Health administration scholar Avedis Donabedian included the same organizational elements as Friedmann in his model for regional medical organization: functional hierarchy of institutions, central location of higher-order functions, and administrative agencies to reintegrate the differentiated functions.[30] Health planners applied economic geography's central place theory, which described regional distribution of business firms, to design what they considered to be an ideal functional and spatial plan for regional health care delivery systems.[31] Yet some medical geographers came to question whether central place theory's tenet that "market forces should dictate thresholds and ranges for each level of service" was an appropriate determinant of health service organization.[32]

Strategies of Regional Reform

Regional health planning sought to integrate medical institutions horizontally, differentiate them into levels of specialization requiring vertical reintegration, and organize regions as designated production and market areas for the highest specialty level—usually academic medical centers (AMCs). As in industry, system-wide regulation or management endeavored to allocate resources, expand productivity, and control capital investment and competition. Originating in large-scale industrial production, these organizational strategies conferred certain economic dynamics on medical institutions and shaped their collective market structure.

Consolidating Hospitals and Medical Groups

The national health planning program picked up the refrain of unnecessary duplication of services as a means of promoting multi-institutional delivery systems. Rorem portrayed group practice as the "private counterpart of community planning," necessary for the "*appropriate* use of buildings, equipment and supplies."[33] The ALPHA Center for Health Planning, one of the planning program's technical assistance centers, explained to the appropriately named "health systems agencies" (HSAs) that multi-institutional linkages could be accomplished either by operational arrangements such as regionalization, affiliation, and shared services or by organizational connections such as contract management, mergers, and hospital chains.[34] Planning policies promoted regional oligopolistic or shared-monopoly delivery systems by means of hospital consolidation.[35] Waving one of the first "merger mania" newspaper articles about the hospital consolidations of the 1980s, the director of another technical assistance center in effect asked a group of concerned planners (myself included), "But isn't this what we wanted?" A good case can be made that the multiplication of services was indeed excessive in terms of efficacy and population need, but the ongoing charge of unnecessary duplication was as much an oligopolistic strategy in medicine as it was in industry.[36] Large—often academic—hospitals appreciated that preventing specialty service multiplication reduced competitive threats to their services.

Health planners as well as administrators of the larger hospitals assumed that consolidation would enhance hospital productivity and economy of scale.[37] With origins in mass production, belief in the economy of scale was deeply embedded in twentieth-century organizational thought. Health planning's official dictionary, in fact, defined *large scale* as a component of efficiency.[38] Yet empirical studies did not consistently find lower unit costs with larger scale (due in large part to larger hospitals' greater technologic intensity). Health economist S. E. Berki summarized his comprehensive review with the wry remark that the literature demonstrated that hospital economies of scale "exist, may exist, may not exist, or do not exist, but in any case, according to theory, they ought to exist."[39] If scale was not consistently associated with lower unit costs, however, research dating back to the CCMC had found that it correlated with higher utilization, higher income per bed, higher profit margins, and less "idle capital."[40] Later studies would link greater hospital scale with higher financial ratios such as higher investment per bed, operating surplus, operating margin, and return on equity.[41] Financial measures such as these signified the real meaning of economy of scale. Consolidation to improve these criteria favored the private and highly specialized institutions and tended to target the financially weakest hospitals, which (not surprisingly) tended to be those serving the poorest populations.[42]

Ironically—since so many hospital administrators strenuously battled planning's consolidation efforts—so-called market strategies drove hospital consolidation farther than planning ever contemplated. Administrators of the larger hospitals then acknowledged that consolidation could constrain competition, expand market power, control production, promote full capacity utilization, and maximize the capital and technology that the system could absorb.[43] While planning promoted operational arrangements, in the ALPHA Center's terms, competitive managed care preferred organizational linkages. Accounting firms, financial experts, and management consultants in the 1990s advised individual hospitals to combine with their neighbors, merge into systems, sell to profit-making corporations, or institute joint ventures.[44] Such consolidation had a snowball effect. Integration of one group of hospitals in a region prompted competitive mergers and acquisitions among its remaining hospitals, resulting in a set of regional systems comprising fewer, larger, and more complex hospitals. By the end of the century 40 percent of U.S. hospitals belonged to systems (that owned their assets), and 32 percent belonged to networks (that did not own their assets).[45] Although they promoted consolidation in the name of competition, market reformers had regional oligopolies in mind.[46]

Consolidation strategies applied also to physicians, in the form of group medical practice. Following the Committee on the Cost of Medical Care's failed attempt to expand group practice, CCMC economist Walton Hamilton worked with the U.S. Department of Justice on its anti-trust suit against the District of Columbia chapter of the American Medical Association (AMA). The Department indicted the chapter and some of its leaders—including Arthur Christie and Olin West, signers of the CCMC minority report—for conspiracy to restrain prepaid group practice.[47] Longtime group practice supporters Michael Davis and Hugh Cabot testified at the grand jury hearing. The government's case supported "free and fair competition between new forms of organization for medical service and older types of practice."[48] Such a view was consistent with Hamilton's concept of "regulated competition."[49] The Supreme Court's ruling for the government treated medicine as a business, "subject to the same free enterprise regulations as other areas of commerce and industry."[50]

Despite the Supreme Court's decision in its favor, group practice (outside of academia) grew slowly, and organized medicine continued to fight it. National health planning promoted systems of organized physician groups, tracing its preference for such groups to the CCMC.[51] Health administration professors advised planners that, by expanding operational scale, hierarchic divisions of labor, and worker management, group practice represented a higher level of industrial development in medicine.[52] Concurrent with health planning's efforts, physician-reformer Paul Ellwood proposed to the Nixon administration that the federal government subsidize organized medical groups, which he renamed "health maintenance organizations" (HMOs).[53] Elwood (in the great rhetorical reversal) ascribed a market ideology to what had been considered progressive reform. Advising President Carter, economist Alain Enthoven described a similar concept of bundling HMO-type organizations into regionally competing units.[54] Both Ellwood and Enthoven participated in formulating the Clinton administration's Health Security Plan, which was based on a strategy of managing competition among HMO-type or managed care organizations.[55] Competitive managed care systems continued to develop after the demise of the Clinton proposal.[56] Like planning before them, managed systems sought to differentiate and then reintegrate facilities and services of different levels of specialization and technologic intensity.

Integrating Hospitals and Academic Group Practices Vertically

Regional medical organization and academic clinical practice fed each other. Organized faculty practice plans grew out of full-time programs and their specialty department-based clinical practice. Medical schools such as the University of Chicago constructed hospitals in the 1920s with foundation funding and supported them with clinical services. At the University of Iowa specialty departments such as obstetrics (but not the more remunerative specialties like surgery) employed departmental chiefs on a full-time basis, and its financial office collected fees from their private practice.[57] Academic leaders envisioned their institutions at the apex of hospital levels systems. Stanford's Ray Lyman

Wilbur supported Dawson's concept—reformulated in 1942 in Michael Davis's *Medical Care*—of a regional organization centered around teaching hospitals.[58] Surgeon General Parran's levels system similarly differentiated teaching hospitals with full specialty services from district hospitals, rural hospitals, and health centers.[59] Following Parran's testimony, the U.S. Senate issued a report that identified the academic medical center as the most appropriate foundation for group practice as well as for regional hospital organization.[60] Parran's design placed the academic medical center at the center of its region and at the top of the levels hierarchy, with linkages to district and community hospitals.[61] Parran's Public Health Service colleague Joseph Mountin subsequently served on an American Public Health Association subcommittee that proposed a national health program based on salaried academic group practices coordinated with community hospitals in their regions.[62]

Faculty practice and regional organization grew significantly in the 1950s, although not so much as they both would in the 1970s.[63] Academic medical centers established themselves as regional specialty hospitals and affiliated with community hospitals thriving on Hill-Burton funds in order to develop specialty markets and control competition for them.[64] They defended their clinical services in terms of their right to compete with private practice. Predictably, the American Medical Association responded to the growth in academic service by raising once again the specter of "corporate practice of medicine."[65] The AMA's critique of corporate organization and its preference for the existing entrepreneurial, private practice organization was conservative, by definition. Reformers designing an opposing (corporate) model called it progressive.

Progressive physician E. Richard Weinerman was one of a number of activists who promoted academic clinical services and their vertical integration with other hospitals. He called systems in which academic centers coordinated the stratified personnel and institutions in their areas "functional," or "regional," group practices.[66] With his impeccable progressive credentials—refusal to sign a loyalty oath in the McCarthy era sidetracked his career considerably—one of his colleagues found it difficult to believe that Weinerman "fully accepted the financial incentives concept" that he applied in a national health insurance proposal.[67] Weinerman attributed "higher net returns due to increased operating efficiency" to medical centers' regional organization and their potential to use production and quality control methods.[68] But such economic concepts were not anomalies in Weinerman's thinking; twenty years earlier he had credited regional medical organization and group practice with maximizing system-wide efficiency and economy.[69] He had also depicted the fabric of group practice as "woven from the warp of individualism and the woof of productive organization."[70] I have selected an exemplary health care reformer to show how progressive reformers adopted organizational structures and managerial methods from the economy. Their primary goal was not individual gain, nor, in many cases, was it institutional profit. Their goal was progress, and to many leaders progress was consistent with the growth of academic medicine. Like the majority on the Committee on the Costs of Medical Care, progressive reformers defined the problem as an individualistic, entrepreneurial practice that had not kept up with the economic organization of the time. Accordingly, they envisioned a (corporate) institutional form of organization as the solution. Academic reformers furthered expansion of their own clinical departments as the answer to the cultural lag in medicine.

Health planning promoted academic medical center–based regional organization and described its levels system as a form of vertical integration. The National Council on Health Planning and Development advised that vertical integration enhanced system-wide productivity in medicine as it did in industry.[71] Citing Britain's Dawson report as well as the CCMC, one health services textbook defined *regionalization* as a "division of functions among hospitals, clinics, and medical personnel based on vertically integrated levels of specialization and intensity of services."[72] Other advocates commended that regionalization offered to medicine the same economic benefits that vertical integration offered to business.[73]

Medical schools vastly augmented their clinical services in the 1970s and 1980s with financing from Medicare, Medicaid, and the regional medical programs. Some schools suddenly beheld a new "service mission"; others were continuing a long-standing tradition.[74] Academic organizations such as the Association of American Medical Colleges earnestly promoted the idea that regionally oriented–academic systems would make the "benefits of scientific medicine quickly accessible and available in every community."[75] The University of Iowa built a new hospital for its faculty practice plan and a three-level statewide system to funnel patients into it. Iowa "jettisoned" its image as an indigent care hospital in the 1970s and looked to Medicare and other private admissions to support its new "tertiary care mission."[76] In a somewhat different approach Johns Hopkins established a joint venture with an insurance company to develop a group health plan in Columbia, Maryland, a planned upscale community.[77] Academic medical centers became big businesses at this time if they hadn't done so already.[78] Clinical practice became medical schools' single most important revenue source in the 1980s, providing over 50 percent of their income by the end of the century.[79] Their practice plans enabled some teaching centers to convert to or sell themselves to for-profit corporations. Even when they weren't accountable to corporate stockholders (and most were not), academic medical centers had to make money or risk being downgraded in the bond market. For financial reasons academic medical centers experienced strong pressures to integrate with community hospitals—at least until 1998.

The level-of-care system manifested the strong overlap between professional and market dominance. Applying concepts of scientific management to hospital systems, architects of regionalization counseled each institution to do the work for which it was best suited.[80] Institutional differentiation by level of specialization and technologic intensity carried an intrinsic economic dynamic. It was well known in industry that differentiation conferred competitive advantages on "higher," that is, more capital-intensive production levels.[81] Economists and economic geographers attributed similar market dynamics to hospital levels systems.[82] Differentiation of three hospital levels reinforced the concept of tertiary care and expanded the market for its services. Enveloping community hospital markets, regional organization worked something like an area-wide assembly line, selectively channeling more complex patients to more complex, generally academic, facilities in order to achieve "optimal use" of their facilities and investments.[83] Academics recognized that levels policies awarded competitive advantages to academic centers and, in so doing, fortified their growing practice plans. Their competitive advantages devolved from the prestige of their position at the top of the hierarchy as well as from the differential allocation of resources and technology inherent in the levels definitions.

Specialty leaders used levels differentiation to restrict duplication of tertiary-level services and protect their practice plan markets. Health services researchers at Stanford University, a pioneer in open-heart surgery, for example, recommended restricting open-heart procedures to a small number of high-volume centers.[84] Open-heart surgery became a focus for specialty-specific regional policy efforts and did in fact remain one of the more regionalized services: 93 percent of teaching hospitals integrated with academic medical centers had open-heart surgery units in 1997, compared with 74 percent of more loosely linked academic hospitals, 48 percent of other teaching hospitals, and 10 percent of nonteaching hospitals.[85] It is not likely, however, that regional planning was forceful enough to achieve such a distribution. One geographic analysis attributed the actual differentiation of hospital levels equally to regional planning and to market forces.[86]

As national health planning was meeting its end, reform leaders promulgated regional integration as market strategy. Vertical integration of HMO systems, explained a New England Medical Center president, matched a "system of mass marketing with a system of mass production."[87] Vertical, or "virtual," integration, which emphasized contractual relationships over common ownership, continued as the dominant organizational strategy in health care in the late 1980s and in the 1990s. Many elements of integrated delivery systems (one of the several labels of the time) were consistent with those of regionalization. They comprised large corporately structured institutional providers organized by hierarchical levels and horizontally and/or vertically integrated with other institutions.[88] Organizational theorists acclaimed that health care had finally closed the organizational gap and caught up with industry in forming vertical and horizontal linkages.[89] As regionalization advocates had before them, integrated delivery proponents extolled the virtues of their systems to be economy of scale, improved financial performance, and competitive advantage.[90] Some analysts reverted to the term *regionalization* to describe the new integrated systems. They explained that hospitals integrated to manage competitive threats and that regional systems were the product of competition.[91]

In order to expand or even maintain market shares, integrated delivery systems had to (or thought they had to) encompass the full range of tertiary-level services. Many systems sought alliances with academic medical centers to achieve this range. Reciprocally, AMCs endeavored to make themselves indispensable to the new systems. Many academic centers restructured their practice plans and expanded linkages with other providers to create integrated delivery systems.[92] They bought physician practices, organized referral networks, developed strategic business units, invested in joint ventures with manufacturers and insurance companies, established their own HMOs, and/or sold themselves to for-profit systems.[93] Duke University, for example, expanded its long private-practice history, developing a comprehensive, corporate, regional system.[94] AMC-based integrated delivery sought to differentiate academic systems from others by promoting their tertiary-level products. Many aggressively marketed high-intensity services as their key selling points and developed quaternary services as the next rung in the competitive levels ladder.[95]

Institutional integration efforts accelerated throughout the 1990s—until 1998. The spectacular implosion and bankruptcy of the Philadelphia-based Allegheny system, "perhaps the epitome of medical empire building," caused an about-face in academic delivery system integration.[96] Business consultants suddenly reversed their previous advice, recommending downsizing and divestment. The extent to which regional academic hospital systems and their markets would integrate or disintegrate remained to be seen at the end of the century. Whether coordinated by AMCs or not, the levels strategy implied that, once differentiated, levels would have to be reintegrated structurally, or at least managerially.

Organizing Regions as Market and Production Areas

Building horizontally and vertically integrated delivery systems required organizing their market areas. Health planning identified the region as the appropriate geographic area for medical delivery systems. Traditional planning methods defined health care regions as market areas and used commercial trade area maps to demarcate them.[97] Regionalization strategies attempted to stabilize hospital markets by geographically assigning defined populations to defined providers. Health planners in Britain and Europe as well as the United States largely defined regions according to the size of the market required to support academic medical centers and their specialty departments.[98] Economic geography once again provided planning with its rationale, describing a three-level hierarchy of market areas corresponding with the three-level delivery systems. Geographers identified the region as the production/market area that circumscribed a population sufficient to support the highest level of specialization.[99] The ALPHA Center called on economic geography's central place theory to identify market areas for different hospital levels.[100] Consistent with such a use of central place theory, health planning textbooks ascribed the concept of medical service area to retail marketing theory.[101]

To a large extent the national health planning programs mapped health facility planning areas according to dominant hospitals' existing or required markets. The initial mapping of health systems agencies and regions was in fact one of the most important decisions taken in the health planning program. It determined from the beginning which tertiary–level centers were awarded a monopoly, which had to compete with others in the same area, and which secondary centers could aspire to regional center status.

Under both regional organization and competitive managed care, academic administrators consistently estimated that they required one to two million people to support their (sub)specialty services and maintain leadership.[102] Integrated academic systems continued to define regions according to their specialty departments' required revenue levels.[103] Because of their similar population requirements, regional planning and competitive managed care each divided nationwide health care into approximately two hundred regions. A significant theoretical difference between planning and managed competition, however, was the number of delivery systems per region—whether medical systems would enact Brandeis's regulated competition or regulated monopoly. In the name of the "public interest," academic leaders advised in the 1960s that each region should have only one system and that all hospitals not affiliated with it should be closed.[104] Otherwise, they warned, growth of specialty services such as heart surgery would lead to extensive wasteful duplication. Many health planners also saw regional monopoly as a goal of hospital consolidation.[105] As one federal official noted in the time of planning, regionalization ideally established a single "health care corporation" in each geographic area.[106]

In practice, however, regionalization advocates had to acknowledge the reality of competing systems in metropolitan areas. To take one—fairly extreme—example, the Health Policy Advisory Center calculated that New York City in 1970 had seven competing "medical empires" (some with quite tenuous linkages) encompassing more than two-thirds of the hospital beds in the city.[107]

In contrast to the monopolistic approach of regionalization, market reformers and administrators at large community hospitals preferred an oligopolistic model comprising several integrated systems per region. Managed competition explicitly designed shared monopolies, with two to four competing alliances in an area.[108] But its proponents acknowledged that continuing consolidation processes could whittle the number down to monopoly.[109] It seemed likely that policies of regionalization and managed competition would lead to a similar number of huge medical center–based integrated delivery systems with similar market shares. In addition, both strategies treated the complex of health care delivery facilities in an area as an industry to be managed or regulated.

Managing Regional Systems

National health planning in the 1970s borrowed methods of managing multi-institutional regional systems from large-scale capitalist enterprise as a means of actively managing system-wide supply and demand.[110] It promoted these managerial methods in order to integrate hospitals, control their growth, and achieve full utilization of their technologic capacity. Commissioning accounting firms to write educational and training materials, national planning encouraged the use of performance indicators and other business methods from econometrics, operations research, and systems analysis. Planning's technical assistance centers also contracted with accounting firms to train planners in business analytic methods including productivity measures, cost-benefit analyses, demand forecasting, financial ratios, resource requirement projections, and systems analysis.[111] Henrik Blum, a dean of health planning theory, drew on systems theory to justify the three-level structure of regional organization.[112] Systems analysts saw health planning as consciously applying methods of scientific management and engineering to health systems.[113]

Situated at the top of the levels hierarchy, academic medical centers positioned themselves to manage regional hospital systems.[114] Managed competition, by contrast, did not privilege AMCs as regional administrators. Large delivery systems (some of which were academic), large insurance plans, and large purchasers competed for systemic management in the 1990s. In one academic bid for control the Association of American Medical Colleges proposed a "national system of regional medical care" that delegated systems planning, building, and managing authority to academic centers.[115] Commonalities in the major system-wide strategies demonstrated the dominance of business models in twentieth-century health care reform.

Reforming Systems

Reform methods are conventionally portrayed in terms of opposing ideologies of planning (or regulation) versus competition (or the market). But both approaches used both market and regulatory mechanisms: planning encouraged competition, and competitive tactics required planning.[116] Health planning was government driven to the extent that organizational criteria such as minimum volumes and levels of care were built into planning methodologies and "guidelines" (which were mandatory for health systems agencies). The criteria extensively incorporated professional standards, however, reflecting the dominance of specialty and hospital associations.

Ideologically and ideally, planning expressed James Morone's "democratic wish" for health policy.[117] But health facility planning areas were not necessarily congruent with political boundaries, and regional planning was not administered by democratically elected officials. Claims of democratic health planning were based on the provision in the 1974 law mandating consumer majorities on all decision-making committees. The Certificate of Need process particularly illustrates how interested parties dominated health planning and regulation. One New Jersey hospital heavily involved in developing the state's Certificate of Need standards for perinatal services subsequently used the process to seek state designation as the regional tertiary perinatal provider for its area.[118] This was typical practice; the committee that I worked with also included administrators from hospitals competitively applying to purchase MRI machines. Aside from the fact that the MRI and other "technical assistance" committees had no consumers, there was a significant power imbalance in favor of the weightier and wealthier players at the table. The larger and more prestigious providers generally came out on top, even if they didn't get everything they wanted. In addition, many participating consumers were concerned with protecting "their" doctors and hospitals from government interference, and local providers played on these fears.

Building their case against planning, market reformers claimed that consumer choice models were more democratic than planning precisely because regulatory agencies tended to become captured by the industry they regulated—as the Certificate of Need experience demonstrated.[119] Yet the ensuing development of massive insurance plans also concentrated provider power and diminished consumer and community power.[120] "The market" served as an ideology that obscured the actual loci and mechanisms of power.[121] The big players held the power in both planning and market reforms, and it was often the same big players, although there was a shift in favor of corporate payers and finance.

Business interests continued to consolidate their control over health policy in the 1980s, and health planning became significantly more business driven. Ironically, this was partly by its own invitation. Health systems agencies such as the one in Sacramento diligently organized the purchaser coalitions that would shortly replace them. Two-thirds of the initial sixty purchaser coalitions were business dominated.[122] Medical geographers came to warn that, in market systems, organized interest groups such as provider associations and insurance companies controlled medical regionalization.[123] Whether under regionalization or competitive managed care, expansion in business control made it less likely that medical systems would or could direct their operations toward meeting the needs of the population.

Yet a major appeal of regional organization was that it seemed to imply some form of responsibility for the health, or at least the health care, of the people living in an area. Many reformers defined *regionalization* as a distribution of medical services according to need, although it did not in fact build in means to achieve such a match. The health planning program required health systems agencies to document the health status of the people residing in their areas, but the permitted planning methods were seldom designed to match service delivery to those measured needs. Most resource requirement projections were based on the distribution and utilization patterns of existing institutions and, as such, reinforced the status quo.[124]

Alain Enthoven claimed that managed competition could succeed where planning had failed, matching the supply and type of physicians, beds, and specialized facilities to the needs of identified populations.[125] But he proposed no mechanism adequate to the task. Ideologies of competition held that "the market" would best accomplish the match, but their claims were unsupported. Managed care's counting of "covered lives" meant that uncovered lives didn't count. Recognizing managed systems' concern with their own customers rather than populations as a whole, the U.S. General Accounting Office warned against the possibilities of gerrymandering and redlining when establishing regional service areas: isolating areas with high-risk populations and offering them fewer services and/or higher prices.[126]

Regional planning, managed competition, and integrated delivery systems all constructed similar forms of organization.[127] The same strategies of economic organization and the same geographic configurations consistently reappeared, although they did so in the guise of different political and economic ideologies. They all sought to manage physicians and other health care workers in groups, expand institutional scale and capital intensity, differentiate levels of specialization, allocate markets, control competition, and manage regional systems. A crucial distinction between regional organization and integrated delivery systems was the latter's integration of finance with delivery, which strengthened the power of financial institutions in health policy. But they were all business models leading to shared monopoly delivery systems.

The hope of restraining inflation in medical specialization and intensity continued to drive international regionalization efforts. "Post-welfare" systems in Britain's reformed National Health Service looked to market-oriented regional organization for their strategies.[128] Following the Conservative government's version of managed competition, British policy analysts resurrected the "hub and spoke" regional model of vertically integrated levels systems.[129] Models like this had long sought to standardize medical care at the level of academic specialty services.[130] Tri-level delivery systems were organized around teaching hospital services, thus exacerbating the intensity escalation. Superimposed on regional organization across the specialties, certain specialties embarked on their own regionalization schemes. Perinatal regionalization, one of the key specialty regionalization ventures, paralleled regional health planning in its application of business models of organization.

Six

Perinatal Regionalization and Economic Order

Medical care after World War II built on developments of earlier decades. Hospitals grew in capacity and technology, and the number of specialists grew, as did the number of insured patients to support them. In obstetrics and gynecology the baby boom sustained this growth until the "birth dearth" hit. In less than a decade the number of U.S. births dropped precipitously from around 4 million a year to just over 3 million in 1973. The specialty felt the pinch as the total number of births per trained obstetrician fell from around 550 in 1963 to 380 in 1970 and down to 280 in 1973.[1] One academic chief at the time exclaimed that he didn't want to "train any more OBs to go out to middle-class communities to compete with established doctors for the few deliveries and hysterectomies that are left."[2] Despite rising numbers of births after the 1973 nadir, continued growth in specialty training meant that the ratio of births to obstetrician continued dropping; it reached 190 by 1980 and 150 by 1990. The much-vaunted undersupply of obstetricians was not true in the 1970s, and it was not true in the ensuing decades, although distribution continued to be a problem—it tended to exclude inner-city areas. As supply outgrew demand in the birth market, obstetric leaders took steps to protect and expand their turf.

Restructuring the Perinatal Industry

The strategy of perinatal regionalization developed primarily in academic medical centers. It was designed to cope with competitive pressures generated by the stagnant birth market, duplication of technologically complex services in community hospitals, and increasing pressure for academic specialty departments to generate revenues from clinical services. In 1965 obstetric leaders at the American Medical Association's national conference on area wide health planning expressed concern that recent technologic upgrades had failed to boost their hospitals' low obstetric occupancy rates.[3] They turned to planning to accomplish what technology adoption hadn't, although they developed their planning apparatus outside the national health planning program. Shortly after the AMA conference, Harvard Medical School's Duncan Reid proposed a regional perinatal network system to link secondary hospitals to medical schools.[4] Reid was at the time the president of the American College of Obstetricians and Gynecologists, which then inaugurated a national survey of maternity care. The survey found that medical school hospitals were getting only 6 percent of all births and their affiliated hospitals a further 13 percent, leaving over 80 percent of the nation's births outside the university domain.[5] The specialist-dominated AMA Committee on Maternal and Child Care subsequently led the 1970 White House Conference on Children's support for organized perinatal systems. The committee also led the full AMA to support centralized perinatal intensive care and the National Foundation-March of Dimes to fund a committee to design it.[6] In 1976 the resulting Committee on Perinatal Health provided the framework for regional perinatal policy in *Toward Improving the Outcome of Pregnancy.*[7]

Toward Improving became widely accepted as national perinatal policy, due in no small part to a mass inundation of fifty or seventy thousand free copies sent to public health departments and planning agencies[8]—where several crossed my desk. I can report from personal observation that planning staff in the health systems agencies (HSAs) generally accepted it as received truth. The national health planning guidelines incorporated its standards, and local HSAs dutifully wrote them into their regional plans.[9] Public and private consulting firms promoted the standards.[10] Nearly all state public health departments adopted policies of perinatal regionalization over the next two decades, and many enforced their policies with regulation.[11] Even sitting in the midst of this activity, I could not see why the report achieved such unquestioning hegemonic status. The answer seemed to be a combination of medical authority; promotion by prestigious hospitals; assumptions that, if some intensive care was good, more was better; and the fact that it was easier for planners to use available standards than to develop their own. Perinatal medicine continued to promote regional systems in the 1990s, alternately portraying them as compatible with or as competitive with managed care. The March of Dimes reconvened its committee and released a revised document, *Toward Improving the*

Outcome of Pregnancy: The 90s and Beyond.[12] *Toward Improving II* made regionalization more congruent with changes in the economic environment. The American Academy of Pediatrics and the American College of Obstetricians and Gynecologists's joint *Guidelines for Perinatal Care* also continued to promote regionalization.[13]

Perinatal regionalization's strategies of economic organization paralleled those of regionalization in general. The joint *Guidelines* saw regional perinatal care as a "systems approach" that coordinated providers in a geographic area.[14] Leaders in the 1990s explicitly drew parallels between perinatal regionalization and regional industrial organization.[15] Like regionalization as a whole, perinatal regionalization sought to differentiate levels of specialization, consolidate smaller units, allocate regional markets, and manage systems. These components and methods of economic organization sought to control growth, grant competitive advantages, integrate services horizontally and vertically, and maximize utilization of specialty capacity.

Elements of Perinatal Regionalization
Specialty Levels

Perinatal regionalization functionally divided hospitals providing maternal and/or newborn services into levels of specialization and service intensity. The American College of Obstetricians and Gynecologists's 1970 maternity care survey concerned itself with teaching level and unit size.[16] Around the same time in Massachusetts, the Medical Society, regional medical program, Department of Public Health, and Blue Cross collaborated to reformulate state licensing standards for hospital newborn services. The new standards defined two levels of intensive care nursery: *high intensity* providing most intensive care technologies and *highest intensity* providing all intensive care technologies.[17] Perinatal leaders subsequently established the Massachusetts Maternity and Newborn Regionalization Project to build on the licensing activities and promote the project as the prototype of perinatal regionalization.

Like the Massachusetts regionalization project, *Toward Improving* identified three levels of specialization. The joint specialty *Guidelines* further defined them according to level of staff specialization and capital investment.[18] Neonatal intensive care units (NICUs) were the more identifiable entity, and hospitals and perinatal planners designated perinatal level by NICU complexity, often without additional obstetric criteria. Obstetric services thus achieved level II or III recognition by piggybacking onto NICUs. *Toward Improving II* more explicitly renamed levels III, II, and I units as subspecialty, specialty, and basic. It clarified that level III interventions were intended solely for use by subspecialists in maternal-fetal medicine (obstetrics) and neonatology (pediatrics) and were not to be provided by lower-level physicians. Both *Toward Improving* reports identified academic medical centers as the prime location for fully equipped level III centers.

The levels system implied that, once they were differentiated functionally, the three levels would have to be reintegrated managerially. Formal agreements among hospitals providing different levels of care created a contractual form of vertical integration. One purpose of this integration was to channel selected patients to academic tertiary centers. Academic pediatricians went out to train physicians and nurses in community hospitals in stabilizing small and sick newborns for live delivery to their tertiary units. As the National Perinatal Information Center recognized, this kind of outreach was a competitive strategy.[19] By the early 1990s, 75 percent of the hospitals belonging to the Council on Teaching Hospitals (COTH) had a level III neonatal unit, compared with 36 percent of other teaching hospitals and 6 percent of nonteaching hospitals.[20] If each COTH hospital had a level III unit and each non-COTH teaching hospital had a level II (an approximation of regionalization goals), the resulting 1,025 high-intensity institutions would control about half of the nation's births.

Managed care alliances also created multi-institutional systems by linking providers of different levels of care. But perinatal policy leaders called it "deregionalization" when the new alliances disrupted academically-oriented ones. Leaders perceived the changes of the 1990s to be a "threat to academic obstetrics" as well as a threat to its practice revenues.[21] *Toward Improving II* took two somewhat contradictory approaches to defining levels in the managed care era. On the one hand, it tried to establish a quaternary-level status (without actually calling it that) by limiting services such as neonatal cardiac surgery and extracorporeal membrane oxygenation (ECMO) to a few subspecialty centers. Yet it also advised that levels could be "collocated," meaning that the definition of levels need not refer to structural levels but could pertain to operational levels.[22] Tertiary facilities (and only tertiary facilities) could thereby monopolize all of maternity care by theoretically operating all three levels in one institution.

In spite of all the efforts to establish levels systems, there was little evidence that they led to better outcomes. Reports in the literature consistently credited regionalization with the concurrent declines in perinatal mortality. Since the declines were century-long trends, however, they must have entailed other factors. Two major controlled studies did not find better outcomes under perinatal regionalization. A North Carolina study did not find significant differences in mortality rate declines between areas with regional perinatal programs and those without, nor did a study of eight Robert Wood Johnson Foundation–funded regions.[23] Rather than question whether regionalization worked, however, the foundation investigators attributed similar outcomes in program areas and control areas to a spread of regionalization throughout. Although such an explanation is plausible, it circularly assumes the validity of the research hypothesis rather than using the research findings to reexamine it. *Toward Improving II* and other subsequent policy statements misleadingly credited the foundation study with demonstrating efficacy of perinatal regionalization. Yet it simultaneously recognized that the 1980s saw no improvement in nationwide perinatal health status, despite the growth of regionalization.[24]

Two negative studies by no means provide conclusive evidence that perinatal regionalization didn't work. They do bring into question, however, the value of regionalization and the nature of its ultimate goals. Examining higher levels of care as a separate element, there also never was sufficient evidence to support perinatal leaders' claims that they provided more effective care for the majority of women and babies (as further discussed in chapter 8). Nevertheless, academic perinatal leaders continued to believe in the levels system, some simultaneously recognizing that their institutions stood to benefit economically from it.

Subspecialists designed levels systems as a means of limiting competitive proliferation of high-intensity services and distinguishing their own work from that of "general" specialists. Administrators at the New Jersey hospital trying to use the Certificate of Need process to achieve level III designation (mentioned in chapter 5) described the tremendous competitive pressure to get the "franchise" implicit in perinatal center designation.[25] Whether or not leaders appreciated it, hierarchic levels have inherent economic dynamics and institutional differentiation awards competitive advantages to the "higher"-level institutions.

Family physicians had grounds for accusing perinatal regionalization of restricting competition from family medicine and consigning the entire birth market to specialists.[26] *Toward Improving* relegated level I hospitals and their family physicians to rural areas (where specialists do not locate). Levels definitions also prohibited competition from freestanding birth centers. The joint *Guidelines* pronounced that such alternative settings were "not encouraged" but that, if they did exist, they should meet level I standards.[27] In other words, they should not be alternative. With little economic or professional power, however, level I institutions and practitioners offered little competitive threat to level III providers. The main threat came from level II.

Academic leaders conceded that perinatal regionalization had problems with competition for regional center status from the beginning.[28] Offering a somewhat lower service intensity to healthier babies, the level II category appears to have been a political compromise to allow larger community hospitals in on the intensive care deal but restrict their competition with academic medical centers. As leaders had feared, however, the academic monopoly on the highest-intensity care did not hold. Academics called the encroaching growth of intensive care services in community hospitals the "level II problem." The levels system spurred rather than quelled regional wars of escalating levels of intensity. It inadvertently formed a ladder that community hospitals could use to climb the levels hierarchy. Policy leaders predicted in the deregulatory environment of the late 1980s that community hospitals would continue to invest in high-tech perinatal equipment, regardless of existing levels policies.[29] Managed care plans encouraged competitive growth of level II units; even smaller hospitals felt compelled to seek level II status so they could compete for managed care contracts.[30] Level III providers criticizing these activities again raised the specter of duplication and fragmentation of services.

The perinatal levels system reenacted and reinforced the socioeconomic stratification in American society. Maternity services continued to account for a large portion of indigent and uncompensated care. Social activists of the 1960s had used disparities in infant mortality to illustrate inequitable distributions of health and wealth. But tertiary leaders turned the argument on its head, claiming that their services could "mitigate the socioeconomic influence on perinatal outcome."[31] Some were trying to stifle a (health care) revolution thought to be imminent. Some explicitly supported regionalization as a substitute for national health insurance.[32] Many were undoubtedly genuinely concerned about the socioeconomic inequities. At the same time, they were aware that they could use their concern as a socially and politically acceptable justification for allocating more resources to their own institutions and practice plans. Intentions notwithstanding, claims that regionalization would mitigate inequities in perinatal care were not subsequently supported.

Not only did perinatal organization not ameliorate inequities, the levels system itself built in socioeconomic discrimination. Perinatal regionalization had no requirement that level II or level III hospitals must accept indigent high-risk patients, even from their own regions.[33] Although a number of academic medical centers did treat indigent populations, their practices varied considerably. In general, private academic centers' practice plans accepted many fewer indigent patients than public ones did.[34] In California in the early 1990s, for example, nearly 70 percent of labor and delivery revenues for university hospitals (most of which were public) came from the state's Medicaid program, compared with 20 percent for large nonteaching hospitals.[35]

Level II status offered higher standing and revenues to larger urban and suburban hospitals catering to privately insured patients. With more money and more political clout, these hospitals were more successful in attracting subspecialists, building intensive care units, and achieving level II designation than many public hospitals serving poorer, higher-risk populations. Perinatal planners for Oakland, California, for example, identified larger voluntary hospitals as the most suitable facilities for level II services.[36] Yet the voluntary hospitals were not located where most of the low-income, high-risk population lived; the county hospital was located there. Despite the fact that half of the county's neonatal deaths and 85 percent of its black neonatal deaths occurred among Oakland residents, the county hospital serving the high-risk population had a hard time getting funds for neonatal intensive care.[37] The local Health Systems Agency (where I was working) acknowledged Oakland's high perinatal mortality rates and the strong community efforts to alleviate them as significant health and political issues. But the methods it was required to use did not and could not take the high mortality rates into consideration when defining the need for perinatal services in the area. Inequality was not just a matter of "access"; it was embedded in the structure and function of perinatal levels systems. As Murray Milner described (for hospitals in general) in *Unequal Care,* inequality was not just an unfortunate consequence of the functional differentiation of hospitals; it was also a basis for it.[38] The levels system also escalated standards for what qualified as an "obstetrics service" and increased the number of patients required to achieve revenues sufficient to cover the high overhead and operational costs.

Minimum Volume and Service Consolidation

Academic leaders as well as system rationalizers had long insisted that larger services were better and more cost-efficient. When demand could not keep up with supply during the Depression, New York City's United Hospital Fund sought to control multiplication of competing maternity units.[39] To the same end, hospital councils in the 1950s tried to impose minimum volume requirements on maternity units. The Philadelphia Hospital Council, directed by former Committee on the Costs of Medical Care staff C. Rufus Rorem, proposed a minimum volume standard of two thousand births a year.[40] The New York Academy of Medicine's Committee on Public Health Relations similarly promoted large maternity units, equating greater availability of specialty, technical, and financial resources with higher quality and cost-efficiency.[41] As in industry, the committee held, larger hospital units could better accrue revenues exceeding their expenses. In the early 1960s John Thompson and Robert Fetter—who would later achieve their fifteen minutes of fame for formulating diagnosis related groups, or DRGs—used methods of industrial engineering to conclude that larger maternity services were more cost-efficient because they could attain higher occupancy rates.[42] Thompson and Fetter's study bolstered the Hospital Review and Planning Council of Southern New York's call for a minimum volume standard of two thousand births a year on the grounds that it would lead to more efficient system-wide capital investment.[43] The American College of Obstetricians and Gynecologists solidified the two thousand birth standard in its 1974 *Standards for Obstetric-Gynecologic Services*.[44] *Toward Improving* similarly budgeted two thousand births for level II and III units so they could expand their capital investments and recover their operational costs.[45] All of these policy efforts promoted a minimum volume of births on economic grounds. The national health planning guidelines initially followed the two thousand birth standard but, due to a vehement outcry from smaller hospitals, reduced the figure to fifteen hundred births and applied it only to level II and III hospitals.[46] Insurers in the managed care era sought out hospitals that could contract to provide high-volume services at reduced rates.[47]

Consolidation of obstetric services was implicit in the minimum volume standards as well as explicit in perinatal regionalization policies. Community hospital administrators became more amenable to obstetric consolidation in 1965, when they came to measure opportunity costs of maintaining low-occupancy obstetric units instead of filling beds with higher-paying Medicare patients.[48] In many consolidations teaching hospitals gained the obstetrics units of non-teaching hospitals. The American College of Obstetricians and Gynecologists advised Congress in 1971 that maternity service consolidation was a "national need."[49] A subsequent Ross Laboratories conference defined perinatal regionalization in terms of merging or "phasing out" smaller maternity and newborn units.[50] This kind of consolidation benefited obstetric providers by reducing competition and helping them raise occupancy rates at least to the financial break-even point.[51]

"Why should an agency try to close maternity services?" rhetorically queried the Boston University Center for Health Planning of its own activities the year after *Toward Improving* came out.[52] Its report never exactly answered the question, but it seemed to be improving the financial positions of the surviving services. In response to growing fiscal problems of the 1970s and in synchrony with the federal health planning program, public and private authorities intensified their efforts to consolidate maternity services. The Boston Regional Health Planning Council promoted further consolidation (elimination, actually) of community hospital maternity services in order to support the academic services connected with the city's three medical schools.[53] As a public health scholar later affirmed, Boston's academic medical centers "used their financial and market strength to drive community hospitals out of business," and, consequently, Massachusetts residents were more likely than residents of other states to be inappropriately hospitalized in tertiary centers.[54]

Perinatal leaders must have been aware of the profound impact that minimum volume standards could have had in constricting maternity service availability. The American College of Obstetricians and Gynecologists's national maternity study had found that three-quarters of U.S. obstetric services in 1967 had fewer than a thousand births per year and that more than 90 percent did not meet the proposed minimum volume standard of two thousand births.[55] Consolidation and its consequent closure of maternity units did reduce service availability in a number of states, especially those with significant rural populations. Nearly a quarter of Alabama's obstetrics services closed in the second half of the 1980s, eliminating all maternity care in eleven counties.[56] Although obstetricians tended to blame an inadequate supply of specialists and their liability problems for what they called an "obstetrics crisis," the contraction in Alabama's services occurred despite an increase in the number of practicing obstetricians and a decrease in malpractice claims. Even in the more populous state of California, implementation of a fifteen hundred birth minimum volume standard in 1990 would have closed or consolidated 77 percent of the obstetric services in the state.[57]

Nationally in the 1990s, even achieving an average (rather than minimum) of fifteen hundred births per unit would have required reducing the number of maternity services to 2,670; a two thousand births per unit average would have further reduced the number to 2,000. The actual count of existing obstetrics services decreased from around 5,340 in 1967 to around 3,810 in 1993.[58] A good case can be made that many middle-class urban and suburban areas did have an oversupply of obstetrics services relative to need, but the reductions generally occurred in the underserved, not the overserved, areas. Perinatal leaders supported such service consolidation on the grounds of quality and cost-efficiency, but the evidence supporting both assumptions was meager.

Perinatal leaders used size and technical level to measure what they called "level of sophistication" of their services. Providers, payers, and planners alike were certain that bigger services were better as well as cheaper. They often cited evidence from open-heart surgery services that quality was associated with size, but findings from one specialty area do not necessarily apply across other procedures and specialties. The Robert Wood Johnson Foundation called it "axiomatic" that larger perinatal services provided higher-quality care.[59] California's influential Maternal and Child Health Data Base studies similarly advised planners that there was "unambiguous statistical proof" that larger maternity services had better outcomes.[60] But its studies were predicated on the assumption that babies with the same birthweight (taking into account multiplicity, sex, and race) were at equal risk of dying and that differences in outcomes could therefore be attributed to the hospital care they received.

Researchers came to recognize, however, what some clinicians must have known all along: not all babies with the same birthweight are equally sick.[61]

The Congressional Office of Technology Assessment summarized research on volume and outcome in hopes of convincing consumers to choose larger hospitals.[62] But its evidence was poor concerning perinatal care. Available empirical research did not provide sufficient evidence to support policies of minimum number of births on the basis of outcome.[63] Consistent with this lack of evidence, the perinatal leadership came to downplay minimum volume standards. The joint *Guidelines* affirmed in 1983 that outcomes were not necessarily influenced by facility size or by birth volume, and *Toward Improving II* did not use minimum volume standards.[64]

Other policy initiatives, however, continued to promote high-volume perinatal care. A 1984 consumers' guide advised pregnant readers in Minnesota's Twin Cities to select hospitals with at least fifteen hundred births a year.[65] Reflecting its perinatal center membership, the National Perinatal Information Center continued to recommend minimum volume standards on the grounds of clinical skill and economy of scale.[66] On finding lower neonatal mortality rates in larger tertiary-level NICUs, academic researchers argued—without further evidence—that the beneficial outcomes might also be attributable to the presumably accompanying high obstetric volume.[67] Despite the inadequate evidence connecting better outcomes to obstetric service size, academic tertiary-level providers continued to affirm that larger, consolidated obstetric services were "inherently safer and more efficient."[68] They were apparently generalizing findings for very-low-birthweight babies in NICUs to obstetric services as well as assuming economies of vertical integration and scale.

In addition to the dearth of evidence concerning efficacy of larger obstetric units, evidence concerning their cost-efficiency was also slim. Demonstrating the certainty of their assumptions if not the validity, training materials from the Harvard School of Public Health and the Boston University Center for Health Planning claimed that economy of scale in maternity services was well documented.[69] They drew graphs to demonstrate their claims, but the curves were based on economic theory; there were no actual cost figures in them. A few studies did measure actual costs. Out of five such studies Thompson and Fetter's found an inverse relationship between volume and unit cost, up to around two thousand births;[70] two studies found U-shaped cost-volume curves;[71] and two found increasing unit costs with size.[72] Some researchers maintained that potential economies of scale were offset by the close association of size with complexity and capital intensity. Yet *because* this association exists and does lead to higher costs, it is misleading to "correct for" increased complexity. In brief, empirical studies did not consistently demonstrate an economy of scale in terms of lower unit costs in larger maternity services. It seems that Berki's conclusion on hospital services in general (quoted in chapter 5)—that economy of scale may or may not exist but according to theory it ought to exist—pertained equally to perinatal services. Despite the lack of evidence, however, faith in economy of scale remained strong. It was consistent with twentieth-century economic thought, and it justified consolidation to benefit larger hospitals. Malpractice lawyers continued to echo doctors in claiming "distinct economic and quality returns to scale up to very large numbers of deliveries."[73] Such an affirmation in itself tended to make large scale a legal standard of care. Whether or not there was an economy of scale, however, larger perinatal services had to encompass wider market areas.

Regional Market Areas

Policies of regionalization designed regions as catchment areas around academic medical centers and drew boundaries that included sufficient population to support the centers' specialty units.[74] Embarking on a project of regional hospital organization in the 1940s, the Commonwealth Fund defined a region as an area capable of fully absorbing all the services provided by a specialized medical center.[75] The Commission on Hospital Care similarly geared up for the Hill-Burton program by mapping regions in Michigan according to the population needed to support hospital specialty departments.[76] Defining regions in this way was consistent with precepts of economic geography that, the more capital-, specialty-, and equipment-intensive production units were, the larger their markets had to be. Health planning agencies of the 1970s consciously applied methods of economic geography in defining regional markets for specialty services such as obstetrics.[77] Designated perinatal regions ranged tremendously in size, depending on the density and purchasing capacity of the population and the number of centralized high-intensity centers they had to support.

Mapping *Toward Improving's* monopolistic vision of one tertiary care center per region, it was not difficult to calculate that its definition of regions as areas encompassing eight to twelve thousand births worked out to about 320 tertiary-level centers. Since perinatal policy saw little need for level I facilities, this regional definition projected approximately four level IIs averaging two thousand births for every one level III. But the 4:1 ratio neglected the competitive dynamics of multiple perinatal centers in the same city, where nearly every major center tried to build a level III service. *Toward Improving II* acknowledged this competition. Managed competition of the 1990s also mapped regions as market areas. Both regionalization and managed competition implied a significant expansion in intensity and contraction in the total number of maternity services, and both would have entailed extensive system-wide management.

Systems Management

The actions required to designate levels of care, consolidate services, and allocate markets required some form of system-wide regulation or management; that was agreed. Who should manage the system was the contentious issue. The American Medical Association's Committee on Maternal and Child Care initially proposed that medical society specialty committees serve as the primary maternal and child health planning authorities for their areas.[78] Academic medical centers, in contrast, envisioned themselves as the regional managers, and *Toward Improving* assigned them the lead role in coordinating perinatal systems. Perinatal leaders were quite successful in keeping perinatal planning separate from the national health planning system. They continued to use branches of government in which they had established a dominant policy role. California's Maternal and Child Health office, for example, funded a perinatal planning project that competed with the local health systems agency and accorded its instigator's service regional perinatal center status.[79]

Perinatal policy makers partially acceded to the growing market ethos of the 1980s. The professional *Guidelines* promulgated a more laissez-faire approach, affirming that each hospital could identify its own level of service intensity.[80] There remained, however, a clear call for some sort of system-wide management or regulation. Combining market and planning approaches, the National Perinatal Information Center proposed that hospitals could choose their own levels but be required (by an unnamed agent) to meet certain minimum volume, technologic, and revenue standards for their chosen level.[81] *Toward Improving II* potentially added another layer of bureaucracy when it proposed establishing local, state, and national Perinatal Boards (under professional control) to manage perinatal systems and the competition among them. It recommended that the boards employ techniques of industrial management to assess needs, designate levels, allocate resources, develop networks, coordinate patient flow, expand financing, and monitor quality.[82] But it turned out to be insurance companies (under less professional control) that took on many of these managerial roles as part of managed care contracting.

Regionalization and competitive managed care each actively integrated perinatal delivery systems. Under both, tertiary facilities linked with secondary ones in their regions, seeking out the more financially stable hospitals. "The dollars are in the suburbs," a Detroit-based academic perinatologist advised his colleagues.[83] He recommended cooperating with suburban hospitals in order to generate practice plan income and improve university hospitals' "competitive position." Some perinatal leaders in the 1990s extolled managed care as the best way to vertically integrate perinatal services and manage their revenues.[84] They pointedly appreciated that managed care's integrated delivery systems were oligopolistic.[85] Developing regional systems for their professional and economic advantages, perinatal medicine missed the opportunity to develop systems according to population need.

Perinatal regionalization seemed to promise levels of service intensity commensurate with the population's needs. Leaders commonly asserted that levels of patient risk drove perinatal levels. Yet the National Perinatal Information Center recognized that perinatal regionalization was designed to provide high-intensity care to "as large a proportion of the population as possible."[86] Professional opinion on the proportion of birthing women requiring high-intensity care varied extensively. This variation tended to reflect the capacity of the existing system in any single area and the professional's position in it. Subspecialists tended to recommend that large proportions of birthing women use level III facilities, general specialists advocated greater use of level IIs, and family physicians and rural systems managers supported continuing high use of level Is for low-risk women.[87] Leaders in Massachusetts and California, where the supply of secondary- and tertiary-level services and specialists was high, advised that all births should occur in such high-intensity services.[88] An alternative approach, more common in rural areas, took level I more seriously. Leaders in North Carolina, for example, proposed that 4 percent of the state's births should take place in level III hospitals and an additional 12 percent in level II services, leaving the remaining 85 percent for level I hospitals.[89]

If policies varied among regions, actual utilization varied even more. In North Carolina, three years after the published policy that 85 percent of its births should occur in level I units, 23 percent actually did; 49 percent of the state's births occurred in level II and 28 percent in level III units.[90] Reports from different perinatal regions across the United States and Canada in the 1980s described an immense variation in actual levels distribution; for every one level III hospital there were 2 to 11 level II hospitals and 2 to 119 level I hospitals.[91] The proportion of births actually occurring in the level III services in the same regions (where the data appeared in the paper) ranged from 6 to 36 percent, and the proportion occurring in level Is ranged from 17 to 73 percent. Such a wide variation among planned perinatal regions suggests that the use of different levels of care was related more strongly to provider supply and aspirations than to epidemiologic measures of population need.

Probably the most important health benefit that perinatal regionalization had to offer was its potential to transfer the births of very-low-birthweight babies (less than fifteen hundred grams)—the group that benefited the most from neonatal intensive care, as chapter 8 shows—to the hospitals providing it. A large portion of women going into very early labor as well as those delivering babies with major malformations (together accounting for an estimated 3–4.5

percent of all births) can be anticipated and could logistically be transported to tertiary perinatal centers for delivery.[92] If rural systems such as Iowa could figure out how to transport such births across the state to the single university-based tertiary center, certainly urban areas could do the same.[93] But competing neonatal intensive care units in children's hospitals (which don't have obstetrics services) and those in level II hospitals objected to maternal transport policies that would bypass their institutions. Reported regional variations of very-low-birthweight births actually occurring in level III services in the 1980s and early 1990s ranged from 33 to 86 percent.[94] Even in states considered highly regionalized, such as Washington, the proportion of very-low-birthweight births occurring in tertiary-level hospitals tended to plateau in the 1990s.[95]

At the high end of the birthweight scale, increasing proportions of full-sized babies came to be born in level II and III services as they continued to multiply. Some of the shift in very-low-birthweight births to tertiary care was due to lower-level services consolidating with larger ones or climbing the intensity ladder themselves. The number of level I hospitals in North Carolina, for example, declined from sixty-eight in 1974 to thirty-seven in 1994, while the number of level II hospitals expanded from nineteen to forty-five and the number of level IIIs nearly tripled from five to fourteen.[96] By 1995 nearly two-thirds of the nation's hospital births occurred in self-identified high-intensity settings: 26 percent in level III units and 37 percent in level IIs.[97] Delivering so many babies in intensive care settings intensified medical intervention in birth and newborn care.

Level II growth in particular was not driven by population risk. Statewide distribution of level II NICUs in California in the mid-1980s did not match distribution of need as measured by actual perinatal mortality, expected perinatal mortality, or distribution of very-low-birthweight births; level III services did better in this regard.[98] Researchers at the end of the century judged that neonatal intensive care capacity was not distributed according to known needs. Neither NICU beds nor neonatologists in the 1990s were preferentially located in areas where more low-birthweight babies were born.[99] Perinatal regionalization in general did not succeed in quantifying levels of intensity according to levels of population need, although this was a frequently stated goal of regional policy and its risk assessment tools.

Even had the political will existed, available risk assessment instruments could not have designed an evidence-based perinatal system. They varied too much. The Institute of Medicine found that different risk assessment instruments led to estimates of high risk ranging from 6 to 55 percent of all pregnancies.[100] Regional policies based on the higher estimates would obviously

try to channel a large proportion of birthing women into high-intensity services. Applying one well-known instrument, the San Diego health systems
agency planned regional high-intensity capacity on the basis of estimates that
60 to 90 percent of patients at every obstetric service in the region were high
risk.[101] Levels systems and the availability of high-risk services configured concepts of risk as much as the other way around. The proportion of birthing
women deemed high-risk also varied by country and tended to reflect their
countries' perinatal systems.

Globalization of Regional Perinatal Models

The United States was not the first to apply strategies of perinatal
regionalization, nor was it the most successful, but it may have been the most
influential. The first *Toward Improving* followed Canada's *Regional Services in
Reproductive Medicine* by several years.[102] Britain had taken a leadership role
in regional organization and theory from the time of the Dawson report. In
the mid-1940s planners in the Oxford region designed a comprehensive maternity system with three types of maternity services: local centers providing
normal midwifery, larger general hospitals, and university and medical school
consultant units. A leading American obstetrics journal published a description of this system in 1971.[103] Britain's National Health Service (NHS) managed tertiary-level services on a regional basis and applied principles of
regionalization to its organization of perinatal services. British Paediatric Association standards delineated three perinatal service levels, and NHS planners worked closely with specialists to identify them.[104] As in the United States,
British planners affirmed that consolidation, or "rationalisation," of services
would achieve a more efficient use of intensive care capital and staff.[105]

In addition to efficiency motivations, Britain's maternity care consolidation
was professionally motivated; it was aimed in large part at phasing out competing general practitioner delivery units. The South East Thames Regional
Health Authority, for example, developed policies in the late 1970s to shift births
from general practitioner units to consultant units with a minimum of twenty-
five hundred births.[106] The authority claimed that this consolidation would increase the productivity of hospital midwives, who delivered most of the nation's
babies. The North West Thames Regional Health Authority similarly adopted
policies that no maternity unit should be "isolated" (from specialty units), that
every maternity unit should have a special care neonatal unit (equivalent to
level II), and that there should be no freestanding birthing centers.[107] The authority responded to the no-growth budgets of the 1970s by establishing a minimum volume standard of fifteen hundred to two thousand births per unit and
proposing service consolidation to achieve this volume. It also pronounced that

"home deliveries are to be discouraged," although in the recent past the NHS had operated a highly effective midwife-attended home birth service. These regional reports from Britain held that larger units promised more efficient personnel use, more cost-effective use of services, more intensive supervision of labor, and greater career prospects (for the consultants). They provided inadequate data to support these conclusions, and they did not seem to consider that the more intensive and more complex facilities would cost more per birth.

In the context of a relatively stable number of births, regional policies led to the closure—by a little over a decade later—of a third of the maternity units in England existing in 1973. By 1996, 87 percent of the country's babies were born in units with two thousand or more births.[108] Some perinatal leaders had recognized, however, that there was no clear evidence that higher volumes led to more cost-efficient or safer maternity care. Noting widespread acceptance in 1985 of the idea that "far from being beautiful, small is both ineffective and inefficient," editors of the *Lancet* acknowledged that there was insufficient evidence to support the assumption that larger hospitals or those with higher levels of staff training had better obstetric outcomes.[109] Nonetheless, perinatal specialists and planners continued to develop policies of regional organization and promote larger and higher-intensity services. In the early 1990s the Thames Regional Perinatal Group endorsed a "three-tier regional structure" of neonatal services in the names of quality and efficiency.[110] Regionalization was widely accepted by the end of the century as the global model for perinatal system organization, although some researchers charged that countries often adopted it "without evidence of improved outcomes."[111]

In sum—although it only partly achieved its organizational goals in the United States—perinatal regionalization was a business model of organization that endeavored to manage personnel, technology, capital, and markets in order to control competition and restructure the perinatal industry. All four strategies of regional perinatal organization: designated levels, minimum volumes, assigned regions, and managed systems served to channel large proportions of birthing women and their babies to high-intensity centers. The number of women and newborns receiving high-intensity care did not necessarily correspond with available knowledge about needs, nor did the women and babies most in need necessarily obtain the higher levels of intensity. System-wide reform strategies led toward similar regional systems. If fully implemented, they would have severely constricted the availability of perinatal services, particularly low-intensity, low-risk care. In so doing, they would have further escalated service intensity. Returning to connections between institutional developments and clinical activities, the final part of this book examines three ways in which business models and strategies in perinatal care warped clinical intervention.

Part III
The Economic Production of Childbirth

The crisis is that continuing intervention is not leading to continuing improvement in maternal and fetal outcome.
—Mortimer G. Rosen, MD, 1990

Seven

Competing for the Birth Market

Providers, Procedures, and Paradigms

As the economic organization of specialty medicine described in chapters 2 and 3 shaped medical intervention in the first third of the century, economic developments in the last third continued to shape childbirth intervention. Competition, multiplication of strategic business units, corporate organization, financial management, and quality management continued to inflate capital and technologic intensity in maternal and neonatal care.

Competing Providers and Treatments

Different providers used medical interventions differently in their competition for the birth market. Obstetricians developed routine technological and surgical procedures to differentiate their specialty and confer competitive advantages upon it. Family physicians competed either by adopting specialty procedures themselves or by developing alternative low-intensity strategies and philosophies. Midwives and independent birthing centers also took a lower-intensity approach. Each competing profession developed concepts of risk that paralleled its position in the levels system and its intervention activities.

Competing Physicians

Joseph DeLee and his contemporaries made significant strides in the 1920s toward raising the economic value as well as the academic status of obstetric procedures. The specialty continued to use technological and surgical procedures to demarcate its professional boundaries and to enhance its competitive position. Columbia's Howard Taylor attributed his specialty's relatively low prestige and revenue levels in the 1950s to its "limited repertory" of procedures.[1] Obstetricians at the time were stung by a relative value scale—prepared to determine physician payments—assigning complete obstetric care a relative weight of 70 compared to 850 for urology's transurethral resection.[2] They doubted that urology's procedure was 12 times more complex, used 12 times more resources, or had a 12 times higher risk. They might have wondered whether penises were deemed 12 times more important than babies, although there is little evidence that they thought of such questions at the time. When the relative value scales of the 1990s continued maternity care's low ranking, obstetricians did pick up the feminist argument so often used against them and accused the scales of gender bias.[3]

Periodic appraisals of professional progress found that procedures contributed significantly to job satisfaction in obstetrics and gynecology.[4] Ob-gyns recognized that their specialty's status suffered from the fact that they spent a large portion of their office time providing primary care (prenatal and annual check-ups) to well women.[5] They also (partially) recognized that marketing was "not only tailoring one's offerings to the market, but also enlarging the market for what one has to offer."[6] In the mid-1980s they broadcast the "worrisome news" that the specialty's surgical workloads and market shares were declining.[7] Yet ob-gyns at that time accounted for a large share of the surgical market: they were spending the same number of hours in surgery and performing the same number of surgical procedures per week as general surgeons.[8] Five of the top six inpatient operative procedures in the mid-1990s were from the obstetrics and gynecology repertoire: episiotomy, repair of obstetric laceration, cesarean section, artificial rupture of fetal membranes, and hysterectomy, in descending order.[9] Pregnancy and birth accounted for at least 18 percent of all inpatient surgical procedures in addition to a large number of nonsurgical procedures such as electronic fetal monitoring (EFM). The concentration of obstetric procedures at the top of the list was due in part to the shift of other specialties' procedures to outpatient settings. Yet obstetrics and gynecology also topped all other specialties in the number of diagnostic and therapeutic procedures ordered or performed during office visits. Thanks in large part to Pap smears, mammograms, and prenatal ultrasound, ob-gyns (or their office staff) performed 236 tests, procedures, or therapies per 100 patient visits, compared with 199 for the second most procedurally prolific area, cardiovascular medicine.[10] But—once again comparing their procedures with those of the male urogenital system—ob-gyns felt that their "invasive services" were underrated and underreimbursed.[11]

In addition to the demand limitation inherent in the finite number of births, ob-gyns restricted their practice socioeconomically. Although the expressed goal of the Medicaid program was to "mainstream" low-income women and children, two perinatal systems continued to operate. The first was the individual entrepreneurial system of fully trained private practice specialists for insured patients; the second was the industrial system of trainee-staffed institutional services for Medicaid and uninsured patients. Patients in the first system, as an American College of Obstetricians and Gynecologists' (ACOG) administrator put it, were women with the "opportunity to choose."[12] Low-income women lacked the opportunity to choose because private ob-gyns did not choose to locate their offices in low-income areas or accept uninsured patients; nearly half (44 percent) of practicing obstetricians in the 1980s rejected pregnant Medicaid patients.[13] Private health insurance in the early 1990s covered just over half of all deliveries,[14] and doctors and maternity services competed for that half. The women and babies in the other half constituted a large portion (27 percent) of what hospitals called their uncompensated care problem.[15]

Command of surgical and technological procedures conferred competitive advantages on obstetric specialists over general practitioners and family physicians. Academic medical centers invented family medicine in the late 1960s as a broad primary care field requiring residency training. This new field enabled their practice plans to compete with community physicians by providing primary care in addition to secondary and tertiary care. Family medicine itself, not surprisingly, thought *family* included the birth of babies. It claimed that childbirth was crucial for its professional identity, satisfaction, income, and procedural expertise—although it somewhat self-defeatingly tended to call it obstetrics.[16] With some justification family medicine accused the ob-gyn specialty of obstructing its maternity care practice. Obstetrics and gynecology succeeded in codifying many of its specialty standards in licensing and reimbursement requirements and in hospital privileging.

Performance of intrapartum (during labor) procedures played a pivotal role in the competition between obstetrics and family medicine. Since specialties never did succeed in controlling the performance of procedures by regulatory or voluntary means, the obstetrics profession tried to accomplish the deed with hospital privilege standards. In the early 1980s the American College of Obstetricians and Gynecologists proposed delineating hospital privileges by procedural complexity.[17] Some hospitals' ob-gyn committees even denied obstetric procedure privileges to the very family physicians they trained to perform them.[18] Challenging this kind of specialty dominance, the American Academy of Family Physicians took the stand in the 1990s that hospital privileging should not restrict use of diagnostic or therapeutic procedures. Consistent with the free market ethos of the times, family physicians defended their use of obstetric procedures in terms of their "right" to practice obstetrics and perform procedures without restrictions in trade.[19]

In practice and in philosophy family medicine developed two different approaches to birth intervention. Family physicians choosing the first approach competed with obstetricians by adopting their technological and surgical procedures.[20] In the second approach they characterized themselves as specialists in normal birth, *the* appropriate providers of low-intensity care to low-risk women.[21] It averaged out that family physicians did have lower intervention rates than obstetricians. For comparable risk patients (with comparable outcomes) family physicians were less likely than obstetricians to use forceps, episiotomy, labor induction, oxytocin augmentation, and epidural analgesia.[22] Cesarean section also became a significant policy issue for the profession. Some family physicians argued that cesarean section capacity was essential to their professional identity; others clearly believed it was not their role to perform it. At the end of the century 26 percent of family physicians with hospital privileges delivered babies, claiming around 15 percent of the birth market; 20 percent (of those with hospital privileges) used labor augmentation, 19 percent used labor induction, 12 percent used forceps, and 4 percent performed cesarean section.[23]

Consistent with their lower-intensity approach, family physicians saw "family-centered" childbirth as a natural in maintaining their stake in maternity care.[24] Although *family-centered* also implied participation of birthing women and their families in decision making, it was a multifaceted strategy that reflected various interests and encompassed competing agendas. Birth activists promoted the concept to challenge medical structures and interventions. Some of them also used it to glorify the family and women's traditional place in it. Hospital administrators used family-centered as a marketing device to expand their share of the local birth market. Obstetricians used it to confer "sensitivity" on their high-tech interventions.[25] The obstetric view generally prevailed. A specialty-oriented interprofessional task force proclaimed that the major changes required by family-centered care were attitudinal and that facilities offering it should continue to meet specialty standards.[26] While it definitely mitigated some of the more inhumane features of hospital labor and delivery, such as leaving women alone during labor, family-centered childbirth also served to strengthen acceptance of high-tech birth. Family medicine's low-intensity approach put it in a competitive relationship with midwifery.

Competing with Midwives

Both obstetrics and family medicine saw midwifery as a competitive threat. A report prepared for the Federal Trade Commission observed that "the obstetric scene in the 1970s made obstetricians and nurse-midwives competitors for the low-risk births" and that many obstetricians were unwilling to "relinquish the low risk mother, the obstetrician's 'bread and butter.'"[27] Yet chapter 2 described how a minority line of thinking within obstetrics had long sought to envelop midwives within the specialty division of labor. Howard Taylor echoed the scientific management thinking of Lewellys Barker and Robert Latou Dickinson when he urged obstetricians in the mid-1960s to employ nurse-midwives to take over obstetrics' "simple and repetitive" tasks.[28] In this way, Taylor maintained, specialists could sequester technical procedures and achieve "surgical virtuosity." In his presidential address to the American College of Obstetricians and Gynecologists, Duncan Reid advocated the use of nurse assistants or nurse-midwives to perform routine care. Calling it a "team," or "group," approach to obstetrics, Reid held that such an approach would permit the specialty to attain a larger share of the birth market.[29] A few years later ACOG advised Congress to train more allied health personnel to attend normal deliveries under obstetricians' supervision.[30] Academic obstetricians came to recognize that allocating simpler tasks to lower-level employees enhanced their own productivity and decreased their costs.[31] As midwifery took a stronger hold, the obstetrics specialty increased its efforts to control the profession by defining certified nurse-midwifery as a category of hospital personnel that worked in hospital obstetrics departments. ACOG correspondingly advised that nurse-midwives should not be allowed to engage in independent private practice.[32] By 1990 only 14 percent of active nurse-midwives had their own practices; 25 percent worked for physicians, and most of the rest were employees of hospitals, academic medical centers, and HMOs.[33] The obstetric team, as ACOG defined it in 1995, was directed by a physician who employed the other professional team members.

The socioeconomic stratification of the birth market offered another means of reducing competition from nurse-midwifery—with the added benefit of reducing obstetricians' responsibility for indigent care. Hospitals and academic practice plans increasingly hired nurse-midwives to provide lower-tier care to their lower-tier patients. A large portion of births attended by certified nurse-midwives in the 1980s occurred in hospitals serving indigent populations.

Nurse-midwives even provided much of the high-risk care for low-income women at hospitals such as Cook County in Chicago and the University of Southern California (USC) in Los Angeles.[34] Some hospitals, including USC, constructed freestanding birthing centers specifically to provide low-cost nurse-midwifery care to indigent women.[35] Consistent with their own insured clientele, private obstetricians rationalized that nurse-midwives were particularly well qualified to treat Medicaid, rural, and "hard-core" women.[36]

As in family medicine, there was a tension within midwifery between legitimizing the profession by performing obstetric procedures or by developing its own less intensive approach. Direct-entry, or "lay," midwives as well as some certified nurse-midwives—particularly those delivering out of hospital—developed noninterventional models of maternity care. In general, hospital-based midwives used more medical procedures than nonhospital midwives. Certified nurse-midwives in one study induced labor in 26 percent of their hospitalized patients, applied continuous electronic fetal monitoring in 46 percent, and performed an episiotomy on 36 percent.[37] Pointing out that many hospitals allowed registered nurses to start intravenous fluids, manage oxytocin delivery, place fetal scalp electrodes, and interpret EFM recordings, some nurse-midwives sought practice privileges to place intrauterine pressure catheters; inject local anesthesia; and perform amniotomy, amnioinfusion, episiotomy, and manual removal of the placenta.[38] Some had even greater technological aspirations, seeking training in vacuum extraction, paracervical block, circumcision, ultrasound, external cephalic version, and cesarean section assisting. Like physicians, these midwives viewed levels of technologic skill as levels of professional achievement.

On average nurse-midwives used obstetric interventions considerably less frequently than did physicians on patients of comparable risk. Nevertheless, their intervention rates were significant. High-tech settings seemed to promote high-tech midwife intervention even on patients identified as low-risk. Nurse-midwives in one academic medical center used continuous electronic fetal monitoring on 34 percent of their low-risk patients, episiotomy on 24 percent, and oxytocin induction and/or acceleration on 22 percent; physicians' rates for comparable patients were 100, 76, and 56 percent, respectively.[39] At Boston's Brigham and Women's Hospital in the mid-1990s midwives performed episiotomy on 21 percent of their patients delivering vaginally for the first time, compared with 33 percent for faculty/resident staff and 56 percent for private practitioners; epidural rates were 50 percent for the midwives, 75 percent for the staff, and 77 percent for private practitioners; oxytocin induction rates were 14, 27, and 29 percent, respectively; and oxytocin augmentation rates were 34, 38, and 40 percent.[40] The interventional hierarchy was always the same, although the midwives did not always greatly distinguish themselves from the two groups of physicians. Comparing low-risk deliveries in the state of Washington, nurse-midwives used continuous EFM on 47 percent of their deliveries, family physicians used it on 58 percent, and obstetricians on 62 percent.[41] Episiotomy rates for low-risk vaginal deliveries were 30, 58, and 60 percent, respectively, and labor induction or augmentation 26, 40, and 42 percent. These comparative birth intervention rates expressed the competition among different birth attendants in the birth market, whether or not the attendants consciously employed interventions as a competitive tool.

Midwifery's lower intervention rates did not disadvantage women's or their babies' health. Midwife-attended births in hospitals, birth centers, and homes consistently demonstrated excellent outcomes.[42] The most authoritative compendium of perinatal effectiveness data advised that "routinely involving obstetricians" and even "routinely involving doctors in the care of all women during pregnancy and childbirth" fell into the category of "forms of care unlikely to be beneficial."[43] American obstetricians undoubtedly pointed out that the source of this advice was Britain, where midwives were the primary birth attendant.

The obstetric specialty's stifling of private practice midwifery was related more to its competitive threat than to any potential threat to the health of women and babies. Yet the profession continued to react vehemently against freestanding birthing centers, independent midwives, and home birth. Taking his cue from obstetricians who saw home birth as child abuse, syndicated columnist Charles Krauthammer called it "criminal self-indulgence." He compared its advocates (perhaps not inappropriately) to Luddites who sabotaged the machines ruining their livelihood by—according to his version—throwing their wooden shoes (sabots) into them. But, he sneered, "they didn't throw their children."[44] Although Krauthammer's attitude demonstrated an obstetric hegemony at the end of the century, economic pressures as well as patient choice were forcing a growing acceptance of midwifery. Insurers began to see nurse-midwives as a "better 'buy'" than obstetricians.[45]

Yet there are potential political and economic ramifications of shifting a large market to any professional domain, be it midwifery, family medicine, specialties, or subspecialties. With more money, power, and patients, midwives might continue to "upgrade" their profession, their technological capabilities, and their interventions. In other words, they might start behaving like obstetricians. There was already precedence for midwives hiring a range of nurses, aides, and doulas; shifting less technical care to them; and maintaining for themselves the more professionally and economically rewarding procedures. Additionally, midwives in private practice are subject to the same entrepreneurial pressures as private physicians. It is not that midwives necessarily would promote an industrial division of labor or behave as entrepreneurs but that institutions and financial incentives could pressure them in those directions.

Competing Birthing Centers

In addition to midwives, freestanding, or nonhospital, birthing centers offered a major structural reform and a potentially serious competitive threat to doctors and hospitals. Consequently, the obstetrics profession tried to impose stringent evidentiary requirements on them. It demanded that birthing centers demonstrate safety and efficacy—a good idea, of course, but never required of the profession's own institutions and practices.[46] One public health officer claimed in 1976 that it was "heretic" even to investigate *whether* out-of-hospital deliveries could be performed safely and economically by qualified alternative staff.[47] When such heretical studies were finally carried out, however, they found equivalent or better outcomes for low-risk women in birthing centers compared with tertiary-level hospitals.[48] Responding to these studies, a representative from the American College of Obstetricians and Gynecologists contended that hospital-based services were still preferable because of the potential for "catastrophic" outcome.[49] The comment had some validity: the rare event of a baby dying during the labor process was rarer still in fully equipped units.[50] Yet such a rare event did not justify providing high-intensity care for all birthing women.

Freestanding birth centers on the whole offered a significant therapeutic alternative to medical birthing. They had lower technological levels and lower intervention rates than hospitals. When the episiotomy rate for low-risk patients at Mount Sinai Hospital was 78 percent, for example, the rate for matched patients at the New York Maternity Center Association was the considerably lower 47 percent, although it was still nearly half of its births.[51] Other interventions in the two facilities showed wider differentials: oxytocin augmentation rates were 60 percent at Mount Sinai and 9 percent in the Maternity Center; EFM 97 and 21 percent, respectively; intravenous drip 97 and 20 percent; epidural 56 and 5 percent; and forceps 44 and 6 percent. The national birth center study similarly found that, compared with low-risk women in hospitals in the early 1990s, independent birthing centers averaged lower rates for anesthesia, continuous EFM, labor induction, labor augmentation, intravenous infusion, amniotomy, episiotomy, and cesarean section (upon transfer to hospitals).[52]

To compete with freestanding centers (as well as with home birth) hospital administrators worked with obstetricians to establish hospital-based alternative birthing centers, known as ABCs. The Women's Institute for Childbearing

Policy in New England, an outgrowth of the birth movement and the women's health movement, attributed the development of many ABCs to hospital marketing departments.[53] Noting the many local billboards advertising hospital-based birthing centers, a business journal on the other side of the country enthused that "the business of birth is big and competitive in the Puget Sound area."[54] Hospital administrators in Seattle and other cities designed ABCs as strategic business units to attract upscale populations.[55] Obstetricians designed ABCs as attractive labor-delivery-recovery rooms complete with all the usual equipment—concealed behind curtains. In Washington State 46 percent of hospital ABCs in the late 1970s had oxytocin induction "options," 71 percent had electronic fetal monitors, and 75 percent had the capacity for oxytocin augmentation.[56] The American Academy of Pediatrics and the American College of Obstetricians and Gynecologists' joint *Guidelines for Perinatal Care* declared that hospital birthing centers should operate under standard specialty protocols.[57] Hospital-based ABCs became known as the plant-hanging-from-the-intravenous-stand model. It seemed that any serious attempt to provide alternatives to high-tech birth would have to go outside the hospital, and even that strategy could be subverted.

Some enterprising obstetricians, especially in California it seems, equipped their private offices with the latest technology and operated them as for-profit birthing centers.[58] Nationally, 59 percent of freestanding birth centers in the mid-1980s were for-profit ventures. Envisioning a growth industry, developers planned chains of birth centers. Although women's health activists had long promoted expanding out-of-hospital birthing centers, they hadn't pictured them as fast-birth franchises. The entrepreneurs' timing was apparently wrong, however; cost-based reimbursement declined, and the threat of birth center chains did not materialize at that time.

Competing with Patients

Obstetricians were competing not only with other professionals and institutions; they were competing with patients for control of birth. Many observers assumed that the birth activists won the battle when they opened up the doors of the labor and delivery room to supportive people of their choice and successfully expanded childbirth education, prepared childbirth methods, breastfeeding, and rooming-in. These activities did significantly humanize the birth experience, although it did not hurt that hospitals at the same time were employing market strategies of customer satisfaction. Obstetricians later claimed credit, however, for a revolution in maternity care, as did nurses, who claimed credit for instituting "sweeping changes" cloaked "in the guise of consumer demand."[59] But patients, doctors, and nurses tended to overstate the impact on medical intervention. Interventional intensity escalated in the decades during which labor and delivery became more humane. Some feminists conceded "two mainstreams" in birth: more humanistic treatment in parallel with greater technology use.[60] The total obstetric intervention rate grew from 94 procedures per 100 deliveries in 1980, to 110 in 1985, and to 166 in 1990, holding at that level through the 1990s.[61]

Competing Paradigms and the Marketplace of Ideas

Academics, activists, and physicians tended to assume that doctors' belief systems explained their clinical practices. Obstetricians at Britain's London Hospital attributed interventional variation to differences in "attitude," dividing colleagues into "active" and "conservative" groups.[62] They found that when the active group induced 20 percent of its labors, the conservative group induced 9 percent, and, when the active group used cesarean section on 12 percent, the conservative group did so on 9 percent. But their study demonstrated larger differences over the three-year time span than between the active and conservative groups: the conservatives' 1978 cesarean section rate was higher than the actives' 1975 rate.

Finding that doctors and patients in the United States as well as Britain held "conflicting paradigms" or "competing ideologies" about birth, researchers assumed that the conceptual differences explained different intervention patterns.[63] But arguments attributing obstetric intervention to the "emergence of interventionist ideology as the dominant belief system influencing ob-gyn practice" were tautologous.[64] The different paradigms were real, but they did not necessarily cause the existing practices; they coevolved with them. The development of clinical organization, clinical interventions, and paradigms reinforced one another. Cautioning midwives against swallowing medical theory whole, sociologist Barbara Katz Rothman observed that "it is not that birth is 'managed' the way it is because of what we know about birth. Rather, what we know about birth has been determined by the way it is managed."[65] Such interactiveness means that reform can't just change attitudes in order to change practice; in fact, reform can't significantly change attitudes without changing settings and practices.

The two-hour rule exemplified the reciprocal relationship between paradigms and practice. In the context of growing cesarean section and waning forceps use, a 1977 study challenged the "dogma" of setting a two-hour time limit between full cervical dilation and birth—the limit that played such an important role in reinforcing earlier forceps use.[66] Calling two hours "arbitrary," the study advised that it was not appropriate to terminate labor just because the preordained period of time had elapsed. Extending this line of reasoning,

British obstetric anesthesiologist J. Selwyn Crawford rejected the concept of labor stages altogether. Crawford was a strong proponent of epidural analgesia administered throughout labor and therefore not keyed to stages. He correspondingly maintained that there was no evidence that labor was itself harmful, that the concept of stages served no therapeutic purpose, and, furthermore, that it led to unnecessary interference in birth.[67] "Labor is continuous," pronounced American minimal intervention advocate Michelle Harrison, reacting to her residency training in obstetrics: "I no longer believe in the second stage of labor."[68] Midwives observing home births similarly came to believe that women's labors normally unfolded at "individual" and "highly variable" rates—although they, too, had ideas of too long.[69]

Both acceptance and rejection of stages reflected practitioners' clinical intervention preferences. Despite the recognized lack of evidence supporting the two-hour rule, it remained operational and appeared as an American Hospital Association quality indicator in the late 1980s.[70] Based on such indicators, lawsuits claimed that a second stage longer than two hours was "prolonged" and a breach of standards.[71] The norm at the end of the century seemed to be a one-hour rule—upped to two hours when epidural analgesia was used—after which a diagnosis of "failure to progress" was likely.

The paradigms of birth as pathologic versus birth as normal were in part competitive strategies. They also reflected the practitioner's position in the levels system.[72] Ob-gyns continued to use their mastery of female reproductive pathology to promote their profession over their competitors. Recognizing that the vast majority of births were normal in the sense of resulting in healthy mothers and babies, obstetric leaders honed in on a pathologic potential of birth, commonly asserting that a diagnosis of normal was possible only in retrospect. This implied that only obstetricians—qualified to deal with pathology—were qualified to deliver babies. Enlarging the market for what the obstetrics profession had to offer meant selling the concept of high risk along with its interventions. Challenging the professionalization of direct-entry midwives in Minnesota, a woman obstetric pathologist enumerated twenty-five thousand risk factors in a random sample of five thousand hospital births.[73]

Obstetric competitors conceived countervailing concepts of low risk that justified their own birth attendance and therapeutic strategies. Specialists retorted that the concept of low risk was meaningless.[74] Although the paradigms of pathology and risk differed a great deal therapeutically, they were all market-oriented. Competitors held that birth was a natural process that could be guided by the relevant competing group: family physicians, nurse-midwives, lay midwives, or birthing women themselves. Most family physicians strategically placed themselves at the normal end of a "philosophical spectrum" ranging from pathological to normal.[75] One family physician criticized that birth had been "perverted into a pathologic product in need of technology," and would return to normal only when women left their "hospital-trained obstetricians to seek safe alternatives in childbirth."[76] Midwives also criticized the pathology model in the process of claiming normal childbearing as their professional domain. Home birth advocates in turn claimed an alternative model based on an "epistemological system that assigns primacy and goodness to the Natural."[77] Nor were patients exempt from viewing risk in terms of location in the levels system. Birthing women tended to minimize the risks and magnify the benefits of the birth services they used, whatever level they were.[78]

Not all obstetricians insisted on a high-risk model, however. One specialist preferring a maternity system in which obstetricians delivered only high-risk cases correspondingly criticized the "expecting trouble" model that defined all births as potentially high-risk.[79] Some obstetricians appropriated concepts of normality. They used them, for example, to stake their claim on "natural childbirth." "Women gain as technology becomes part of natural birth," the *New York Times* headlined in 1988.[80] The accompanying article featured the obstetrics chief at the New York Hospital-Cornell Medical Center, who pronounced natural childbirth "alive and well" but asserted that it had become a "marriage of biology and technology." Due to his department's growing use of epidural analgesia, the chief changed its definition of natural childbirth to encompass all births in which the woman was awake and delivering vaginally. Obstetricians working in managed care settings also developed a "new paradigm" of normality, otherwise known as "wellness."[81] Their wellness paradigm was consistent with managed care's economic incentives to minimize resource consumption, just as the pathology model had been consistent with fee-for-service incentives to maximize it. Like the concept of pathology, the concepts of "natural" and "wellness" reflected practitioners' positions in the perinatal system and their intervention practices.

Feminist critique of the pathology model was closely related to their analysis that doctors "medicalized" birth in their quest for hegemony.[82] Identifying patriarchal dominance had great appeal to those of us in the *Our Bodies, Ourselves* group who knew from personal experience in the 1960s how our (at the time almost always male—and private) doctors' control of our reproduction controlled our lives. Feminist scholars went on to claim that doctors used medical technology to "reinforce the subordinate role of women" in society.[83] A British view near the end of the century linked labor induction with controlling deviant laboring women as well as deviant labor.[84] Feminist critics specifically charged male physicians with using birth interventions to control reproduction and reproducing women and to expropriate childbirth. The dominance thesis remained a major interpretation of obstetric intervention in both North America and Britain, although it was stronger among activists and social scientists than historians.

It was unclear at the end of the century the extent to which the recent influx of women into medicine had changed clinical practices. Studies tended to show little difference between the sexes when specialization and length of practice were taken into account. Women ob-gyn residents were (only) slightly less likely than their male colleagues to use forceps in birth, although the difference was statistically significant.[85] Women physicians (including obstetrician-gynecologists) did tend to spend more time per patient visit, however, leading feminists to hope for higher levels of communication with them and managers to disparage them for not being as productive as their male colleagues.[86]

The concept of "medicalization" is useful in describing doctors' dominance behaviors, but I do not accept the reification inherent in turning a descriptive concept into a "powerful force in American society."[87] Critical studies of birth intervention emphasized medical concepts and relationships at the expense of analyzing its institutions. Explanations of medical intervention must also consider the economic organization of medicine. Medicalization was in large part a market strategy. Specialties actively developed new clinical procedures and new markets for them by reclassifying life processes and social issues as medical problems amenable to medical solutions.[88] The specialty of obstetrics and gynecology claimed the female reproductive system as its market niche. Consequently, ob-gyns had a particular impact on women's lives. Many of them undoubtedly thought this was a good idea. But they were also performing over a million neonatal circumcisions a year;[89] did that mean they were seeking to control male sexuality too?

It may sound considerably more mundane, but the obstetrics and gynecology specialty medicalized birth in much the same way that the dermatology specialty (considerably later) medicalized tough toenails. The American Academy of Dermatology placed an advertisement in the *American Journal of Public Health* identifying thick, tough toenails as a medical problem that dermatologists could treat.[90] In pathologizing tough toenails, the specialty was seeking to expand its patient base and compete directly with podiatrists as well as health aides for trimming the elderly population's hardening toenails. Obstetricians' pathologizing of birth similarly aided them in their competition with family physicians and midwives. The competition contributed more than the pathologizing to birth intervention patterns, including the use of cesarean section. Most obstetricians recognized that the huge cesarean section expansion in the 1970s was not due to any sudden change in beliefs about pathology of birth or new information demonstrating benefits of the operation.

The Great Cesarean Section Escalation

Cesarean section grew in safety and in favor during the 1950s, thanks to developments in antibiotics, blood transfusion, surgical technique, and growth of the profession of obstetrics.[91] Echoing DeLee's forceps rationale, a Beverly Hills obstetrician credited cesarean section with enhancing the prestige of the profession by elevating birth to the status of surgical operation.[92] The national cesarean section rate suddenly escalated from 5 percent in 1965 and 6 percent in 1970 to 25 percent of all births in 1988.[93] Nearly one million women (plus one million babies) a year were experiencing birth as a major surgical procedure. Professional and citizen interest groups alike charged that "for almost one in four babies to be delivered operatively is a national disgrace."[94] The section rate declined slightly after its 1988 peak, leveling off at 21–23 percent, where it hovered for the remainder of the century.[95]

If 25 percent cesarean section was the answer, what was the question? The obstetrics profession initially assumed that the cesarean rise was scientifically justified. Out of forty-one investigations completed by federally funded Professional Service Review Organizations early in the expansion, only one judged any sections to be unwarranted.[96] By 1980, however, obstetric leaders convened a consensus conference to address the cesarean section problem. It was striking that conference participants found it necessary to admonish their colleagues that decisions to use cesarean section should be "based solely on sound medical judgment."[97] Reports such as the consensus conference concluded that there was a serious lack of evidence to support the high cesarean section use. In the managed care environment of the 1990s a large number of papers emerged in the medical literature questioning the benefits of cesarean section and emphasizing its risks.

Many researchers expected studies of indications recorded in clinical records to explain cesarean section use. Ideally, indications for a treatment are specific conditions shown to benefit from that treatment. Yet obstetricians had long noted that the increased safety of cesarean section had allowed indications for it to broaden beyond the clinical evidence of its necessity.[98] Leaders in the 1980s echoed an earlier charge that obstetricians too often retrospectively identified indications for cesarean section after they performed the procedure. Warren Pearse, executive director of the American College of Obstetricians and Gynecologists, predicted that "a labor of 16 hours that ends in vaginal delivery will probably not carry prolonged labor as a complication diagnosis; the same labor that ends with cesarean section will."[99] The diagnostic incidence of *dystocia,* a catch-all term meaning "abnormal labor," similarly expanded and contracted with the use of cesarean section (and several other interventions). Harvard ob-gyn professor Benjamin Sachs suggested that clinical practice changes caused the rise in the diagnoses of dystocia, rather than the other way around.[100]

Investigators asked what, if not science, had propelled the great cesarean section expansion. They offered a plethora of factors, although none provided a complete explanation, and it was not clear how they could all fit together. The obstetrics profession itself tended to blame growing cesarean section on what it called its liability crisis.[101] In an editorial in the *New England Journal of Medicine* at the height of the inflation, two Park Avenue obstetricians proposed routine cesarean section at term as a form of preventive medicine—against lawsuits.[102] The specialty was in fact enduring an upward spiral of lawsuits, monetary awards, and insurance premiums. Obstetricians' earlier hubris was coming back to haunt them: in capturing the middle-class birth market, they had claimed that they and only they could prevent damaged babies with their delivery techniques—although evidence came to show that most damages occur prior to labor. Obstetricians should not have been too surprised when parents of damaged babies held them accountable for their claims. The lawsuit was a major recourse most parents had to help pay for lifelong care for disabled children—and a surfeit of lawyers was willing to represent them on contingency fees. Nearly three-quarters of all ob-gyns reported that they had been sued at least once by the mid-1980s.[103] Quite a few of them claimed that they intended to give up obstetrics because of their liability problem or at least reduce their "high-risk" practice, the very clinical situation they were specially trained to treat. Despite their claims, however, the subsequent declines in obstetric practice were only slightly higher than usual. Nor did they give up the more lucrative gynecologic surgery, despite the fact that it accounted for as many lawsuits as birth. Although obstetricians overstated their liability problem and used it as an excuse for routine intervention and turning away indigent patients, they had actually lost in court only 3 percent of the lawsuits closed by 1987.[104]

Investigators came to question the extent to which the liability situation drove cesarean section use. Different studies found different associations: negative, positive, and none at all.[105] If there were a connection, it accounted for only a small proportion of the rise in cesarean section. The liability issue did serve other purposes, however. Despite a much lower incidence of lawsuits initiated against family physicians delivering babies, the obstetrics profession used the liability issue to bolster its competitive position over family medicine.[106] Contributors to the Institute of Medicine's Committee to Study Medical Professional Liability and the Delivery of Obstetrical Care advocated adoption of national standards for obstetric practice.[107] It is more than likely that the committee expected specialists to lead any such national standardization efforts and institute their own practice standards.

Technologic and operative procedures such as cesarean section served as instruments of professional achievement. Ob-gyns in part used cesareans in the 1970s as they had earlier used forceps: to establish their professional identity. Obstetricians at Chicago's Lying-in Hospital complained that continued use of forceps in the 1980s invited professional derision—ironic in light of the role of the hospital's founder, Joseph DeLee, in promoting routine forceps in the first place.[108] The growth of the profession contributed to the escalation in cesarean section: growing numbers of obstetricians were performing cesarean sections on a limited supply of patients. Studies in some geographic areas found cesarean section growth to be partly driven by physician supply; studies in other areas did not.[109]

Competition among hospitals contributed to the cesarean section escalation. Cesarean section boomed in a time of competitive hospital growth and diminished somewhat in a time of competitive downsizing, with academic hospitals leading both trends. With rates as high as 8 percent in 1958 and 9 percent in 1968 (when it was 5 percent nationally), the cesarean section rate at Columbia's Sloane Hospital continued to rise ahead of national rates, to 14 percent in 1972 and to 22 percent by 1977.[110] There was a gradient in cesarean section use by hospital complexity and size early in the escalation, but smaller hospitals kept pace just a few steps behind larger ones. Middle-sized community hospitals used their cesarean section capacity as a marketing device. In Oakland, California, I saw a young pregnant woman wearing a T-shirt advertising the double entendre, "cesarean is a cut above," followed by the name of a local voluntary hospital. To black, low-income Oakland residents, cesarean section may have been a symbol of the mainstream obstetrics that often excluded them. National cesarean section rates in 1986 were 25 percent for white women and 22 percent for "other" women.[111] Cesarean section rates at prestigious hospitals serving affluent populations matched those at academic medical centers early in the boom and often rose considerably higher by the end. Already 12 percent in 1970, the section rate at Cedars Sinai Medical Center peaked at 31 percent in 1987.[112] Rates at the Huntington Memorial Hospital, also in the Los Angeles area, went even higher, peaking at 39 percent in the same year. On average, however, the smallest hospitals had caught up with and often exceeded the larger ones in their cesarean section rates by the early 1990s.[113]

Related to competition among hospitals, the American College of Obstetricians and Gynecologists initially promulgated standards that required the structural and staffing capacity to perform cesarean section within fifteen minutes (from decision to incision) for hospitals admitting high-risk patients.[114] Ostensibly established for the baby's sake, the fifteen-minute standard granted a competitive edge to teaching hospitals with in-house staff. Later professional *Guidelines,* however, identified thirty minutes as the recommended standard.[115] The prevalence of private practice in the United States meant that most hospitals had no responsible in-house obstetrician and that the thirty-minute standard better fit their organization. Obstetricians in Britain's National Health Service, where most hospitals did have resident specialty staff, supported the fifteen-minute standard and challenged the American compromise.[116] Both timing standards in both places related more to competitive factors and existing organization than to evidence of women's or babies' health needs.

The rise in use of cesarean section also coincided with the growth of neonatal and obstetric intensive care, and section rates were initially higher in hospitals with intensive care units.[117] Electronic fetal monitoring, the emblematic technology of obstetric intensive care, particularly seemed to contribute to the cesarean section escalation. Early studies found higher section rates associated with EFM use, although, as EFM became more widely used, the association declined.[118] By the 1990s researchers concluded that, if there was an association between cesarean section and EFM use, it was small.[119] Some recognized that the effect could also relate to the intensive care setting rather than EFM use itself.

The cesarean section escalation amplified its market distribution. For-profit, proprietary hospitals had the highest cesarean section rates nationally in the early years of the expansion, followed closely by voluntary hospitals and not so closely by public hospitals.[120] Near the height of the boom, cesarean section rates in New York State for women *with no identified risk factors* were 29 percent in proprietary hospitals, 23 percent in voluntary hospitals, and 18 percent in public hospitals.[121] There was a clear relationship between cesarean section and a population's socioeconomic and insurance status. In California, when the cesarean section rate for births financed by low-income programs was 16 percent, it was 23 percent for births covered by the Medi-Cal (Medicaid) program and 29 percent for births covered by private insurance.[122] Researchers at the end of the century concluded that the "risk of Cesarean delivery was still greatest in low-risk pregnancies."[123]

Doctors' and hospitals' economic incentives also played a role in cesarean section expansion, but not as much as many economists insisted. After contending for most of the century that medicine was an exception to the productive economy because as a profession it was driven by service and not by economic incentives, clinicians and researchers did an about-face in the 1980s and adopted market theories wholesale. In part they blamed middle-class consumers for demanding more cesarean sections.[124] On the supply side the growing numbers of economists working in health services research explained clinical intervention in terms of physicians' wallets. They pointed out that a long labor incurred opportunity costs for physicians, serving as an incentive for them to shorten it.[125] They related the cesarean section expansion to obstetricians' efforts to maximize billable procedures as well as their own professional satisfaction. A National Bureau of Economic Research study hypothesized that obstetricians performed more cesarean sections to maintain their income levels when faced with declining fertility rates of the 1970s.[126] The study did find a correlation, although it explained only a small portion of the cesarean section growth during the time period. The increment that obstetricians received for cesarean section could only have explained a portion of their rise in income level. Obstetrician-gynecologists' mean net income after expenses (including liability insurance) rose from $55,000 in 1973 to $181,000 in 1988; after cesarean section rates had plateaued, their average income further rose to $229,000 by 1997.[127] While greed was not unknown to the obstetrics profession (as these income levels suggest), it was too simplistic to conclude that obstetricians performed more cesarean sections between 1971 and 1988 to fill their wallets or fewer afterward to cut their alleged losses under managed care. Market explanations such as these reduce professional, institutional, and socioeconomic complexities to a factor of individual gain and give a false hope that reform need only address doctors' financial incentives.

Hospitals had greater charge differentials and gained more revenues from high cesarean section rates than did obstetricians. Average hospital expenditures and revenues for cesarean section in 1987 were nearly double those for a normal delivery.[128] At the peak of the boom cesarean section generated 40 percent of hospitals' income from childbirth. *Hospitals* magazine warned administrators that cesarean section reduction programs such as the one at Chicago's Mount Sinai Hospital cost the hospital one million dollars in lost revenues in its first two years—and that, unlike Mount Sinai, not every hospital would be able to cover its losses by expanding volume.[129]

In sum, a convergence of professional, institutional, organizational, demographic, and economic factors shaped both the escalation of cesarean section and its (small) decline. Although the rise entailed many factors, there was little evidence of benefit to women or their babies.[130] Examining a single intervention can be misleading, however, as interventions wax and wane in popularity, demonstrate wide practice variations, and are linked with other interventions, sometimes in a cascade effect. Interventions such as induction, acceleration, and pain relief seemed to increase cesarean section rates.[131] The many variables involved in cesarean section seemed to be interrelated in ways not always decipherable by available statistical methods, and they were not equally pervasive across all geographic areas or institutional settings. In the quantitative environment of the 1990s it took great courage for one perinatologist/lawyer to suggest that the cesarean section expansion may have been influenced by factors that did "not readily lend themselves to statistical analysis."[132] To add to the complexity, there was a simultaneous worldwide dynamic of cesarean section increase but at different levels and at different rates of growth. Ranging from 2 to 6 percent in 1970, measured international rates in developed countries grew to range from 6 to 23 percent in 1985.[133] In Britain, where some obstetricians proudly pointed out that their 1993 cesarean section rate was half that of the United States, with better outcomes, the section rate further rose to 19 percent in 1997–1998 and was expected to reach 20 percent by the year 2000.[134]

Competition played an important but not a solitary role in shaping cesarean section and other birth interventions in the United States in the 1970s and 1980s. The obstetrics, family medicine, and midwifery professions designed intervention strategies that distinguished their services and their institutions from those of their competitors. They correspondingly conceived concepts of pathologic and/or natural birth that paralleled their institutional and interventional developments. The simultaneous development and competitive growth of neonatal and obstetric intensive care intensified medical intervention on laboring women and their babies. Policies of perinatal regionalization promoted this high-intensity care as the standard of care and sought to attain its "maximal utilization."[135]

Eight

Capital Intensive Medicine and Academic Practice Plans

Intensive care units (ICUs) and their respective subspecialties exemplified tertiary care and provided the rationale for the three-level regional systems. Packaging subspecialists, nurses, and machinery into a dedicated hospital space, ICU innovation was more organizational than technological. ICUs used organizational innovation itself as a competitive strategy. Academic leaders recognized that ICUs applied "science, technology, and specialized expertise to the production and marketing of new patient services."[1] Their diagnostic and therapeutic interventions played an important role in the growth of subspecialties and enhanced their financial contributions to academic practice plans.[2] Historian Julie Fairman concluded that neither new technology nor new therapeutics drove the development of one of the first ICUs in the country (in a community hospital); rather, intensive care was a strategy that "fit the economic goals of the hospital."[3] Intensive care growth had financial as well as clinical consequences. It institutionalized a quantum leap in the capital intensity of hospital care and a quantum leap in its medical intensity.

Administrators worked with specialty leaders to organize multiple subspecialty-based intensive care units as revenue centers for their hospitals and practice plans. The internal medicine department at the University of Iowa, for example, recognized that its ICU significantly enhanced departmental revenues.[4] By the mid-1980s intensive care accounted for an estimated 20 percent of all inpatient costs (and, roughly, revenues) in the country.[5] The growing numbers of hospital administrators trained in business management increasingly pressured clinical specialty directors to expand or contract their services for economic purposes. They came to expect each department to become "self-supporting"—that is, able to support its existence with revenues generated from selling its clinical and research work. They regarded interdepartmental cross-subsidization as unbusinesslike and a "taxation" on high-revenue departments. The high-revenue departments were happy to concur with this view. Cardiology and cardiovascular surgery stood as the gold standards for other subspecialties to emulate. Although obstetricians strove to convince their administrators that investment in obstetric intensive care was at least as important as investment in coronary intensive care,[6] cardiology maintained the lead. Cardiologists generated an average of $639,000 in hospital inpatient revenues in 1987, compared with $372,000 for obstetrician-gynecologists.[7] Perinatal subspecialists expected their intensive care leadership to improve their departments' competitive position and attract higher-ranking graduates and research funding as well as clinical revenues.

Intensive care units functioned as strategic business units—although such business language was not used initially to describe them. Like strategic business units in the corporate world, ICUs were designed to enhance reputations, volumes, revenues, and market shares. When business language did become the mode, marketing consultants explicitly advised hospitals that such strategic business units would help them develop product lines on the basis of projected returns on investment.[8] ICUs conferred initial competitive advantages on academic medical centers and their practice plans, but the innovation spread rapidly. Ten percent of U.S. hospitals had one or more ICUs by 1960, nearly 50 percent did by 1970, and 80 percent did by 1980.[9] By 1990 ICU admission rates were ten times higher for hospitalized patients in the United States than in Western Europe. The tremendous ICU growth and utilization related more to competition than to evidence of population need.[10] Neonatal and obstetric intensive care units were part of this market- and revenue-oriented expansion.

Intensive Care Nurseries
Competitive Expansion
Neonatal intensive care units (NICUs) modeled themselves along the lines of other subspecialty intensive care units, but they also had their own antecedents. Following similar developments in France, Joseph DeLee set up an incubator station for premature infants in the Chicago Lying-in Hospital in 1900.[11] DeLee experimented with a variety of ventilation techniques, intervening at least as aggressively on tiny babies as he did on their mothers. Although he closed his incubator unit due to lack of funding, other hospitals obtained funding to open their own. Thanks in large part to the post–World War II Hill-

Burton construction program, "preemie" units became a standard of care for larger maternity services.

Academic medical centers and their pediatricians developed neonatal intensive care units and the subspecialty of neonatology in the 1960s. Funding groups such as the Robert Wood Johnson Foundation and the National Institutes of Health supported the earlier units.[12] NICUs came of age, however, in the context of growing academic practice plans, and they sold their services to sustain their growth. NICU development made newborn insurance coverage an economic and political issue. Since most insurance plans at the time excluded them, the American Academy of Pediatrics and the Health Insurance Association of America collaborated to write state legislature bills mandating newborn coverage in existing insurance policies.[13] Governmental programs such as Maternal and Child Health and Medicaid subsidized NICU utilization for uninsured populations. Economic and professional competition amplified their growth. It did not take long for their builders to envision regional systems of fully-equipped NICUs.[14] Fueled by the (relatively) generous reimbursements, the number and complexity of NICUs grew rapidly. The national number of tertiary-level neonatal units (level III) multiplied from fewer than 20 in 1965 to between 300 and 400 in 1980, around 600 in 1985, 700 in 1988, and over 750 by 1991.[15]

Yet, as early as 1970, clinical directors in San Francisco complained about NICU overdevelopment. They charged that the city's neonatal units were jeopardizing babies' health by treating them "too intensively."[16] The directors advocated closure of two of the four then existing NICUs, but there were apparently no volunteers. Recognizing that NICUs were "money-makers and prestige-builders for hospitals," neonatologists implied that (other) hospitals developed them for these purposes.[17] NICU adoption did pay off, and most units maintained healthy profit margins. Actual NICU costs in Florida in the early 1980s (before the state limited payment with prospective pricing) represented only 70 percent of the fees that hospitals charged for them.[18] NICUs continued to grow and pediatric departments in academic and other large hospitals became dependent on their revenues.[19] A 2002 *New England Journal of Medicine* editorial attributed NICU "overgrowth" to a "market-driven health care system with inadequate public planning."[20]

Functional Division of Labor

Subspecialty-based intensive care units functionally divided their work and their workers along scientific management lines, as had their parent departments earlier in the century. Academic NICU directors delegated a hierarchy of tasks to a hierarchy of salaried fellows, residents, nurses, and technicians.[21] The most highly trained board-certified neonatologists—generally the most technically proficient physicians—did not personally perform much of the medical work. They established treatment policies for the unit and supervised the fellows in training. Neonatal fellows in turn spent much of their time supervising pediatric residents. Pediatric residents—most of whom did not intend to subspecialize in neonatology, and many of whom did not like it—performed the bulk of the medical work in the NICU.[22] But residents and fellows came and went; nurses were the mainstay of day-to-day work in the intensive care unit.

Nursing historians identified intensive care units' organization of nursing as their most distinctive feature.[23] The organization conformed with precepts of scientific management as well as with the needs of medical subspecialization. NICU nurse practitioners at the top of the nursing hierarchy performed at a high level of technological capability as well as responsibility. Taking over procedures previously entrenched in the physician's domain, they performed endotracheal intubation, umbilical catheterization, lumbar puncture, and intravenous drug administration. In addition to their nursing functions, NICU work required nurses to diagnose, prescribe, and treat—the basic definition of physicians' work.[24]

Nursing's extended functions in the NICU conflicted with traditional power, status, and competency hierarchies in medicine. As one neonatologist recognized in the mid-1970s:

> Some of the nurses who have been in the house a long time are so very good they frighten the house officers [residents and interns] to death. They can do procedures better than the house officers; they have much better clinical judgement. They can determine more accurately when a baby is sick, and what the right move is in terms of changing ventilator, changing settings, or oxygen. It isn't just technical expertise; they know more physiology! This is very threatening to the insecure house staff. They shouldn't feel that their medical degree is being challenged by a nurse. You recognize the problem—that the doctor just out of medical school says, "Gee, I've got an M.D. and this person is an R.N. and knows more than me," and that's a very threatening situation.[25]

According to this neonatologist, the challenge to the medical hierarchy was a threat, and its solution seemed to be continuing exploitation of nursing expertise without permitting it to realign the hierarchy.

Managed care continued the division of labor in the neonatal intensive care unit. NICU staffing trends in the 1980s and 1990s confirmed one of house officers' worst fears: they could be replaced by nurses. Hospitals without pediatric residency programs as well as hospitals that had downsized their training programs maintained their NICUs by hiring nurse clinicians to perform most of the medical functions. Studies of these units found the nurses' performance to equal or better the performance of residents.[26] Regardless of whether doctors or nurses performed the tasks, however, neonatal intensive care increased medical intensity in neonatal care.

Levels of Clinical Intensity

By definition, intensive care inflated the capital, technologic, and labor resources consumed in a day or episode of clinical care. Admission to the intensive care unit was a major therapeutic decision in itself. Intensive care did not just shape clinical intervention; the intensive care structure was itself the clinical modality. Neonatal intensive care units served as the template for extending clinical technologies to newborns. They applied assisted respiration and continuous biochemical and electronic monitoring procedures to tiny babies. Staff attached machines to the baby (or the baby to the machines) as a matter of routine. The machines were devices for monitoring physiological functions and delivering water, sugars, salts, heat, and air. Machines also administered a wide array of drugs through a wide array of catheters and infusion pumps. Babies themselves became input-output machines reminiscent of dog preps in the physiology lab in medical school.

Mechanical ventilation, one of the most invasive ICU interventions, became a defining technology for neonatal intensive care. Regional perinatal policy held that only level III units should provide long-term mechanical ventilation, but level IIs competed by expanding their own ventilatory capacity. Some neonatologists accused ventilatory "aggressiveness" of escalating despite inadequate evaluation.[27] The sudden rise, and partial fall, of neonatal extracorporeal membrane oxygenation (ECMO)—circulating the baby's blood through an oxygenation machine outside its body—was a case in point for competitive expansion of intensive treatment of small babies in the face of inadequate data on effectiveness. Once one medical center announced its ECMO capacity, others defining themselves as cutting edge followed suit. The national number of neonatal ECMO units multiplied to exceed one hundred in the 1990s before the procedure declined in favor (and in revenue).[28] ECMO proponents emphasized the intensity and invasiveness of standard NICU mechanical ventilation in order to defend their own (highly intensive and invasive) technology.[29] Other neonatologists supported less invasive ventilatory techniques on grounds that damage resulting from ventilation could itself require ECMO.[30] Uncertainty regarding ECMO effectiveness combined with a declining economic environment contributed to its decline. By the late 1990s some neonatologists called the procedure an "established therapy," while others considered it an "adverse outcome."[31]

NICUs provided the framework for using other hospital technologies besides ECMO on very small babies. Enthusiasts saw premature babies as "untapped potential" for technologies such as near-infrared spectroscopy, magnetic resonance imaging, magnetic resonance spectroscopy, positron emission tomography, pulmonary function monitoring, and total body electrical conductivity measurements.[32] Academic neonatologists applying procedures such as these defined themselves as practicing at the "leading edge of technology and medical knowledge."[33] They used the high-intensity technologies in their clinical research and in their clinical work in order to advance (in) their field. Neonatology came to advertise itself as a subspecialty that challenged the limits of life itself. Nonetheless, its researchers did not show neonatal intensive care to be as effective as its practitioners often claimed.

Evaluation of Efficacy

Fetal, neonatal (the first month of life), and postneonatal (two to twelve months of age) mortality rates declined, at various rates, throughout the twentieth century. It was socially and politically significant at the time of NICU building that professional concern about neonates—the NICU clientele—supplanted concern about the rest of infant mortality, which related more to socioeconomic factors. Neonatal mortality rates did in fact fall more rapidly between 1965 and 1980 than in the decades preceding or following. Many obstetricians, neonatologists, and researchers at the time attributed this more rapid fall to simultaneous changes in the type of obstetric and neonatal care provided, identifying technologically "aggressive" interventions in particular.[34] The evidence supported that conclusion only for very-low-birthweight babies. NICU promoters neglected nonmedical explanations for declining mortality rates. Social, economic, and demographic changes such as availability of contraception and legalized abortion, expansion in primary care and nutrition programs, and a more equitably shared economy were also likely to have had an impact.

In its beginning many journal articles on neonatal intensive care confined themselves to exuberant descriptions of their authors' brand-new NICUs and their declining mortality rates. Although these articles demonstrated a widespread professional certainty regarding the effectiveness of neonatal intensive care, a few neonatologists challenged this certainty. John Sinclair warned in 1981 that NICU effectiveness had not been empirically demonstrated.[35] "If the supportive evidence is as weak as I charge," William Silverman queried around the same time at a conference on "Benefits and Hazards of Hospital Newborn

Care," "how has it come about that the militant approach to the care of the newborn has gained such wide acceptance?"[36]

Accumulating evidence over the next two decades showed that neonatal intensive care did prevent the deaths of some babies, but it also demonstrated that conclusions about its efficacy had been widely overgeneralized. The Congressional Office of Technology Assessment (OTA) criticized that the enthusiastic case reports from individual hospitals and physicians did not offer statistical validation of efficacy.[37] Pooling data from the reports in a meta-analysis, the OTA concluded that NICUs did improve outcomes for low-birthweight infants (weighing less than 2,500 grams at birth—about 5.5 pounds).[38] In fact, however, the accompanying data in its 1981 report and in its 1987 follow-up provided evidence for such a conclusion only for the small category of very-low-birthweight infants (weighing less than 1,500 grams).[39] The California Maternal and Child Health Data Base studies similarly credited tertiary-level NICUs with reducing mortality rates among low-birthweight babies and similarly supported its conclusion only for very-low-birthweight babies.[40] Most reports on NICU efficacy (including the major random controlled trial) selectively studied very-low-birthweight populations or showed a significant effect only for that group.[41]

Consistent with the NICU-based studies, most infants weighing over 1,500 grams and nearly all infants weighing over 2,000 grams were surviving long before the invention of neonatal intensive care. Combining available studies, authors in 1921 claimed neonatal survival rates of 89 percent for infants weighing 2,000–2,500 grams at birth and 59 percent for those weighing 1,500–2,000 grams.[42] Combining data from 1922 to 1949, the incubator unit at Chicago's Michael Reese Hospital reported comparable survival rates of 91 and 82 percent, respectively.[43] Consistent with these reports, population-wide studies found that 95 percent of babies in the birthweight category 2,001–2,500 grams were surviving in 1950.[44] The fact that those survival rates rose to 98 percent in 1980 did suggest an intensive care benefit for a small proportion of babies in the group.[45] It was a fallacy, however, to extrapolate the improved outcomes among very-low-birthweight babies to the 98–99 percent of babies with higher birthweight or to conclude that hospitals providing higher levels of intensity provided more effective neonatal care in general or more effective obstetric care. Growing numbers of neonatologists came to agree with Silverman, who reprimanded his colleagues in 1998, charging that "uncontrolled explorations of new treatments in neonates have not been curbed appreciably," despite the burgeoning popularity of health services research.[46] Another problem with NICU evaluation was that it primarily investigated short-term survival. One academic at the end of the century accused perinatal regionalization of abandoning its long-term follow-up policy, holding that "only a tiny fraction of very-low-birth-weight survivors are followed up rigorously and evaluated across the domains of health, growth, development, and behavioral outcomes."[47]

The evidence from the outcome studies strongly suggested that many babies were receiving intensive care treatments that they did not need and that could possibly harm them. Babies in neonatal intensive care units were subjected to many intensive and invasive procedures that could themselves lead to physical and possibly psychological damage. A 1989 *Ms.* magazine article quoted a paper from the AMA (the American Medical Association) journal maintaining that "in any setting other than an intensive care unit, a daily routine that involved restraining neonates in bed, placing plastic tubes…into various body orifices, and pricking the feet with needles…would be considered torture."[48] Although they became increasingly familiar with iatrogenic complications from NICU care,[49] neonatologists did not generally broadcast them until a replacement technology became available. Then they could concede negative aspects of the technology it replaced—like the ECMO proponents who used complications of mechanical ventilation as a marketing tactic for their newer technology. Ethical concerns focused on inequitable access to NICUs and on futile care of seriously ill and extremely low-birthweight babies, certainly important issues. But ethicists seldom addressed harming babies. They tended to ignore NICU overadmission and overtreatment of larger and healthier babies, a more common, if considerably less dramatic, situation.

Mismatch between Supply, Use, and Evidence of Benefit

Given high levels of financial reimbursement and professional certainty, the supply of NICUs in large part drove their utilization.[50] Already six per one hundred live births in 1977, NICU admission rates in California rose to nine in 1980 and to ten in 1990.[51] In the decade of Medicaid limitations and managed care, this rate slipped down to nine in 1995.[52] California's rates seemed to parallel national NICU admission rates. The high-level perinatal centers listed by the National Perinatal Information Center alone admitted 18 percent of their 1984 inborn live births—or 8 percent of the nation's births—to their neonatal intensive or intermediate care units.[53] It is unlikely that such a high proportion of babies needed intensive care. Although the United States had a much greater supply of neonatologists and NICU beds than Canada, Australia, and the United Kingdom, it did not have better neonatal outcomes.[54]

Overestimating the effectiveness of neonatal intensive care, neonatologists overestimated the need for it. They also differed widely among themselves. They variously recommended that between 2 and 6.5 percent of all newborns required intensive care and that an additional 0.4 to 8 percent needed an intermediate level of intensity.[55] The empirical evidence summarized in the previous section suggested that the lower figures were more appropriate. The findings that NICUs improved mortality rates primarily among babies weighing less than 1,500 grams at birth did not prove the necessity of intensive care for many higher-weight babies. Since very-low-birthweight babies represented only 1.2 percent of all babies born in the early 1980s—although that proportion had risen to 1.5 percent by the late 1990s—and the next higher birthweight group (1,500–1,999 grams) represented an additional 1.3 to 1.5 percent of births, the outcome evidence by birthweight supported admitting only about 3 percent of all newborns to intensive care units.[56] Data on NICU benefits for acutely ill larger babies were considerably more meager. Many larger babies admitted to NICUs had major congenital defects, some of which were incompatible with life. National Apgar scores (a simple 1–10 rating of a newborn's condition) also suggested NICU overuse. Throughout the 1990s only 1.4 percent of newborns had a five-minute Apgar score lower than 7, the point experts agreed was most likely to identify babies with potentially serious problems.[57] The fact that perinatal leaders came to evaluate regionalization programs in terms of very-low-birthweight babies and that researchers singled out this group for their efficacy studies speaks to their recognition that very-low-birthweight babies constituted the primary population needing NICU treatment.

Because actual NICU admission rates in many areas were considerably higher than the estimated 3–4.5 percent of babies with very low birthweight or major malformations,[58] it appeared likely that NICUs admitted larger, healthier, lower-cost babies to balance the extremely high costs of the smallest babies. Neonatal programs also used NICUs for surveillance. Some neonatologists in the early years proposed admitting all newborns to transitional-level NICUs until they were decreed healthy (a policy that conflicted with the contemporary rooming-in movement).[59] Nearly half of the babies admitted to one tertiary-level academic NICU around 1980 were low-cost admissions with no major risk factors.[60] Newborns admitted for evaluation purposes in another academic NICU in the 1990s accounted for 2 percent of the unit's work hours but 7 percent of its revenues.[61] It is understandable that doctors and parents want to ensure that their babies aren't suffering from treatable conditions, but, as authors noted, there was considerable potential for NICU overtreatment. Physicians and nurses initially judged around 60 percent of the neonatal admissions at two other tertiary-level units to be low-risk or mildly ill, an appraisal that turned out to be accurate.[62] Focusing on the equal prognostic accuracy of doctors and nurses, the investigators did not question why babies who appeared healthy and turned out to be healthy were admitted to the NICUs in the first place.

Managed care augmented concern about excessive neonatal intensive care utilization. While the evidence did support reduced NICU supply and use, it was not at all clear the extent to which the managed care reductions were appropriate. It looked as if they exacerbated socioeconomic inequities. Proportionately fewer NICU resources were spent on newborns who were uninsured or covered by Medicaid programs.[63]

Despite the dearth of evidence supporting prevailing NICU growth and utilization, neonatal intensive care units provided economic and professional success stories for neonatologists and their hospitals. Aspiring to this level of success themselves, academic obstetric leaders duplicated the structure and functioning of neonatal intensive care but with even less evidence of efficacy.

Intensive Care Obstetrics
Intensive Care and Academic Subspecialization

Academics built perinatal centers that combined neonatal and obstetric intensive care units. Blueprints and photographs of gleaming new equipment-saturated centers filled an entire journal issue in the mid-1980s.[64] Obstetric subspecialists upgraded the technologic and staffing level of their labor and delivery suites, consciously modeling their new units on neonatal (as well as coronary) intensive care. They worked with pharmaceutical, supply, and equipment companies and their affiliates, such as Ross Planning Associates and the Robert Wood Johnson Foundation, to develop clinical units with expanded capacity for consuming drugs, supplies, and equipment.[65] They built in technologies for continuous intrauterine pressure measurement, electronic fetal heart monitoring, and epidural analgesia. In the process they constructed obstetric intensive care units (OBICUs), the subspecialty of maternal-fetal medicine (also known as perinatology), and the concept of fetal intensive care.

As teaching departments became more dependent on clinical practice revenues, one academic obstetrician projected a need for innovative subspecialty services (which he called better "mouse traps") to attract more patients.[66] Management consultants similarly targeted perinatal care as fertile ground for innovative product lines.[67] Defining product line development as "rebundling already available services into a package to which consumers could relate," they advised that consumers could relate better to delivering babies . . . than barium enemas, for example.[68] High-risk diagnostic and intensive care units for women and infants proved to be highly successful product lines for their academic centers. *The Rise of a University Teaching Hospital* demonstrated how the University of Iowa's intensive care strategy particularly propelled practice plan growth in its obstetrics and gynecology department, which by the 1980s was supplying more hospital admissions than any other department.[69] Academic departments hired increasing numbers of subspecialists and fellows to staff their intensive care units and work for their practice plans. By the mid-1990s more than half of the faculty members in ob-gyn were subspecialists; they contributed a large portion of their time and earning capacity to their institutions' practice plans.[70] Maternal-fetal medicine fellows in most programs spent at least 30 percent of their time providing patient care.[71]

As in neonatal intensive care, obstetric intensive care functionally divided labor and placed subspecialists at the top of the hierarchy. Specialists and subspecialists recognized that assigning tasks to trainees and nurses enhanced their own productivity.[72] *Teamwork* often meant substituting nurses for physicians in routine care, but it did not necessarily mean nursing authority to match the enhanced responsibilities. Nursing organizations, including the one set up by the American College of Obstetricians and Gynecologists, officially concurred with the college's pronouncement that the specialist was the team manager. The obstetrician was the "chief executive officer," whose role included setting standards, monitoring task distribution, and supervising all team members.[73] Nurses were to take care of the patient, plot the progress of labor on a graph, and perform procedures under protocol or direct orders.

It did not take long for community hospitals to build competitive high-intensity obstetric units of their own. After the number of trained subspecialty fellows increased to fill the faculty slots in academic centers, perinatologists—like their neonatal colleagues—moved to establish intensive care units in community hospitals. By 1984, 576 high-risk centers responded to and were listed in the National Perinatal Information Center's *Perinatal Center Directory*.[74] Although nearly 40 percent of the country's births that year occurred in the named centers alone, they aspired to a still higher share of the birth market. Using brand-name marketing tactics, perinatal leaders placed articles describing their high-tech capabilities and their "miracle babies" in popular books, magazines, and newspapers.[75] One book specifically advised its pregnant middle-class readers (high- and low-risk) to choose perinatologists practicing at the high-tech hospitals named in the *Directory*.[76]

The Special Interest Group for Community Hospital-Based Perinatologists, composed of nonacademic members of the Society of Perinatal Obstetricians, published a manual in 1989 on how and why to continue to upgrade the level of "sophistication" of their departments. "'High risk obstetrics' is currently a buzz word and many patients will seek the subspecialist," a private practice perinatologist advised the interest group.[77] And many patients (particularly middle-class ones) did participate in creating the demand for high-intensity maternity care. A community hospital ob-gyn chief affirmed that the "discriminating consumer" was more likely to select a hospital with a complete range of services.[78] Not surprisingly, academic perinatologists criticized the competitive perinatal center development in community hospitals. "We have seen and trained the enemy," lamented one chief, rephrasing *Pogo,* "and they is us."[79] The competitive growth vastly increased the use of intensive care birth interventions such as electronic fetal monitoring (EFM).

Electronic Fetal Monitoring

Serving as the structural basis for obstetric intensive care, electronic fetal monitoring was the initial defining technology for the subspecialty of maternal-fetal medicine. Edward Hon, Edward Quilligan, and Richard Paul pioneered electronic fetal monitoring in the 1960s and 1970s as they moved from Yale to the University of Southern California.[80] Hon engineered the technology and founded Corometrics Medical Systems to produce it commercially; he also conducted the company's research and development studies, managed its marketing seminars, and supported its technology in court.[81] Feminist scholar Judith Kunisch alleged that over 50 percent of Corometrics stock was held by "the very men who worked so hard to promote the product as a standard of obstetrical care."[82] Kunisch also linked EFM to medical patriarchy. Calling it a "story of male dominance in defining the birthing of infants," Kunisch argued that men had dominated EFM development, manufacturing, marketing, investment, and utilization. But her story of the merger of business and medicine to create a more intensive standard of obstetric care was more thorough and more compelling.

Telling a different gendered story, nursing historian Margarete Sandelowski held that in practice, nurses dominated EFM use. Because they cared for women during the long hours of labor, obstetric nurses became the experts in EFM use, according to Sandelowski, and companies such as Corometrics marketed the technology to them.[83] After targeting nurses in academic centers initially, Corometrics defined the EFM market as every birth in the country. Corometrics as well as other EFM manufacturers regularly packaged additional technologies such as intrauterine pressure measurement into their machines, thus rendering their older equipment obsolete.[84] *Contemporary Ob/Gyn,* a journal with a reputation for advertising and promoting technology, kept the profession apprised of each feature. The new features not only created a constant market for new machines, they also expanded interventional intensity as nurses hooked up all the built-in technologies to the patients.

Consistent with his EFM leadership role, Quilligan defined a major role of the perinatal subspecialist to be developing and testing new procedures and technologies.[85] Listing interventions purportedly for subspecialist use only, perinatologists linked their professional identity with testing and using "powerful" drugs and "invasive" techniques.[86] Companies such as Corometrics and Utah Medical Electronics funded academic obstetrics departments to use and test their new machinery.[87] While testing was certainly necessary and (according to my biases) probably better when performed in academic settings, there was a fine line between using a technology to investigate its benefits and hazards and developing it as a new standard of care.

Continuous EFM rapidly became accepted as standard obstetric procedure. As usual, academic hospitals tended to adopt it first, but community hospitals did not lag far behind. EFM use rates at Columbia's Sloane Hospital rose from 2 percent of their births in 1970 to 85 percent just five years later.[88] Starting with a policy of 100 percent electronic monitoring, the University of Utah achieved 88 percent in its first year.[89] Perinatal leaders recognized that their intensive care equipment—like other hospital technologies—had to be used to capacity in order to amortize the costs.[90] A decade after EFM entry into the market, 77 percent of surveyed U.S. physicians believed it should be used for all labors.[91] National use estimates varied considerably in the early years, but it appeared that around 48 percent of all births were monitored electronically by 1980, 73 percent by 1990, and 84 percent by 1998.[92] Ironically, routine EFM took hold more slowly at the University of Southern California, where most maternity patients were indigent.[93] Nationally, EFM use was consistently higher for private patients than for uninsured ones.[94]

Obstetricians appreciated EFM for the scientific respectability it brought to their specialty, but its growth was not driven or even justified by scientific evidence of efficacy. Promoters had shown EFM technology to work in terms of measuring fetal heart rate patterns, but they had not shown it to work in terms of improving birth outcomes. Research obstetrician Arnold Haverkamp told a U.S. Senate committee that the March of Dimes and the National Institutes of Health had each questioned his initial grant proposals to evaluate electronic fetal monitoring on the grounds that the technology was already known to be necessary and effective.[95] And, indeed, this knowledge was a constant refrain in the literature of the 1970s. Quilligan and Paul asserted that EFM use could lead to 50 percent reductions in mental retardation and in perinatal mortality and morbidity.[96] Within a decade, however, researchers had rejected such claims.[97]

Only one out of twelve random-controlled trials conducted by the mid-1990s had found any benefit of continuous EFM over nurses' monitoring intermittently with a stethoscope (called "auscultation"). A number of investigators criticized the continuing routine use of EFM in the face of "overwhelming evidence" that it did not improve outcomes.[98] In a festschrift for Quilligan, longtime EFM supporter Barry Schifrin acknowledged that the technology had not lived up to initial expectations, but he held out for as-yet unidentified "potential benefits."[99] Schifrin was probably correct in claiming that worldwide EFM use in the 1990s demonstrated continuing professional confidence in the technology.[100] In a paper entitled "Technology Follies" obstetrician David Grimes charged that the academic prestige of EFM advocates had contributed significantly to the initial use of the technology and that its continued routine use despite lack of supporting evidence was a matter of letting "sleeping dogmas lie."[101] The profession itself tended to blame the liability/malpractice situation for excessive EFM use, but this was a circular argument. By definition legal negligence is a breach in the standard of care, and obstetricians had defined EFM as the standard of care. EFM development and use shaped malpractice law as much as the other way around.[102]

Social scientists sometimes blamed excessive use of EFM and other obstetric intensive care machinery on medical models of birth as a mechanical process. They maintained that doctors perceived birth pathology as a mechanical breakdown of labor (or the laboring woman's body) and assumed that they could use engineering techniques to repair the malfunction. Referring to EFM as well as to the active management of labor, British sociologist Ann Oakley held that the mechanical model "informed much of the technological innovation in obstetrics."[103] American sociologist Barbara Katz Rothman attributed EFM's wide acceptance to its fit with a mechanical/industrial paradigm, which she also called "the ideology of patriarchal society."[104] Pointing out that many critics used the imagery of industrialization and mechanization to oppose routine birth intervention, literary analyst Tess Cosslett held that they often didn't recognize how profoundly the rhetoric of natural childbirth had influenced their own thinking.[105] My argument—not based on assumptions of what is natural—is that medicine constructed an industrial organization of birth, thus contributing to an industrial discourse about it.

Professional development and commercial marketing of technology reinforced the mechanistic and pathologic paradigms. EFM manufacturers in particular promoted pathologic models of birth. A perinatal nurse working for Corometrics advised that labor was inherently dangerous and that all labors should therefore receive high-risk care—that is, electronic fetal monitoring.[106] Assuming that EFM patterns deviating from the statistical norm correlated with physiologically deviant babies, obstetricians called the non-normal patterns "fetal distress." They then found it problematic when more than 40 percent of babies with the diagnosis turned out to be perfectly healthy.[107] Admitting that the term *fetal distress* itself encouraged inappropriate birth intervention, the American College of Obstetricians and Gynecologists recommended replacing it with *nonreassuring fetal status.*[108] A nonreassuring improvement, it did contest the implication of a specific disease entity. *Fetal intolerance of labor* was another nonspecific but impressive-sounding term that came to be used to support EFM and other intensive obstetric interventions.[109] EFM supporters in the 1990s continued to call the birth process "extremely treacherous."[110]

While mechanistic and patriarchal paradigms were indeed prevalent, EFM's continued use was based on more than birth paradigms or dogma. Operating intensive labor units equipped with monitoring devices in itself reinforced mechanistic and pathologic paradigms of birth. Advising his colleagues to embrace an "intensive care orientation," Quilligan acknowledged that intensive care was not just a concept; it was embodied in fully-equipped intensive care units.[111] Its mechanistic and pathologic paradigms were just as much a result as a cause of EFM use. As investigators of another obstetric technology concluded, the introduction of a technology entailed a "mutual adaptation of technique and intellectual problems," or reconceptualizing pathology in terms of the new technology.[112]

Continuous electronic monitoring became a part of the normal structure and function of labor and delivery units. New and upgraded perinatal centers built electronic monitoring into the architecture. Banks of monitors in central nursing stations displayed the electronic data emanating from every labor bed. Since nurses had previously listened to babies' hearts with a stethoscope, EFM use meant one more substitution of human skill and human contact with technology. EFM reduced nurses' personal relationships with women in labor and their ability to provide labor support and coach women in pain control methods. Requiring fewer nurses to oversee the data output, EFM expanded nursing as well as physician productivity. Ironically, obstetricians came to wonder whether EFM itself contributed to fetal distress or at least whether the hands-on process of nursing care alleviated it, but they didn't change their dependence on the technology.[113] Clinicians perceived nurse auscultation as "impractical" in the competitive managed care environment.[114] Hospitals and managed care plans mandated routine EFM use in the interests of cost-efficiency.

In summary, perinatal intensive care units, their diagnostic and treatment modes, and their conceptual models codeveloped. Labor and delivery suites as well as nurseries became intensive care units by incorporating electronic monitoring and other technologic devices. Academic research showed neonatal intensive care to be effective in lowering mortality among very-low-birthweight infants (especially when born in academic or other tertiary-level units).[115] But this effectiveness was inappropriately generalized to larger babies and even to birthing women, who did not, for the most part, experience better outcomes in higher-level services. In raising the capital intensity and price of maternal and newborn care, intensive care units raised the financial contributions of the obstetric and pediatric specialties to their hospitals and academic practice plans—and consequently raised their costs to society. Neonatal and obstetric intensive care units developed *as* strategic business units and their technologic procedures developed *as* product lines. They upped the capital ante for competing in the business of maternity care, and they upped the intensity of medical care delivered. Active management of labor was another high-intensity birth intervention shaped by developments in the economics and the economic organization of medicine.

Nine
Managing Birth
*Managed Care and Active
Management of Labor*

Managed care flourished in the 1980s and 1990s as a contractual combination of physicians, hospitals, and insurance. Its antecedents included contract medicine in the first decade of the century, private group clinics in the 1920s and 1930s, organizations such as Kaiser Permanente in the 1940s, and health maintenance organizations (HMOs) in the 1970s. Both government and industry dressed health maintenance organizations in the "rhetorical garments of private enterprise and the free market,"[1] but, like their predecessors, HMOs embodied a corporate organization of medicine.[2] Health administration professors acknowledged this organization when they advised the national health planning program to favor group medicine on the grounds that it paralleled industrial development. They appreciated that its extensive divisions of labor, substitution of capital for labor, and review processes permitted group medicine to maximize specialist productivity and "streamline the productive process."[3] The key features of managed care were corporate organization, financial management, and clinical process management.

Elements of Managed Care
Corporate Organization
Academic practices strengthened their corporate forms of organization in parallel with HMOs. Johns Hopkins described its 1973 decentralization of managerial functions to specialty departments as an industrial organization.[4] Academic medical centers increasingly organized their clinical care along man-

aged care lines. By the 1990s, 40 percent of U.S. medical schools organized their practice plans as multispecialty group practices.[5] Their goal was to offer a comprehensive range of services and successfully compete for managed care contracts. Teaching units continued to divide clinical work into teams composed of subspecialists, specialists, specialty nurses, and a range of other nursing and technical personnel.[6] They assigned much of the detail work to nonphysician personnel, which accounted for a large proportion of employed nurse-midwives. Obstetric leaders were beginning to see doulas, or supportive birth companions traditionally from the woman's culture, as effective, cost-efficient labor room staff.[7]

Private physicians' groups similarly organized corporate independent practice associations (IPAs) and other abbreviations, turning their practices into managed care organizations in the process. Physician-owners of perinatal IPAs, for example, hired other perinatal specialists as employees, developed patient care protocols, managed the group financially, and deselected physicians who didn't meet their clinical or economic performance criteria.[8] Entrepreneurs subsequently invented physician roll-ups, which bought and consolidated medical practices to create investor-owned physician groups. Although many did not do as well financially as their creators had hoped, a *New England Journal of Medicine* editorial observed that the firm Pediatrix, employing nearly six hundred perinatal subspecialists in 185 neonatal intensive care units, remained financially successful during the turbulent 1990s.[9]

Financial Management

As early as the 1930s, hospital administrator A. C. Bachmeyer criticized some hospitals for reporting back to their physicians the number of patients they had referred and the revenues each had generated.[10] Beginning with diagnosis related group (DRG)–based reimbursement for Medicare patients in 1983, government and private payers wrested control over price from providers. This payer revolt challenged the open-ended, cost-based reimbursement systems that had financed so much medical care expansion. It shifted much of the financial risk from payers to providers, who in turn intensified their use of financial management methods in order to cope with it. Financial management in specialty departments was consistent with the expectations that each specialty had to cover its expenses with revenues generated from the sale of its research and clinical work. It was a short step from self-supporting departments to requiring that every service and every clinician in the department had to support themselves by selling their services.

Financial analyses and other managerial methods reinforced business values in hospital operations. They focused the attention of administrators—by then calling themselves chief executive officers, chief financial officers, and chief operating officers, like their self-identified counterparts in industry—on performance in terms of profitability, capital structure, and productivity.[11] Financial ratios pressured hospital administrators to use their technologic capacity at its highest possible level. Managing financial risk meant downsizing services with lagging revenues, even in academic medical centers. Like other chief financial officers, academic financial managers sought to reduce bed capacity, expand admissions, and upgrade technologic capacity to improve financial performance.[12]

DRGs facilitated the ongoing development of hospital product lines based on specialty and subspecialty procedures. Coming out of statistical control theory, which offered a method of industrial quality control, DRGs enabled hospital administrators to identify which patient conditions and product lines brought in the highest revenues and direct their service development and marketing efforts accordingly.[13] They also contributed to clinical process management by presupposing that each DRG represented a package of standardized practices. A surgeon credited DRGs with treating patients as if they were on production lines, discharging them as soon as possible following their procedures.[14]

Clinical Process Management

Managerial mechanisms to control clinical processes grew exponentially in academic centers and other managed care organizations. Clinical process management—also called quality management—explicitly embraced methods from the industrial and managerial revolutions. Its techniques were based on methods of hospital industrial engineering and operations research, themselves grounded in Frederick Taylor's scientific management. Some quality managers of the 1990s had been the hospital engineers of the 1960s. Both industrial engineering and quality management sought to control production, management, and information.[15] They designed ways to streamline patient flow and enhance staff productivity primarily at the departmental level. In the obstetrics and gynecology department at Stanford University Hospital an operations research project in the mid-1960s reduced costs by accelerating the flow of patients through the labor and delivery unit.[16] Industrial engineers earlier and quality control managers later drew patient flow diagrams with the intent of enhancing productivity.

The field of industrial quality management sciences (IQMS) further applied industrial process management to medical performance and, like Taylor, called it science. Quality control gurus in the 1980s and 1990s promoted IQMS techniques such as continuous quality improvement (CQI) and total quality management (TQM) in an attempt to standardize clinical production.[17] Hospital administrators, subspecialists, and pharmaceutical companies such as Burroughs-Wellcome and Ross Laboratories worked together to develop practice guidelines, clinical process protocols, and research networks in many specialty areas, including perinatal intensive care.[18] Increased productivity was the primary goal of the practice guidelines and other forms of clinical management.[19] Academic practice plans were not excepted, measuring "clinical productivity" by revenues generated and applying corporate strategies to maximize throughput.[20] Besides augmenting speed, IQMS methods sought to reduce procedural variation, an activity they equated with improving quality. Applying the statistical methods designed to control variation and enhance productivity in manufacturing, IQMS methods focused the attention of researchers, managers, and policy makers on variations in clinical practice. They treated institutional as well as regional variation in health care delivery in perinatal and other specialty areas as the "fat" that its methods sought to reduce.[21] Since procedural variation tended to be higher for interventions carrying greater professional uncertainty about their benefits, quality management tried to concretize certainty. Trimming the fat also required streamlining medical delivery. In obstetrics IQMS protocols built in the use of oxytocin to control and streamline delivery.

Oxytocin Development

Oxytocin induction and acceleration of childbirth labor enacted clinical process methods of managed care. Oxytocin use accelerated during the managed care era, although the drug had a longer history. American and British obstetricians had long experimented with various ways of administering the hormone oxytocin—the desired active agent of posterior pituitary extract—in different ways during the course of the twentieth century. The first wave of use in obstetrics (discussed in chapter 3) was followed by harsh condemnation. Obstetricians used a 1940 symposium to censure excessive use of the extract. Joseph DeLee drew upon his typically colorful metaphors to accuse pituitary extract of creating an "exploding" uterus, making a "projectile" of the baby, and blasting it through the cervix.[22] DeLee also criticized pharmaceutical companies for marketing the extract without approval from the American Medical Association's Council on Pharmacy and Chemistry. But other academic obstetricians around the same time worked with the companies to formulate preparations that they hoped would ameliorate the extract's known harmful effects.[23]

Pituitary extract enthusiasm entered its second wave in the mid-1940s, when Duncan Reid of Harvard and Nicholson Eastman of Johns Hopkins each conferred their imprimatur on it—on the condition that only specialists use it. Reid was the more fervent advocate, advising routine use upon any evidence of uterine inertia.[24] Obstetricians subsequently referred to Reid's and Eastman's articles as encouraging their own use of pituitary extract. British obstetrician Geoffrey Theobald's innovation of delivering the extract by intravenous drip furthered its use for labor induction as well as acceleration. Already an advocate of labor induction, Theobald's unit used oxytocin drip to induce 14 percent of its deliveries in the early 1950s and to accelerate 3 percent of them.[25] Synthetic oxytocin (Pitocin ®) became commercially available in the mid-1950s, further contributing to its use.

Academic obstetricians forged the mechanisms for labor induction and acceleration and guided their midcentury use. Some favored oxytocin for acceleration, others for induction. They used pituitary extract primarily on their private patients; residents delivering in ward services did not use the drug regularly. Johns Hopkins used oxytocin acceleration on 4 percent of its ward patients and 12 percent of its private patients, a figure that Eastman called excessive.[26] Standard obstetric practices at Columbia's Sloane Hospital followed a similar pattern: induction rates were 20 percent for private patients, while they were close to zero for ward patients.[27] All Sloane obstetricians performed elective (not medically indicated) inductions, and they all cited patient convenience as their primary reason. Inferring that they actually meant physician convenience, the editor of the series defended the practice, reassuring readers that obstetricians' preference for daylight obstetrics was nothing to be ashamed of. The obstetrics literature at the time was "replete with articles extolling the virtue" of labor induction; faculty at the University of Pennsylvania averaged a 14 percent elective oxytocin induction rate in the 1950s, with individual obstetricians' rates peaking at 61 percent.[28] A Philadelphia-trained obstetrician later noted:

> Ed Bishop was the champion of elective induction of labor. In the early 1960s, it had become quite fashionable for a Philadelphia matron to choose her labor day. With the house organized, her hair done, and her partner having the day off, she arrived at the hospital for epidural anesthesia, amniotomy, and oxytocin administration. Several hours later a baby had arrived and the mother was ready for visitors, looking rested and happy. Bishop realized that for this scheme to work someone needed to quantify what most experienced obstetricians knew, when the cervix was "ripe" and induction would be short and easy.[29]

Thus was elective induction of Philadelphia society the incentive for the Bishop score, although the ease of the process for the "matron" might be taken with a grain of salt. Efficiency was one of the identified virtues of induction. The management group that applied industrial engineering methods to maternity care and later invented DRGs suggested using operations research methods to expand elective labor induction and achieve a more efficient use of hospital facilities.[30] Despite the attempts to standardize obstetric practices, however, hospitals and physicians continued to vary in their oxytocin use. A small sample of academic hospitals alone found induction rates for white patients in the early 1960s ranging from 2 to 14 percent and augmentation rates ranging from 1 to 34 percent.[31]

Much as academic obstetricians would like to have monopolized oxytocin use, they could not control its spread beyond academia or even beyond their specialty. When board-certified specialists were electively inducing 12 percent of their patients in 1967, the national maternity care study showed that generalists were inducing 6 percent of theirs.[32] The following year 7 percent of all births in New York City were induced, and 22 percent were augmented.[33] The literature was soon replete with papers promoting prostaglandin as another induction agent. Industry and academia worked together again to develop the hormone for clinical use.[34] The Upjohn Company, a prostaglandin manufacturer, provided technical assistance and samples to a large number of clinical investigators and funded the research of some of them.[35] Upjohn also supported and disseminated research comparing hospital costs of using different chemical induction agents. One such Upjohn-funded study in Britain concluded that labor induction could save hospitals money by enhancing staffing and other efficiencies in their labor and delivery units. Two U.S. studies, in contrast, found induction to be less cost-efficient due to increased epidural and/or cesarean section rates.[36]

In sum, scientific and technologic developments, institutional and professional growth, and commercial incentives all advanced oxytocin use at midcentury. Whereas oxytocin administration was primarily a special procedure for private practice obstetricians in the United States, it developed as managed care process within Ireland's and Britain's health systems.

Active Management of Labor: Dublin

Like intensive care, active management of labor was more managerially than technologically induced. Kieran O'Driscoll formulated the strategy of managing labor with oxytocin acceleration when he became master at Dublin's high-volume National Maternity Hospital in 1963. O'Driscoll's method incorporated structural, financial, and procedural elements that collectively came to be called managed care in the United States. It divided labor functionally, budgeted resources, and controlled clinical and biological process in order to enhance efficiency. O'Driscoll's management shifted decision-making control up the staff hierarchy to fully trained specialist consultants.[37] This meant less responsibility for lower-ranking doctors, including registrars—specialists in training serving as hospital staff, equivalent to residents in the United States—as well as for the midwives, who actually delivered most of the babies.

In addition to centralizing management in the consultant's office, O'Driscoll purposely designed active management of labor to be a cost-efficient clinical procedure. Its goal was to accelerate the speed of labor in order to manage patient flow, unit staffing, and costs efficiently. O'Driscoll claimed that assigning a student midwife to each laboring woman permitted each fully trained midwife to cover 622 deliveries per year (obviously not providing much personal care themselves). Such a level of productivity, he boasted, vastly exceeded that of other maternity services.[38] In the 1993 edition of his book O'Driscoll called active management a "prime example of the application of principles of cost efficiency in contemporary medical planning, where good medicine and sound economics are seen to complement each other."[39] He did not say why he thought good medicine and economics were necessarily complementary.

O'Driscoll gauged efficiency in individual labors by the rate of dilation of the cervix of the patient's uterus. If the cervix did not dilate at a rate of at least one centimeter per hour after the patient's admission to the labor unit, active management protocol required an amniotomy, or artificial rupture of the amniotic sac. If amniotomy did not achieve the mandated rate, the protocol then required the midwife to initiate a high-dose oxytocin regimen.[40] By the early 1970s, 55 percent of primiparae (women giving birth for the first time) at Dublin's National Maternity Hospital were receiving oxytocin stimulation.[41] Apparently not registering routine amniotomy and oxytocin acceleration as intervention, O'Driscoll and his colleagues claimed that active management ensured normal progress in labor and incurred "very low intervention rates."[42]

Active management's use of cervical dilation rates to schedule labor intervention was based on the diagram that obstetrician Emanuel Friedman invented at Columbia's Sloane Hospital in the 1950s.[43] The Friedman partographs, partograms, or curves, as they were variously called, graphed cervical dilation against time—although clinicians came to add other variables, such as uterine contraction strength and descent of the baby—further subdividing labor and further multiplying stages. Friedman depicted partographs as requiring minimal skill to use, meaning specifically that obstetric specialists could assign the tasks of measuring cervical dilation and filling in the graphs to nurses. Physicians could then monitor the graphs (rather than the patients) to make their intervention decisions. This use of partographs further separated thinking from doing in the obstetrics unit, deskilling nurses, midwives, lower-level doctors—and, arguably, obstetricians themselves.

Partographs' mechanistic approach reinforced the specialty's scientific management analysis of birth as a series of steps in a production process. Although he called his own analogy "somewhat oversimplified," Friedman viewed the patient in labor as a "complex machine" in which the ratio of work output to energy input was a "measure of the efficiency of the mechanical device under study" (presumably the uterus, rather than the body or the woman).[44] Extending the metaphor of the body as machine into a production metaphor, anthropologist Emily Martin attested in *The Woman in the Body* that the partograph subdivided a woman's labor "like factory labor . . . into many stages and substages."[45] The partograph served as a performance indicator in an engineering model of birth. Partographs portray variation in the biological processes of birth, and active management sought to reduce this variation. A pharmaceutical company distributed free partograph forms with the brand name of its oxytocin product emblazoned on them, the obvious implication being that obstetricians should use its product in labors that fell behind accepted norms.

O'Driscoll's minimum cervical dilation speed limit of one centimeter per hour was consistent with Friedman's definition of normalcy. Yet Friedman's norms came from teaching hospitals (he was by then at Boston's Beth Israel Hospital, which used oxytocin acceleration in 14 percent of its labors); thus, the norms were artificially fast.[46] On the other hand, a potential benefit of the Friedman curve was that it normalized slow dilation rates in early labor and could thereby restrain pressures to intervene surgically or pharmaceutically at that time. Friedman's own labor management was called "more or less conservative" by some of his colleagues because he did not advocate routine acceleration of below-normal rates.[47] Yet he diagrammed an "ideal" labor by selecting the "best" 40 percent of his hospital's primiparae; he then advised that oxytocin could help many of the remaining 60 percent achieve similar partographic success.[48] This kind of advice belies the statistical meaning of norm as the average in a population around which there is a normal variation. It also tends to define success in childbirth in terms of curves on a graph.

One of the simpler reasons O'Driscoll's active management worked economically and medically was that it redefined labor. It limited delivery unit admission to women in what Friedman called the active phase of labor and started the clock at that time. This restricted admission policy left women in early labor without medical or nursing support. It also reflected O'Driscoll's disinterest—unlike his British colleagues—in admitting patients who were not in labor in order to induce it.

Induction and Active Management: Britain

When Britain's National Health Service (NHS) was established just after World War II, midwives attended about 90 percent of the nation's births, many of which took place in the home.[49] The obstetrics profession promoted a national policy of 100 percent hospitalization of birth in its 1970 Peel report, when specialist and hospital capacity had grown to the point of being able to accommodate such a policy.[50] Salaried staff in NHS hospital consultant units were organized by "firm" and built on a functional division of labor within each firm.[51] One consultant traditionally headed one firm and managed its workforce, dividing the work among a hierarchy of medical and nursing staff. Registrars occupied the middle level, and house officers with little or no specialty training occupied the bottom medical rung. Although midwives continued to deliver the majority of babies as birth moved from the home to the hospital, the new location situated them more firmly in the medical hierarchy.

Consultants' relatively small numbers, their position at the top of their firms, and their upper-class, private practice, Harley Street heritage meant that they were more likely to define their work as truly consultative and less hands-on than their American counterparts. Medical and midwifery trainees performed the routine obstetric work, while the intermediate-level doctor waited on call to assist.[52] Registrars performed most of the urgent instrumental and operative procedures. Obstetrics consultants were more likely to define their work in terms of elective procedures scheduled during working hours. Labor induction particularly suited this definition of consultant work. The policy of hospitalizing every birth may also have created an induction incentive—women had to go to the hospital to have their labors started. Induction rates expanded from 8.3 percent in 1962, reputedly peaking in 1974 at 39 percent in England and Wales and at 48 percent in Scotland.[53] The reported rates then declined, plateauing at 17–18 percent from 1985 to 1994, before they rose again to 20 percent in 1994–1995.[54]

Obstetrics consultant Alexander Turnbull contributed to the induction boom by adapting the automatic infusion pump to deliver oxytocin. Medical supply companies subsequently plunged into the infusion pump business, marketing the machines widely for obstetric use.[55] Turnbull developed concepts of oxytocin "titration" corresponding with the functioning of infusion pumps. By *titration* he meant an incremental and precise increase in the oxytocin dose until uterine contractions reached a particular frequency and strength.[56] Known to beginning chemistry students as reaching an exact point in a chemical reaction, the term implied greater physiologic precision than the procedure actually entailed and imbued oxytocin use with the aura of an exact science. Turnbull and colleagues promoted oxytocin for its contribution to maximizing efficiency in the work of the uterus and in the work of the maternity unit. His firm induced in the morning with the intent of delivering by evening, thus reducing birth labor and staff labor to one working day. Turnbull was far from the only ob-gyn consultant who appreciated induction for its contribution to efficient scheduling and rationalized workloads.[57] An article in the *Sunday Times* called induction a "production line system where women have their babies by clockwork."[58]

As insinuated in the *Sunday Times,* Britain's high induction rates met with considerable criticism from both inside and outside of medicine. In her book *The Dignity of Labour?* sociologist Ann Cartwright showed that induction use varied by type and size of hospital as well as by patient class—despite National Health Service policies of equal and free access to services.[59] Cartwright used the variations to imply that the high induction rates were not medically justified. Other health services researchers were coming to similar conclusions. Turnbull collaborated with Iain Chalmers on a study finding that Turnbull's "active approach" of inducing 27 percent of his patients had no health advantages (or disadvantages) over the approach of a less active team with a 9 percent induction rate.[60] After founding the National Perinatal Epidemiology Unit, Chalmers broadened his purview to all of medicine in the Cochrane Collaboration. The two efforts were milestones in the development of evidence-based medicine.

Although high induction rates were widely criticized, the accuracy of the data was questionable. While, on the one hand, official British data may have underreported labor induction, on the other hand, it did not distinguish between oxytocin induction and its use to augment labor contractions, possibly leading to overreporting of induction. Data analysts estimated that the reported rate of 31 percent in 1980 roughly signified a 20 percent induction rate and an 11 percent augmentation rate.[61] Other studies, however, supported higher induction rates. A 1978 midwife survey reported induction rates of 25 percent and acceleration rates of 18 percent.[62] Postpartum women in Cartwright's surveys reported induction rates using amniotomy and/or oxytocin of 24 percent in 1975, 30 percent in 1984, and 28 percent in 1989.[63] In addition to the likelihood that some births recorded as induced were accelerated instead, oxytocin-induced labors *were* oxytocin-accelerated labors; the infusion was generally kept running throughout labor.

Whether it peaked at 39 percent or a greater or lesser figure, induction was initially the dominant oxytocin intervention in Britain. But oxytocin acceleration was gaining momentum in medical school and specialty hospitals. Initiating an active management policy in 1971, Queen Charlotte's Maternity Hospital in London promoted a "more confident and a more controlled" use of oxytocin acceleration alongside an expansion in epidural analgesia and electronic fetal monitoring.[64] Like Kieran O'Driscoll, Queen Charlotte consultant John Beazley appreciated active management for conferring control over all of labor and delivery on consultants and expediting labor by removing bottlenecks in the flow of patients through the unit.[65]

Consultant involvement in the delivery unit expanded as the supply of consultants expanded.[66] Although the number of live births per employed midwife was relatively stable at around 30 between 1975 and 1998 in England and Wales, growth in the number of trained and employed specialists meant that the number of births available per obstetrician-gynecologist declined from about 260 to 160.[67] Active management fit this expansion by shifting decision making from the hands of midwives (and junior medical staff) to those of consultants. By 1981 an obstetrician reviewing O'Driscoll's book for the *British Medical Journal* pronounced active management to be a "revolution in intrapartum care."[68] A few years later 89 percent of consultant units used a partograph for all women in labor, and 26 percent had a predetermined definition of slow progress, first steps in an active management approach.[69] One unit with an active management policy also had an induction rate of 27 percent.[70] Oxytocin acceleration rates for primiparae varied from 5 percent to over 40 percent of a hospital's births; this variation contributed to the conclusion in *Effective Care in Pregnancy and Childbirth* that active management of labor was not evidence-based.[71]

The active management revolution grew in Britain in the context of national policies and managerial efforts to control hospital costs. The National Health Service had initiated a department-based costing system in 1959.[72] The 1967 "cog-wheel" reports (named after their mechanistic logo) on "Organisation of Medical Work in Hospitals" prompted further use of industrial management methods to control hospital expenditures. NHS managers employed the cog-wheel reports as a model for staffing and scheduling maternity units and using resources efficiently.[73] Yet the government continued to fund significant NHS growth until 1976, when it capped expenditures. This cash-limit policy was later credited as an initial impetus in the development of clinical management methods.[74] The 1983 Griffiths report expanded the use of business management techniques in hospital services, and the Department of Health released the first of its performance indicators.[75] Like their counterparts in industry, performance indicators evaluated clinical services largely in terms of operational and cost efficiencies.[76] Managers used performance indicators to evaluate specialist and nursing staff productivity and resource use in hospital maternity units.[77] In this way clinical audits and performance indicators converged with methods from the industrial quality management sciences to expand birth management.

NHS managerial requirements had a strong impact on maternity service functioning. National policy in 1980 advised that maternity unit directors develop guidelines to standardize the work of junior medical staff across all consultant firms in their departments.[78] Some hospital administrators subsequently organized clinical directorates based on the Johns Hopkins model of department-based management.[79] Department heads and NHS planners continued to consolidate consultant firms in the 1990s in the name of efficient management of hospital personnel. Regional planners as well as the Royal College of Obstetricians and Gynaecologists supported obstetric unit consolidation with the goal of establishing consultant-directed units with fifteen hundred to two thousand deliveries each. Units of this size, they advised, would require only two or three specialist consultants, four midlevel and junior doctors, and forty midwives to deliver all their patients.[80] Not inadvertently, such consolidation would also eliminate independent general practitioner maternity units.

Consolidation of delivery units and department-wide management of consultant firms contributed to a growing tension between consultants' clinical autonomy and their submission to departmental standards. This tension exploded in the case of Wendy Savage, an ob-gyn consultant fired in 1985 essentially for differing from departmental politics and practices.[81] Savage had opposed consolidating the obstetrics unit at Mile End Hospital with its parent department, the professorial unit located at the London Hospital at Whitechapel. She was one of Mile End's "conservative" obstetricians (described in chapter 7) with lower intervention rates than the "active" obstetricians at the Whitechapel unit. In 1982, to exemplify one relevant year, labor induction rates were 7 percent at Mile End, compared to 19 percent at Whitechapel (for patient populations of similar risk and with similar outcomes); augmentation rates for primiparae were 7 percent compared to 18 percent, cesarean section 10 to 14 percent, and forceps 4 to 8 percent.[82] Savage was charged with incompetence on the basis of selected adverse outcomes in her firm and subjected to a hearing. Depicting the dispute in terms of "Who controls childbirth?" she garnered strong support from local women, general practitioners, midwives, and national advocacy groups. She was eventually exonerated by her peers outside of the London Hospital and reinstated.

National politics continued to impact obstetric care in Britain. The Conservative Party's internal market policy of the 1990s was a major leap in organizing the National Health Service along business lines. Inspired by managed competition strategies and strategists from the United States, the internal market split the health care system into corporate providers and corporate purchasers, who were then required to contract with one another in buying and selling services.[83] The contract system expanded clinical management incentives, and childbirth became a favorite target for economic evaluation and management.

The Department of Health's report on *Changing Childbirth* was the other major policy effort that shaped maternity care in the 1990s—ostensibly opposing the active management movement. In the interests of efficient staffing as well as midwives' aspirations for professional autonomy, the report challenged health authorities to allot at least 30 percent of their areas' births to "midwife-led" maternity services.[84] Working in consultant firms had expanded midwives' technical skills; they had come to perform amniotomy and episiotomy, attach fetal scalp electrodes for internal electronic monitoring, and add analgesics to epidural and oxytocin to intravenous infusions.[85] But they were limited in making decisions about when or whether to perform certain procedures, especially EFM use and oxytocin acceleration.[86]

One of *Changing Childbirth*'s announced goals was to reform birth intervention, but its impact in this area seemed to be slight. Programs identified as midwife-led did not necessarily challenge existing obstetric practices. Studies found that midwife-led programs reported birth intervention rates on low-risk women diverging more from one another than from consultant units in their own localities.[87] Although midwife-led programs generally did have lower episiotomy and/or EFM rates, they had only slightly lower oxytocin induction and augmentation rates. One high-intervention midwife-led program induced 24 percent and accelerated 43 percent of its deliveries. Championed by activist as well as midwife organizations, *Changing Childbirth* was, ironically, consistent with managerial ideology. It enacted a managerial cost-control strategy of workload rationalization. From both managers' as well as activists' points of view, it sought to "demedicalize" birth in the sense of substituting nurses (cheaper workers) for doctors (more costly workers).[88]

At the end of the 1990s it looked as if physician-based management had changed childbirth in Britain more than *Changing Childbirth*. Sequential use of prostaglandin to soften the cervix, oxytocin induction, and oxytocin stimulation had become standard practice in many British obstetric units.[89] Active management strategies had also become widespread.[90] A study of economic aspects of different delivery modes supported active management as a substitute for the rising cesarean section rates on grounds that it cost less, used less staff, and shortened labor.[91]

Although the Labour Party repudiated the NHS internal market when it won national election in 1997, it retained its key element, separation of purchasers and providers. The distinction between Conservative "contracting" and Labour "commissioning" was not clear, not at least in the first few years. In addition, the Labour Party expanded the use of industrial quality management sciences methods to control medical practice. It established a National Institute of Clinical Excellence to produce service guidelines and performance measures as well as a commission to manage their implementation.[92] In form and in function NHS organization resembled managed care in the United States (and vice versa).

Actively Managing Labor and Cesarean Section Rates: United States

While British obstetricians were inducing and actively managing births in the 1970s and 1980s, American obstetricians were actively removing babies by cesarean section. Active management of labor did not seem to capture Americans' interest until the high cesarean section rates led to financial and political embarrassment. Subsequently, active management flourished in the dual context of cesarean reduction programs and managed care. Insurers promoted active management protocols to reduce their maternity care costs under managed care. Hospitals shifted their financial and clinical strategies from maximizing production to maximizing productivity. Hospital administrators came to see cesarean section as a resource consumer rather than a revenue generator. Obstetric chiefs hoped that cesarean section reduction programs would improve the bottom line of their departments as well as their position in the competition for managed care contracts.

Projecting from its own experience, one academic group estimated in the mid-1990s that oxytocin acceleration could save the country ninety-three million dollars a year due to faster labors and fewer cesarean sections.[93] Governmental, corporate, and insurance company payers had even higher financial goals. Seeking to reduce the number of cesarean sections they were buying as employee benefits, payers projected a national savings of one billion dollars a year in preventing unnecessary cesarean sections.[94] The Pacific Business Group on Health—whose membership included Bank of America, Hewlett-Packard, Lockheed Martin, and General Electric—established a coalition to reduce corporate health insurance costs.[95] The group joined with providers to organize the California Perinatal Quality Care Collaborative, which applied continuous quality improvement and other industrial quality management science methods to reduce cesarean section.

Taking their lead from HMOs' traditionally lower cesarean section rates, providers applied managed care approaches to control cesarean section. The Kaiser system's cesarean section rate in California, for example, had peaked at 20 percent, compared with 26 percent in both the nonprofit and the for-profit sectors.[96] Clinicians in the managed care era even suggested that the cesarean escalation might have reflected managerial deficiency in the first place.

They noted that the rise began just as the American College of Obstetricians and Gynecologists rescinded its consultation requirement for primary cesarean section.[97] Cesarean reduction programs monitored the performance of individual clinicians and informed them how they compared with their colleagues (and their competitors). The reduction programs also tried to change professional attitudes about cesarean section, although some specialists continued to envision cesarean section as the "'ultimate' in delivery technique," representing "all that could be done."[98] In the sense that cesarean section was the ultimate invasive procedure their specialty had, they were right.

As managed care offered providers a means of controlling cesarean section rates, cesarean section management offered payers a means of controlling providers. Corporate purchasers used public and private data sets revealing hospital- and physician-specific cesarean section rates to shop for low-cost providers.[99] Insurance companies used comparative cesarean section rates as performance indicators in selecting and deselecting physicians and hospitals.[100] Aetna U.S. Healthcare's report cards, for example, compared its contracting obstetricians' cesarean section rates with one another, with specialty standards, and with "company expectations."[101] Reversing the incentives of fee-for-service payment, Aetna and other insurers financially rewarded doctors whose report cards revealed low cesarean section rates.

After the crest of the cesarean section wave, academics attributed the lower rates in teaching hospitals—20 percent in 1990, compared with 25 percent in nonteaching hospitals—to better managerial devices.[102] They pointed out that teaching programs had always used consultation requirements, review conferences, and hierarchical staffing to manage their residents and interns. Experienced in writing clinical protocols for interns and residents, academic obstetricians contracted with managed care companies to write their clinical management guidelines.[103] One group worked with the Utah Medical Insurance Association on a physician manual detailing oxytocin acceleration regimens.[104] These and other methods from the industrial quality management sciences spread rapidly to secondary-level hospitals. By the mid-1990s cesarean section was number two on the list of procedures most frequently targeted by clinical algorithms, practice protocols, critical pathways, and other process management techniques (coronary artery bypass grafting was the number one procedure).[105] One-third of all hospitals surveyed at that time used one or more of these management methods to control their cesarean section rates.

Substituting other obstetric procedures for cesarean section was a major tactic in the process management techniques. Champions for the restitution of forceps once again identified forceps as obstetricians' "primary surgical instrument."[106] But forceps did not take hold this time. The national forceps rate declined from nearly 40 percent in the early 1970s to 5.5 percent by 1989 and to 2.3 percent by the end of the century.[107] Some cesarean reduction protocols offered clinical approaches usually considered "alternative," such as heat packs, birthing balls, and choice of birthing position.[108] Most protocols, however, were considerably narrower. Oxytocin augmentation became the most common substitute for cesarean section, contributing to the century's third wave in oxytocin use.

A pioneering cesarean section reduction program in the 1980s at Chicago's Mount Sinai Hospital turned to a number of tactics, including a "liberal" use of oxytocin. Although its instigators did not call it active management, the program led to a 41 percent oxytocin augmentation rate for all births (not just primiparas).[109] Mount Sinai led the way in hospitals' using their cesarean section reduction programs to advertise themselves as "brand-name, quality hospitals."[110] The University of Texas called on a Dublin expert to help design its active management/cesarean section reduction program.[111] With a 26 percent cesarean section rate as late as 1993, the upscale Cedars Sinai Medical Center in Los Angeles sought to reduce it (with limited success) with high-dose oxytocin and physician feedback as part of its CQI program.[112]

Many active management programs developed as research protocols investigating the effect of such management on cesarean section rates. Although results were inconclusive at the end of the 1990s, it looked as if active management slightly reduced cesarean section use in the United States. Yet researchers often found oxytocin acceleration use to be nearly as high for "conventional care" patients within the investigated institutions as the designated active management patients. One academic medical center used oxytocin acceleration on 70 percent of primiparous patients assigned to its active management protocol and 56 percent of its control patients.[113] Comparable figures in another center were 71 and 66 percent, respectively (with a 36 percent oxytocin augmentation rate in its midwifery service).[114] The extent to which the high acceleration rates among the controls were Hawthorne effects of the studies versus standard obstetric practice in those institutions was not clear. Consistent with the contemporary academic practice, the textbook author who criticized in 1990 that continuing intervention was not leading to continuing improvement identified use of oxytocin on all laboring women as acceptable practice.[115] Yet the World Health Organization Safe Motherhood Unit advised a few years later that there was no scientific evidence that "liberal use of oxytocin augmentation ('active management of labour') is of benefit to women and babies."[116]

Inducing labor and managing it actively were congruent with the structure and function of managed care, if not with scientific evidence. The procedures incorporated hierarchic divisions of labor, departmental management, and industrial quality management sciences methods. Each of these elements streamlined clinical process and enhanced departmental productivity.[117] Perinatal chiefs used IQMS methods to analyze and manage departmental practice patterns, resource consumption, and revenue generation.[118] Quality control in the maternity ward in part meant control of labor; the one-workday labor was a major incentive for elective induction. Like their counterparts in Britain, U.S. obstetricians scheduled amniotomy early in the morning with a goal of delivering by evening.[119] Consistent with the usual intervention patterns by hospital type, when induction rates in Arizona were 31 percent in investor-owned hospitals, they were 21 percent for nonprofit hospitals and 14 percent in government hospitals—a discrepancy not explained by clinical risk factors.[120] Another quality management goal was reduction in the number of days of nursing care after birth, which led to widespread condemnation of "drive-through delivery." Such condemnation was ironic in view of the fact that shortening the hospital stay had long been a birth activists' goal in order to reduce medicalization of the childbirth experience.

As managed care plans and cesarean section reduction programs expanded, national oxytocin acceleration rates rose from 11 percent of all births in 1989 to 18 percent in 1998, remaining at that level through 2000.[121] National growth in labor induction paralleled that of augmentation. Total induction rates (using oxytocin, prostaglandin, and/or amniotomy) grew from 9 percent in 1989 to 20 percent in 2000. In sum, nearly 40 percent of all births at the turn of the twenty-first century were induced and/or accelerated. Acceleration and induction rates seemed to be particularly high in tertiary-level academic centers. The induction rate at Northwestern University's hospital in the mid-1990s, for example, was 28 percent. Northwestern's induction rates of 31 percent in its private service and 17 percent in its resident service showed that two perinatal systems still existed and that academic practice plans continued to contribute to socioeconomic discrimination.[122] The induction rate in another academically affiliated tertiary center reached as high as 44 percent.[123]

Only about one-third of the nation's inductions were performed for maternal or fetal indications, which meant that two-thirds were elected by patients and/or physicians.[124] A 1994 textbook condoned elective induction for the purpose of managing delivery unit as well as patient schedules.[125] Bowing to contemporary practice, the American College of Obstetricians and Gynecologists softened its stance against elective induction for logistic reasons.[126] Obstetricians continued to claim that they induced many labors due to patient request, although it remained difficult to determine the extent to which physician-reported "patient request" actually meant patient request. Doctors had a long tradition of making patient care decisions without consulting patients (or the research evidence, for that matter). Nevertheless, patient request for induction or any other specific intervention raises the difficult policy question of how to balance patient participation in decision making with scientific evidence (and lack thereof) of the procedure's risks and benefits. Physician certainty that the *latest* development signifies irrefutable scientific progress adds another layer of complexity to medical decision making.

Oxytocin use was linked to structural, financial, and procedural elements of managed care in Ireland, Britain, and the United States, although these elements do not fully explain its use in any one place at any one time. Induction of labor and its active management enacted managed care by assimilating its managerial and organizational elements. Structurally, induction and active management built on an industrial-style functional division of labor in hospital specialty departments. Financially, inducing and managing labor allowed the departments to budget expenditures and schedule delivery unit staff and equipment. Procedurally, induction and acceleration embodied industrial quality management processes that divided biological processes into a sequence of steps in linear production.[127] Active management used partographs as quality control flowcharts.[128] With primary goals of accelerating throughput and enhancing productivity in the labor and delivery unit, active management and induction were inherently managerial techniques that enhanced the development of birth as a production process.

This perspective of managed birth is consistent with interpretations linking active management with metaphors of industrial and capitalist production—up to a point.[129] I agree with Emily Martin's association of active management with production metaphors. But, as with other paradigm/intervention associations, it was not that the metaphors drove practices. Oxytocin use itself shaped the metaphors; active management prescribed oxytocin to strengthen uterine contraction and correspondingly diagnosed dystocia as a problem of inadequate contraction. This focus on uterine contraction ignored other factors contributing to prolonged labor, such as resistance of the cervix and birth canal. Metaphors of production were just as much the result of structuring labor and delivery units like production units and using technology to enhance productivity as they were its cause. Like the use of forceps, episiotomy, cesarean section, and intensive care before it, active management theory and practice coevolved with the economic organization of obstetrics. This means that re-forming medical practice requires re-forming this organization.

Ten
Conclusion
Re-forming Medicine, Reforming Reform

Nearly everyone at the end of the twentieth century agreed: something was wrong with the U.S. health care system. There the agreement ended. Some thought it delivered the best medicine in the world—it just excluded too many people and/or cost too much. Others thought it didn't even provide good medicine, let alone good health care, to the people it did include. Some perceived the difficulties to be of recent origin; others saw problems of longer duration. Some turned to business models such as managed care as a panacea; others indicted managed care as one of the major problems. Yet most health care reform efforts accepted prevailing forms of organization and their modes of operation, seeking only means of paying for them. Financial reform is necessary, but it is not sufficient. Without structural change, financial reform can bloat or starve medicine—and, in both cases, lead to inappropriate clinical care.

Twentieth-century medical care was not designed to meet people's health needs—defining design not as intent but as the blueprint itself. Business models shaped American medical organization and practice long before managed care. Medical professions, institutions, and multi-institutional systems throughout the century had assimilated elements of business organization. These elements—including functional divisions of labor, revenue-generating services, strategic business units, and regional oligopolies—acted as powerful forces in shaping clinical processes. They augmented the use of surgical and technologic procedures, running the labor and delivery unit like an assembly line, turning childbirth into an intensive care situation, managing labor pharmaceutically, and admitting well babies to intensive care units. Designing a medical system to meet people's health needs requires reforming medical ethics, structure, process, and reform itself.

Reforming Ethics

Many health care reformers throughout the century were clearly motivated by principles of justice and civil rights. Activists in the 1930s as well as the 1960s challenged contemporary inequities with the slogan that health care was a basic right. The theory of rights specifically holds them above the market; it deems rights inalienable, which means they cannot be bought and sold. Pro-market reformers, in contrast, did not believe in a principle higher than the market. Reformers from both philosophies looked to the field of ethics to justify their views.

Professional ethicists situated themselves on both sides of the question of whether business reforms were ethically justified in health care. Some affirmed that justice and the market were compatible, given Adam Smith's caveats and provisos.[1] As Smith himself put it in *Wealth of Nations* (1776), economic theory holds that the sum of all interactions between sellers and buyers in an unrestricted market creates an optimum situation—although it refers to optimizing aggregate wealth, rather than health or equitable distribution. Other scholars contended that the market was an inadequate basis for ethical health care reform precisely because it exacerbates inequities. A health administration professor charged that the claims that the market optimizes health care distribution "strain credulity."[2] After all, cream skimming—selectively treating wealthier patients or those with more remunerative diseases—is not an aberration of the market; it is how the market works. Its defenders justified the inequities of the 1990s with the ideology that "the market has spoken."[3] As increasing numbers of influential, often academic, providers gained in the marketplace, their ethical theory tended to accommodate their reforms.[4]

A problem with measuring medical reform with the yardstick of ethical theory is that business models warped the yardstick itself. Market champions defined *public interest* in terms of rational choice theory as "expressed by the public itself through its free choices in the marketplace."[5] Not only does such a definition limit public participation in decision making to the role of consumer; it also portrays public interest in terms of some people getting high-cost coronary artery bypass grafts, hysterectomies, or cesarean sections with dubious efficacy, while others do not get low-cost immunizations demonstrated to be highly effective. For the provider "market justice" emphasizes "freedom from collective obligations."[6] This form of freedom allows doctors, hospitals, and insurance companies to avoid collective responsibility for the health of the community.[7]

A number of feminist scholars, in contrast, encouraged the provision of services on the basis of need rather than ability to pay as a "larger social good."[8] They held that the discourse of rights when applied to corporate providers in addition to individual consumers conflicted with governmental responsibility to allocate health care resources according to population need.[9] The property rights ethic, for example, has long limited what government could do, prohibiting a social justice choice when it conflicted with economic growth and profit making.[10] In disputing community action to benefit health if it threatens the economic growth of individuals or corporations, property rights and other economic ideologies threaten evidence-based medicine. Valuing freedom of choice in the marketplace "more highly than equality of outcome," market-oriented theories of justice require that individuals receive only those health care services that they can pay for.[11] When business theory drives ethics in this way, social benefit factors such as meeting health needs and caring become "externalities."

The business model that calls health an externality is predicated on a set of values congruent with its economic heritage. The first is maximizing productivity, or seeking the most intensive use of technology, personnel, and facilities. Efficiency is the same input-output formula as productivity, but it emphasizes minimizing resources spent rather than maximizing goods and services produced. Expanding productivity creates economic growth and is an important factor in profit making. Control, or management, is also necessary for maximizing productivity. The objects of such control are personnel, patients, and productive as well as biological processes. Adding to managerial processes, rules of control are built into the structures of specialization, institutional differentiation, and other hierarchical relations, including the doctor-patient relationship. Control also refers to market control, which includes horizontal and/or vertical integration to manage supply and demand. When these business values predominate, they trump justice and turn human relationships into limited contracts.

The dominance of business principles obscured ethics based on values of health rather than wealth. But some ethicists, reformers, and consumers clung to the idea that society should provide health care on the basis of need. Values of need diametrically oppose tenets of market economics. Economists explicitly denied need as an operational concept, proclaiming that in their model "wants and desires replace needs; marketing replaces needs assessment and epidemiology."[12] A needs model would be based on values of social justice, including equity. But the justice approach often ignores medical appropriateness and runs the risk of equalizing unnecessary intervention. The definition of *need* must also consider effectiveness of the proposed interventions. Quality medical care requires consistency with scientific evidence on improving outcomes. Social justice and equity would also include widespread participation in decision making concerning what would be produced and how it would be produced. This participation would require a form of democratic planning.

The final component of a needs model is caring, a strong therapeutic force in itself. Nursing and other feminist scholars developed ethics of care that were alternative to business ethics. Nursing theory of caring valued egalitarian relationships, connecting with patients, and taking responsibility for one's work. It rejected "atomistic" and "mechanistic" views of the person,[13] which reinforced and were reinforced by the specialty divisions of labor. It saw procedure-oriented specialization as fragmenting patient care and conflicting with caring for the whole person.[14] Feminist ethicists similarly valued mutuality, responsibility, solidarity, and attention to end results.[15] They identified paying attention to needs as a required ingredient of caring.[16] Some explicitly proposed an ethic of care to replace the market ethic, emphasizing that the care ethic could ameliorate existing disadvantages to women.[17] Although justice and care are often presented as an either-or choice, a needs-based model of health care must integrate the two values.

The concept of need is deceptively simple, however. The dominance of market thought means that there is no adequate theory of need for allocating health care resources.[18] Doctors and hospitals tend to define need in terms of their existing or desired capacities. Prevailing concepts of distributive justice legitimize contemporary institutions and accept the "institutional organization and agenda of medicine."[19] Economists had advised the national health planning program against trying to use need in estimating health care requirements.[20] Heeding such advice, planning devoted itself primarily to promoting cost-efficient use of existing institutions and their high-tech services. As a health planner, I supported its efforts to increase cost-efficiency, believing that efficiency is better than inefficiency when meeting needs. But cost-efficiency may well be incompatible with need when it becomes the driving force of medical reform. Cost control can hurt most the financially weakest institutions serving disadvantaged populations. A business management professor in the time of planning advised hospitals and their specialty departments that "no investment decision should explicitly consider social good in the absence of attendant cash flows to the institution."[21] In plain words, if it doesn't make money, don't do it—no matter how beneficial. Health plans of the 1990s called the proportion of revenues they actually spent on actual medical care their "medical-loss ratios."[22] With such a perspective it is clear that values of need do not thrive in professions and institutions built along the lines of business.

Re-Forming Medical Care Structure

Twentieth-century developments and reforms built contemporary features of economic order into the fundamental structure of medical care, and future reform efforts seeking to meet health needs must reappraise this structure. As described in previous chapters, medical specialization in the first half of the century and subspecialization in the second half entailed an industrial-type functional division of labor that fragmented medical work into a series of procedures performed by a series of workers. This form of specialization required an institutional base to define and control ancillary occupations and prevent their competing against specialties for the clinical work. Development of the (academic) hospital specialty department provided that institutional base and set in motion methods to manage the fragmented work and the fragmented workers. Midcentury insurance plans and government programs consolidated earlier gains and subsidized further institutional and technologic growth. This growth reciprocally required an economic organization built to expand in capital and technologic intensity. Specialty leaders bundled their technologies and their personnel into dedicated hospital spaces, inventing specialty-specific intensive care units in the process. The highly capitalized ICUs served as strategic business units, initially conferring competitive advantages on academic medical centers. But the subspecialists they trained went forth and multiplied their services in competing community hospitals. Academics countered with the strategy of regionalization, which—like the integrated managed systems that followed—established regional oligopolies and controlled competition.

Medical care built structures of business organization for many reasons. Many leaders perceived their organizational forms as scientific, or at least as necessary organizational means of adjusting to scientific and technologic developments. Different people had different incentives. Specialists saw that the new organization contributed to their professional growth and control of their institutions. Financiers required efficient use of their capital investment, and hospital administrators had to get their ledgers in the black. But medical development cannot be reduced to individual motivation alone. Medical institutions became economic entities and actors in themselves.[23] Institutional sociologists proposed three mechanisms to explain how so many different types of organization from the Progressive Era onward came to adopt similar organizational forms. All three mechanisms are exemplified in this book: the force of law and its regulatory requirements, imposition of professional norms, and competition.[24] In addition, business strategies and structures carry economic dynamics of their own. Hierarchical and financial management, corporate organization, and regional oligopolies built in the rules and mechanisms of action of the dominant economic order. Finally, the values and assumptions of this order were deeply embedded in twentieth-century thought. Providers, policy makers, and the population at large absorbed the ideologies that the pursuit of self-interest is the highest form of ethics, that competition is the motor of society, that productivity and economic growth are society's most important goals, and that the market has spoken—and has blessed medical inequity, if not inflation.

From the Committee on the Costs of Medical Care's concern that medical care was undernourished and had not achieved its portion of the country's economic pie,[25] reformers came to accuse medicine of "devouring" more than its share of the nation's wealth.[26] After medicine's explosive growth between World War II and the 1970s, the last two decades of the century brought challenge to growth, when governments and private insurers reversed their reimbursement policies and tried to put the health care system on an enforced diet. Payers used managed care to reduce growth in medical delivery and providers used it to cope with the reductions. Nevertheless, uncontrolled growth continued. Reducing sustenance to an obese system (which some people not inappropriately called "rationing") was not a bad thing in itself. It was certainly not necessary for every radiology group to have its own MRI machine to meet population needs for the technology. But the underfed starved more than the overfed.

Health planning's question of how to make intensive care units, imaging centers, and tertiary-level hospitals more cost-efficient conceded the expansion game to the industry from the start. The key reform questions—which health planning recognized but could do little about—are how many of these organizational elements are really needed and what other forms of health care delivery (not to mention an adequate standard of living, another story altogether) might better improve people's health. Most birthing women, for example, do not need and do not benefit from the continuing buildup of high-intensity services.

Re-Forming the Perinatal System

The perinatal medicine example has shown how the business model of medicine warped maternity care and its clinical processes. An intriguing feature of perinatal care is that it is a sector of medical care that could undergo short-term structural and/or financial reform somewhat independently of the rest of medicine—and there were in fact attempts to do so. The early 1990s' (failed) proposal for universal maternity care took significant strides in moving beyond existing financing systems, although it built in existing structures and strategies.[27] If we were able to redesign a perinatal system on the basis of need and efficacy (even one limited to existing professional and institutional categories), couldn't we come up with a system with more equitable access and more appropriate clinical intervention for the dollar equivalent of the 1993 ten thousand dollars a birth—or less?

A needs-based system of perinatal care would require equal coverage for all women in the same services—not a separate welfare system for the poor. Such a maternity care system could perhaps be implemented at the state level. A single-payer insurance system would probably be necessary, and it would have to abolish the fee-for-service payment system. Neither of these (huge accomplishments) would be sufficient, however, to achieve equity and appropriateness. The new system would have a budget—that is, it would not be required to support itself by selling its services—and it would have democratically derived priorities of how to allocate its budgeted funds. Building a needs-based system would require quantifying and redistributing personnel, institutions, and equipment to match service intensity levels with the best available scientific evidence on efficacy and the problems of particular people in particular areas. Recognizing that there is always a tension between the two, it would be important to integrate scientific expertise and democratic process.

Were I one of the participants at the drawing board, I would maintain that the effectiveness literature supported a maternity care system that included midwives as well as independent birth centers and furthermore showed that such a system could enhance equity of access, appropriateness of intervention, and caring. I would sketch a plan in which all pregnant women would sign up (with no out-of-pocket expenses) for prenatal care and delivery with a primary care provider. This provider would refer them to a specialist if serious problems arose. This part of my outline is consistent with the Women's Institute for Childbearing Policy's judgment that there was an "urgent need to replace the present system of front-line, high-technology, acute and specialist care with a *Primary Maternity Care System.*"[28] Such a primary care system includes health promotion, continuity of care, and clinical assessment, and the Women's Institute favored midwives to provide most of it.

Carrying this recommendation into a system-wide approach, there would be a need to employ more midwives and family physicians and fewer obstetricians than were active at the end of the twentieth century. Obviously, such a work power realignment would require significant programs to train new personnel yet not lose the expertise of those already trained. The number of primary care facilities would be expanded to take the majority of deliveries (and they would not be colocated in tertiary care facilities). Consequently, there would be fewer obstetric and neonatal intensive care units. The range of facilities would include independent birth centers directed by—and with licensing standards developed by—midwives and birthing women with consultation from the medical profession. Administratively separate, these centers should be physically close to a hospital for ease of patient transfer. If necessary, a transport system would physically take women in premature labor to an intensive care facility. Ideally, the primary care attendant would remain with the woman upon transfer to provide continuing care and advocacy. Birthing centers would be strictly limited in performing cesarean section and other complex and invasive procedures. In this way much excessive intervention would be controlled structurally, rather than by means of process management or financial incentive. It would be necessary to carry out ongoing scientific evaluation of obstetric and neonatal interventions and ensure that the clinical care provided was consistent with the findings. Costs of such expensive evaluation could be reduced by requiring evidence of efficacy before new procedures and technologies could be used—thus limiting their diffusion from the beginning. These ideas are not new; a system like this could have developed in the United States. Most of the ingredients are there—but in massively different proportions.

Such a needs-based maternity care system unapologetically requires planning and regulation, which are anathema to the free market ideology. It could not satisfy the market values that grant every trained specialist the privilege to a high income in the system, every institution the privilege to grow as large or as technology-intensive as it can, or every consumer the privilege to have any treatment she demanded (and could pay for). For these reasons powerful members of each group would oppose or subvert it. Implementing such a system could incur many risks. Politicians and providers might try to restrict the maternity care budget so they could channel more resources to more profitable services serving wealthier (and more masculine) populations. Its planning would risk capture by the industry. Requiring technical expertise, especially in the evaluation of efficacy, it would continue to run the risk of domination by academic leaders. Finally, it would run the risk of substituting a rigid, impersonal, technocratic system for the injustices, rigidities, and high costs of market and medical dominance.

One might well ask why all this effort and risk would be worth it. But not doing it means condoning the continuing widespread inequities as well as overtreatment and undercare of women and babies. Not instituting overt reform leaves medical care in the hands of the dominant parties. As long as medical institutions grow in technologic intensity, the cost of medical care and the cost of health insurance must continue to rise. The more these costs rise, the more people they price out of the system. Yet instituting a single-payer system without controlling system-wide supply and intensity would bankrupt the new system in no time. This kind of control not only entails structural change; it would require changing clinical processes.

Reforming Clinical Process

Health services researchers came to attribute medical practice changes to many factors, including specialty development, the expanding supply of physicians, institution-based practice, technologic advances, malpractice fears, competition, private profit ownership, inflow of new capital, and medical centers' brand name strategies.[29] Many, but not all, of these factors directly related to medicine's business model. They all contributed to inflating the use of surgical and technologic procedures far beyond their demonstrated efficacy. The high-cost procedures augmented financial as well as professional returns from clinical practice and promoted specialties in academia and in the market.

Managed care's contracting and package pricing for a predetermined number of procedures revealed the importance of procedures in specialty medicine.[30] Academic medical centers and other leading providers even patented procedures from obstetrics and other specialties.[31] The seven million MRI examinations, the million cesarean sections, the half-million coronary artery bypass grafts and hysterectomies, and the numerous other procedures performed each year were the main dishes served in the national medical cafeteria in the mid-1990s. They absorbed a large portion of the nation's health care resources. Since these things do not really pay for themselves, they proliferated at the expense of alternative ways of meeting health needs, including public health, primary care, chronic and long-term care, and caring itself. The much-touted consumer choice did not include a less intensive, less expensive, option, even as procedures proliferated without sufficient evidence that they worked.

Evidence-based medicine, which did examine how well procedures worked, was the great shining hope for clinical reform in the 1990s. Its health services research verified the lack of evidentiary support for many procedures and offered a potential for restructuring medical care according to need and therapeutic effectiveness. It certainly beat the American College of Obstetricians and Gynecologists's 1971 use of an audiometer as an applause meter to judge a professional debate on routine hysterectomy for sterilization (the procedure won).[32] But evidence-based medicine was a double-edged sword. While it was a welcome, if belated, attempt to improve effectiveness of medical care, it gathered momentum for reasons of economy. Prompted by managed care companies and incorporating business management methods itself, evidence-based medicine also served financial interests. If corporate payers had reason to believe that the escalating procedures had not been driven or even justified by scientific evidence, they could question their obligation to pay for them. At the time he wrote his article on excessive procedures, Joseph Califano was chairman of the health care committee of the board of directors of the Chrysler

Corporation and a leader in the corporate effort to reduce (the costs of) employee health care benefits.

Health services research became a powerful weapon in the high-stakes competition for professional and financial control of the medical industry. Analysts supported it as a means of destroying physician "stranglehold" on clinical care.[33] Physicians raised the specter that health services research would be "hijacked" by purchasers and managers.[34] Academic departments and their researchers had in fact long accepted funding from pharmaceutical and equipment manufacturing companies to test their products.[35] In effect, the companies invested in specialty departments, and the departments became increasingly dependent on such funding. Industry sponsored more than half of the nation's health research and development in the mid-1990s, although it increasingly shifted such funding to private contract research organizations.[36] The medical information industry, with goals of its own, also played a significant role in shaping evidence-based medicine. Intellectual property was the commodity of the information age, and health care information became a significant business in itself. Financial experts expected its value (or cost) to reach twenty-five billion dollars by the end of the 1990s.[37]

Evidence-based clinical care was intimately linked to managerial methods. To managers evidence-based meant coupling findings from health services research with methods of industrial quality management sciences (IQMS) to reduce costs and improve productivity. "If you can't measure it, you can't manage it," the basic principle of total quality management (TQM), drove much quantitative analysis in health care.[38] The Joint Commission on Accreditation of Healthcare Organizations (JCAHO) came up with a corollary for choosing quality improvement projects: "If you can't measure it, don't do it."[39] Such a maxim obviously undervalues a wide variety of medical care activities, including caring. In the names of quality and the market (doubly ironically), U.S. medicine was on its way to becoming the "most clinically regulated system in the world."[40]

The vast complexity of the accumulating data, however, belied any claim that the evidence could easily be reduced to sets of best practices. There were scientific difficulties in defining and measuring efficacy, and there were political and economic barriers to using the information. As the accumulating information was increasingly used for competitive purposes, its public availability declined. The Cleveland Health Quality Choice program, a joint academic/industrial venture, divulged outcomes in perinatal and other specialty areas to subscribers only.[41] California's publicly funded Maternal and Child Health Data Base, using vital statistics in the public domain, also became a project of privately shared analyses not available to the public.[42] The health care industry sometimes even resorted to the courts to prevent dissemination of its technology assessment reports.[43] Such a privatization of information contradicted market theory requiring informed consumers.

Competitive use of scientific evidence once again raised questions of evidence for what? and for whom? Use of clinical audits, clinical protocols, and other quality management methods shifted control in medical care and medical policy.[44] Pharmaceutical and biotechnology companies developed "disease management" protocols to maximize use of their products, while managed care providers wrote competing protocols to minimize their own costs.[45] Recognizing that social and economic factors shaped obstetric practice, many of its critics seemed not to see that the same factors molded its research. Obstetrics and gynecology used its clinical research to establish its professional niche and to compete with other specialists, family practitioners, and midwives—and its competitors did the same. Health services research (like all scholarly endeavor) is contingent on professional, social, economic, and historical conditions. It is inescapably conducted by people with personal and disciplinary standpoints from which they (we) formulate research questions, design methodologies, and interpret results. The best we can do is pay attention to these limitations as we carry out and apply the research. I believe that society can choose to start the difficult process of re-forming medical care according to the best available estimates of efficacy and need (while continuing to improve those estimates). Such an endeavor entails not only developing new models of medical organization but also re-forming reform.

Re-forming Reform

This book has concentrated on what should be reformed in medicine, but how it should be reformed is another question altogether. Most progressive medical reformers did not renounce the economic order; they sought to regulate it for purposes of equity and efficiency.[46] Competition, reminded Committee on the Costs of Medical Care leaders Michael Davis and Rufus Rorem, is a "fundamental American tradition." But, they held, "competition must be fair, and it is part of the public's business through the government or otherwise to see that it is fair."[47] Perhaps the most significant change at the end of the century was the repudiation of this liberal social contract that accepted market reforms on the grounds that government could ensure a modicum of fairness. Yet this was inconsistent; few market reformers at that time wanted true laissez-faire. Few would have taken away the enormous role government played in subsidizing medicine by means of product patenting, monopolistic licensing, tax benefits, and paying for people who were over sixty-five or indigent. Widely touted as market reform, managed care was by definition highly regulatory—although most of its regulation was private, rather than governmental. So-called market reform was a selective deregulatory strategy to reduce public services and to privatize policy.

As health planning mistook its consumer-majority committees for democracy, market-oriented reform mistook the reduction of government regulation for democracy, a common fallacy. In the 1930s economist Wesley Mitchell had conceived democracy as the "political complement of economic liberty."[48] The equation of democracy with the market accepts rule by dominant interests as a stand-in for democracy. Neither planning nor the market was democratic in the sense of distributing decision-making power. Both strengthened the hands of corporate providers, purchasers, and insurers; both empowered the larger, wealthier providers and payers to dominate medical policy. As a means of countervailing such power inequities, some ethicists proposed that the "whole community" define health care needs.[49] They were hazy on just how to accomplish this, however. For the community to decide the amount of society's resources to be spent on health care (or even just perinatal care) and how they should be apportioned among providers of different types and levels would require new decision-making processes. These processes would take epidemiological, social, and cultural factors as well as measures of efficacy into consideration in reframing health care delivery.

Feminist scholars engaged in developing theories and practices to enhance democratic participation in decision making. Maintaining that an equal right to vote (difficult enough to achieve) limits political participation to choosing decision makers and does not mean equal decision-making power, feminist political theorists worked on creating means of democratic participation beyond voting and representation.[50] They held out for people's right to participate directly in decision making concerning their work and the other activities they engaged in.[51] Such activities include health care. The women's health movement has long maintained, for example, that women's clinics should be controlled by the women participating in them as providers, as community members, and as patients.[52]

But the hegemony and momentum of a given economic order make it difficult to develop alternatives. The dominance of the business model sentenced reformers to look for better and better forms of business organization and management. Reformers at the end of the century continued to accuse health care of lagging behind business in its economic organization. This diagnosis assumes an inevitable economic evolution, that development per se requires adoption of capitalist-industrial characteristics across social institutions and across countries.[53] One organizational theorist criticized his field for accepting the "state of human affairs in the market-centered society as a given, being unaware of a larger range of objective possibilities."[54] Globalization strove to make the larger range of alternatives impossible.

Corporate, political, and even public health leaders sought to globalize the business model of medicine. Explicitly applying "business processes" and "management culture" to the health sector, agencies such as the World Bank dominated worldwide health care reform at the end of the century.[55] The World Bank's self-defined purpose was to streamline countries' health care systems and reduce their governments' spending on them in order to stabilize their economies for foreign capital investment. Joining the general celebration of capitalism at the end of the century, the business model became a universally accepted blueprint for health care re-organization. It was still incomplete, however, both nationally and internationally. Financiers sought further capital penetration in health care delivery.

I am not offering a new overarching theory or an a priori model of reform. I am just holding out the hope that we can scientifically and democratically match health care delivery to known needs. The chapters of this book have analyzed different aspects of what went wrong with twentieth-century medicine in order to illuminate possibilities for twenty-first-century reform. They have also raised more questions than answers. Pivotal questions remain: How should we define and measure need? efficacy? quality? equity? appropriateness? What blueprints match structure to need? How can they be built? How can they be achieved politically? democratically? Can alternative systems survive within a dominant economic order? To demonstrate the necessity for new ethical concepts, structural forms, clinical processes, and reform methods in answering these questions, I have tried to show how deeply medical care developments and reforms internalized economic ideologies and how they contributed to inappropriate clinical care. Professionalism as well as progressivism portrayed themselves as alternatives to the business model, but they also built in business concepts and structures. Business models so dominated twentieth-century thought that it was difficult to see beyond the existing economic order to conceive of alternative models.

Reform to meet human health needs would be more threatening to existing professions and institutions than most reformers have dared imagine. It would challenge much of what was defined as progress in the twentieth century. Even in the short run the goal of meeting health needs would require developing new modes of finance and organization. In the long run it would require redefining medical occupations and institutions and transforming the fundamental structures, processes, and paradigms of medicine.

Notes

Preface and Acknowledgments

1. Certificate of Need is a regulatory program in which hospitals apply to state government for approval to make large capital expenditures by demonstrating "need" for and cost efficiency of the proposed project.

2. Stanley Joel Reiser and Michael Anbar, eds., *The Machine at the Bedside: Strategies for Using Technology in Patient Care* (Cambridge: Cambridge University Press, 1984), 59.

3. Dolores L. Burke, *Physicians in the Academic Marketplace* (New York: Greenwood Press, 1992), 28–29; Jonathan H. Sunshine, Gerald R. Busheé, and Rajiv Mallick, "U.S. Radiologists' Workload in 1995–1996 and Trends since 1991–1992," *Radiology* 208, no. 1 (1998): 19–24.

4. H. David Banta, *An Approach to the Social Control of Hospital Technologies* (Geneva: World Health Organization, 1995), 12.

5. Quoted in Caroline Whitbeck, "Fetal Imaging and Fetal Monitoring: Finding the Ethical Issues," in Elaine Hoffman Baruch, Amadeo F. D'Amano, and Joni Seager, eds., *Embryos, Ethics, and Women's Rights: Exploring the New Reproductive Technologies* (New York: Harrington Press, 1988), 47–57.

6. U.S. Congress, Office of Technology Assessment, *Nuclear Magnetic Resonance Imaging Technology: A Clinical, Industrial, and Policy Analysis* (Washington, D.C.: U.S. Government Printing Office, 1984), 91.

7. Robert A. Bell, "Economics of MRI Technology," *Journal of Magnetic Resonance Imaging* 6, no. 1 (1996): 10–25.

8. Lawton S. Cooper et al., "The Poor Quality of Early Evaluations of Magnetic Resonance Imaging," *JAMA* 259, no. 22 (1988): 3277–3280.

9. Clark C. Havighurst, "The Changing Locus of Decision Making in the Health Care Sector," in Lawrence D. Brown, ed., *Health Policy in Transition: A Decade of Health Politics, Policy and Law* (Durham: Duke University Press, 1987), 129–167; H. E. Frech, *Competition and Monopoly in Medical Care* (Washington, D.C.: AEI Press, 1996), 151.

One   Introduction

1. "Editorial: The Medical Industrial Complex," *Health PAC Bulletin* (November 1969): 1–2; Arnold S. Relman, "The New Medical-Industrial Complex," *New England Journal of Medicine* 303, no. 17 (1980): 963–970.

2. James A. Morone, "Gridlock and Breakthrough in American Health Politics," in Theodor J. Litman and Leonard S. Robins, eds., *Health Politics and Policy* (Albany: Delmar, 1997), 64–74.

3. Donald W. Light, "The Restructuring of the American Health Care System," in Litman and Robins, *Health Politics and Policy,* 46–63.

4. John M. Eisenberg and Andrea Kabcenell, "Organized Practice and the Quality of Medical Care," *Inquiry* 25, no. 1 (1988): 78–89.

5. Roger M. Battistella, "Hospital Receptivity to Market Competition: Image and Reality," *Health Care Management Review* 10, no. 3 (1985): 19–26.

6. Stephen M. Shortell et al., *Remaking Health Care in America: The Evolution of Organized Delivery Systems* (San Francisco: Jossey-Bass, 2000), 71.

7. John H. McArthur and Francis D. Moore, "The Two Cultures and the Health Care Revolution: Commerce and Professionalism in Medical Care," *JAMA* 277, no. 12 (1997): 985–989.

8. I. S. Falk, C. Rufus Rorem, and Martha D. Ring, *The Costs of Medical Care,* CCMC Report no. 27 (Chicago: University of Chicago Press, 1933), 384.

9. Louis Galambos, "The Emerging Organizational Synthesis in Modern American History," *Business History Review* 44 (1970): 279–290.

10. Robert F. Berkhofer, "The Organizational Interpretation of American History: A New Synthesis," *Prospects* 4 (1979): 611–629.

11. Donald L. Madison, "Preserving Individualism in the Organizational Society: 'Cooperation' and American Medical Practice, 1900–1920," *Bulletin of the History of Medicine* 70, no. 3 (1996): 442–483.

12. Thomas Goebel, "American Medicine and the 'Organizational Synthesis': Chicago Physicians and the Business of Medicine, 1900–1920," *Bulletin of the History of Medicine* 68, no. 4 (1994): 639–663.

13. Charles Rosenberg, "George Rosen and the Social History of Medicine," in Charles Rosenberg, ed., *Healing and History: Essays for George Rosen* (New York: Science History Publications, 1979), qtd. in Nancy Tomes, "Review Essay: The Social Transformation of American Medicine: An Historical Perspective," *Sociology of Health and Illness* 7, no. 2 (1985): 248–259.

14. Joseph A. Califano, "The Health-Care Chaos," *New York Times Magazine,* March 20, 1988, 44, 46, 56–58.

15. Avedis Donabedian, *The Definition of Quality and Approaches to Its Assessment,* vol. 1: *Explorations in Quality Assessment and Monitoring* (Ann Arbor: Health Administration Press, 1980), 80–81. In addition, I use the terms *medical* as inclusive of surgery, *therapeutics* as inclusive of diagnostic procedures, *therapeutic* referring to all clinical activities, not just those known to benefit the patient, and *model* to refer to organizational structures as well as to clinical paradigms.

16. Paul Starr, *The Social Transformation of American Medicine* (New York: Basic Books, 1982), 198.

17. Samuel P. Hays, *The Response to Industrialism: 1885–1914* (Chicago: University of

Chicago, 1957), 10–11; Thomas C. Cochran and William Miller, *The Age of Enterprise: A Social History of Industrial America* (New York: Harper and Row, 1961).

18. Frederick Winslow Taylor, *The Principles of Scientific Management* (New York: Harper and Brothers, 1911).

19. Alfred D. Chandler, *The Visible Hand: The Managerial Revolution in American Business* (Cambridge: Harvard University Press, 1977), 1–12, 281.

20. Robert H. Wiebe, *The Search for Order, 1877–1920* (New York: Hill and Wang, 1967), 295.

21. Samuel Haber, *Efficiency and Uplift: Scientific Management in the Progressive Era, 1890–1920* (Chicago: University of Chicago Press, 1964), ix–x.

22. Glenn Porter, *The Rise of Big Business, 1860–1910* (New York: Thomas Y. Crowell, 1973), 1–25.

23. Chandler, *Visible Hand,* 285–288.

24. Alfred D. Chandler, *Strategy and Structure: Chapters in the History of the Industrial Enterprise* (Cambridge: MIT Press, 1962), 14, 31; Leslie Hannah, *The Rise of the Corporate Economy* (London: Methuen, 1983), 1–7.

25. John C. Burnham, "How the Idea of Profession Changed the Writing of Medical History," *Medical History,* supp. no. 18 (1998).

26. Eliot Freidson, "The Reorganization of the Medical Profession," *Medical Care Review* 42, no. 1 (1985): 11–35.

27. Eliot Freidson, *Professional Dominance: The Social Structure of Medical Care* (New York: Atherton Press, 1970), 167.

28. Madison, "Preserving Individualism," 442–483.

29. William F. Ogburn and Meyer F. Nimkoff, *Sociology* (Boston: Houghton Mifflin, 1940), 345.

30. Porter, *Rise of Big Business,* 4, 61–62.

31. Corinne Gilb, *Hidden Hierarchies: The Professions and Government* (Westport, Conn.: Greenwood Press, 1966), 82–87.

32. Eliot Freidson, *Profession of Medicine: A Study of the Sociology of Applied Knowledge* (New York: Harper and Row, 1970), 116.

33. Theodore Levitt, *The Marketing Imagination* (New York: Free Press, 1986), 50, 61.

34. George Rosen, "The Hospital: Historical Sociology of a Community Institution," in George Rosen, *From Medical Police to Social Medicine: Essays on the History of Health Care* (New York: Science History Publications, 1974), 274–303.

35. Morris J. Vogel, *The Invention of the Modern Hospital: Boston, 1870–1930* (Chicago: University of Chicago Press, 1980); David Rosner, *A Once Charitable Enterprise: Hospitals and Health Care in Brooklyn and New York, 1885–1915* (Cambridge: Cambridge University Press, 1982).

36. Charles E. Rosenberg, *The Care of Strangers: The Rise of America's Hospital System* (New York: Basic Books, 1987), 347.

37. David Rosner, "Heterogeneity and Uniformity: Historical Perspectives on the Voluntary Hospital," in J. David Seay and Bruce C. Vladeck, eds., *In Sickness and in Health: The Mission of Voluntary Health Care Institutions* (New York: McGraw-Hill, 1988), 87–125.

38. Rosemary Stevens, *In Sickness and in Wealth: American Hospitals in the Twentieth Century* (New York: Basic Books, 1989), 239.

39. Rosemary Stevens, "Looking Back to Go Forward: History as Health Services Research," *Journal of Health Administration Education* 9, no. 1 (1991): 1–8.

40. Charles Perrow, *Complex Organizations: A Critical Essay* (New York: Random House, 1986), 52.

41. James D. Mooney, *The Principles of Organization* (New York: Harper, 1947), 185. To attest to their universality, characteristics of organization have been compared to characteristics of organic evolution. But economist John Maynard Keynes and others have argued that organic evolution has itself been viewed through the lens of economic production.

42. James D. Mooney and Alan C. Reiley, *Onward Industry! The Principles of Organization and Their Significance to Modern Industry* (New York: Harper, 1931); Chester I. Barnard, *The Functions of the Executive* (Cambridge: Harvard University Press, 1938); Alfred P. Sloan, *My Years with General Motors* (Garden City, N.Y.: Doubleday, 1963).

43. J. Warren Salmon, ed., *The Corporate Transformation of Health Care: Perspectives and Implications* (Amityville, N.Y.: Baywood Publishing, 1994); E. Richard Brown, *Rockefeller Medicine Men: Medicine and Capitalism in America* (Berkeley: University of California Press, 1979); Howard Berliner, "Medical Modes of Production," in Peter Wright and Andrew Treacher, eds., *The Problem of Medical Knowledge: Examining the Social Construction of Medicine* (Edinburgh: Edinburgh University Press, 1982), 162–173.

44. Starr, *Social Transformation of American Medicine,* 429.

45. Jeff Charles Goldsmith, *Can Hospitals Survive? The New Competitive Health Care Market* (Homewood, Ill.: Dow Jones–Irwin, 1981), 97–106.

46. Robert Heilbroner and William Milberg, *The Crisis of Vision in Modern Economic Thought* (Cambridge: Cambridge University Press, 1995), 106–108; Thomas K. McCraw, intro., in Thomas K. McCraw, ed., *Creating Modern Capitalism: How Entrepreneurs, Companies, and Countries Triumphed in Three Industrial Revolutions* (Cambridge: Harvard University Press, 1997), 1–16.

47. Light, "Restructuring of the American Health Care System," 46–63.

48. Thomas C. Cochran, *The American Business System: A Historical Perspective, 1900–1955* (New York: Harper and Row, 1957), vi.

49. J. D. Kleinke, *Bleeding Edge: The Business of Health Care in the New Century* (Gaithersburg, Md.: Aspen, 1998), 26.

50. Vicente Navarro, *Medicine under Capitalism* (New York: Prodist, 1976), 215–217.

51. W. W. Rostow, *The Stages of Economic Growth: A Non-Communist Manifesto* (Cambridge: Cambridge University Press, 1960).

52. Kleinke, *Bleeding Edge,* 115.

53. Robert A. Bell, "Economics of MRI Technology," *Journal of Magnetic Resonance Imaging* 6, no. 1 (1996): 10–25; U.S. Department of Health and Human Services, "Ambulatory and Inpatient Procedures in the United States, 1995," *Vital and Health Statistics* 13, no. 135 (1998): table 5.

54. Kerr L. White, "Information for Health Care: An Epidemiological Perspective," *Inquiry* 17, no. 4 (1980): 296–312.

55. E. A. Codman, "The Product of a Hospital," *Surgery, Gynecology, and Obstetrics* 18, no. 4 (1914): 491–496.

56. Califano, "Health-Care Chaos," 44, 46, 56–58.

57. Roger M. Battistella and John B. Ostrick, "The Political Economy of Health Services: A Review and Assessment of Major Ideological Influences and the Impact of New Economic Realities," in Theodor J. Litman and Leonard S. Robins, eds., *Health Politics and Policy* (Albany: Delmar, 1997), 75–108.

58. Sheryl Burt Ruzek, "Access, Cost, and Quality of Medical Care: Where Are We Heading?" in Sheryl Burt Ruzek, Virginia L. Olesen, and Adele E. Clarke, *Women's Health: Complexities and Differences* (Columbus: Ohio State University Press, 1997), 183–230.

59. Doris Haire, *The Cultural Warping of Childbirth* (Milwaukee: International Childbirth Education Association, 1972). I use the medical literature to make judgments about levels of intervention at the population level; this book should not be interpreted as advice for the individual giving birth.

60. Nancy Stoller Shaw, *Forced Labor: Maternity Care in the United States* (Elmsford, N.Y.: Pergamon Press, 1974); Suzanne Arms, *Immaculate Deception: A New Look at Women and Childbirth in America* (Boston: Houghton Mifflin, 1975); Shelly Romalis, ed., *Childbirth: Alternatives to Medical Control* (Austin: University of Texas Press, 1982).

61. U.S. General Accounting Office, *Better Management and More Resources Needed to Strengthen Federal Efforts to Improve Pregnancy Outcome* (Washington, D.C.: General Accounting Office, 1980).

62. U.S. Senate, Subcommittee on Health and Scientific Research, *Obstetrical Practices in the United States, 1978* (Washington, D.C.: U.S. Government Printing Office, 1978), 2, 81.

63. Henci Goer, *Obstetric Myths versus Research Realities* (Westport, Conn.: Bergin and Garvey, 1995).

64. Iain Chalmers, Murray Enkin, and Marc J. N. C. Keirse, eds., *Effective Care in Pregnancy and Childbirth* (Oxford: Oxford University Press, 1989); *Pregnancy and Childbirth Module of the Cochrane Database of Systematic Reviews* (Oxford: Cochrane Collaboration, Update Software, periodically updated).

65. Lewin and Associates, *Competition among Health Practitioners: The Influence of the Medical Profession on the Health Manpower Market,* vol. 2: *The Childbearing Center Case Study* (Washington, D.C.: Lewin and Associates, 1981), 13. Wording is that of report writer.

66. Sally Macintyre, "The Management of Childbirth: A Review of Sociological Research Issues," *Social Science and Medicine* 11, nos. 8–9 (1977): 477–484.

67. Naomi Wolf, *Misconceptions: Truth, Lies, and the Unexpected on the Journey to Motherhood* (New York: Doubleday, 2001) and Boston Women's Health Collective, *Our Bodies, Ourselves* (New York: Simon and Schuster, 1973).

68. Helen M. Sterk et al., *Who's Having This Baby? Perspectives on Birthing* (East Lansing: Michigan State University Press, 2002), 142, 167.

69. M. Robin DiMatteo, Katherine L. Kahn, and Sandra H. Berry, "Narratives of Birth and the Postpartum: Analysis of the Focus Group Responses of New Mothers," *Birth* 20, no. 4 (1993): 204–210.

70. Barbara Katz Rothman, *Recreating Motherhood: Ideology and Technology in a Patriarchal Society* (New York: W. W. Norton, 1989), 155.

71. Robbie E. Davis-Floyd, *Birth as an American Rite of Passage* (Berkeley: University of California Press, 1992), 282.

72. U.S. Department of Health and Human Services, "Trends in Hospital Utilization: United States, 1988–92," *Vital and Health Statistics* 13, no. 124 (1996): tables 18, 28; U.S. Department of Health and Human Services, "National Hospital Discharge Survey: Annual Summary, 1994," *Vital and Health Statistics* 13, no. 128 (1997).

73. Joyce A. Martin et al., "Births: Final Data for 2000," *National Vital Statistics Reports* 50, no. 5 (2002): 14–15, 59; U.S. Department of Health and Human Services, "1999 National Hospital Discharge Survey: Annual Summary with Detailed Diagnosis and Procedure Data," *Vital and Health Statistics* 13, no. 151 (2001): 35. The episiotomy figure is less exact and from 1999.

74. Marsden Wagner, "The Public Health versus Clinical Approaches to Maternity Services: The Emperor Has No Clothes," *Journal of Public Health Policy* 19, no. 1 (1998): 25–35.

75. "Trends in Infant Mortality by Cause of Death and Other Characteristics, 1960–88," *Vital and Health Statistics* 20, no. 20 (1993): 3; "Perinatal Mortality in the United States: 1985–91," *Vital and Health Statistics* 20, no. 26 (1995): 15; U.S. Department of Health and Human Services, *Health, United States, 2000* (Hyattsville, Md.: National Center for Health Statistics, 2000), 157.

76. Roger A. Rosenblatt, "The Perinatal Paradox: Doing More and Accomplishing Less," *Health Affairs* 8, no. 3 (1989): 158–168.

77. U.S. Department of Health and Human Services, *The 50 Most Frequent Diagnosis-Related Groups (DRGs), Diagnoses, and Procedures: Statistics by Hospital Size and Location,* Hospital Studies Program Research Note 13 (Rockville, Md.: Agency for Health Care Policy and Research, 1990), table 3.

78. Stephen H. Long, M. Susan Marquis, and Ellen R. Harrison, "The Costs and Financing of Perinatal Care in the United States," *American Journal of Public Health* 84, no. 9 (1994): 1473–1478; U.S. Department of Health and Human Services, *Expenditures for Pregnancy and Infant Medical Care, 1987* (Rockville, Md.: Agency for Health Care Policy and Research, 1994). The government study calculated a total of $27.8 billion, $7,254 per mother-infant pair, in 1987 (which included continuing infant medical care in the first year of life). The RAND (Long) study found costs of $6,850 per mother-infant pair in 1989.

79. Health Insurance Association of America, *Source Book of Health Insurance Data, 1996* (n.p.: Health Insurance Association of America, 1997), 86. The $30 billion and $40 billion figures were calculated by different methods and are not strictly comparable.

80. Sheryl Burt Ruzek, "Ethical Issues in Childbirth Technology," in Helen B. Holmes, Betty B. Hoskins, and Michael Gross, eds., *Birth Control and Controlling Birth* (Clifton, N.J.: Humana Press, 1981), 197–202.

Two   Specialty Departments

1. Daniel Nelson, "Scientific Management in Retrospect," in Daniel Nelson, ed., *A Mental Revolution: Scientific Management since Taylor* (Columbus: Ohio State University Press, 1992), 5–39.

2. William G. Rothstein, *American Medical Schools and the Practice of Medicine: A History* (New York: Oxford University Press, 1987), 187.

3. George Rosen, *The Specialization of Medicine with Particular Reference to Ophthalmology* (New York: Froben Press, 1944), 31.

4. Rosemary Stevens, *American Medicine and the Public Interest* (1971; rpt., Berkeley: University of California Press, 1998), xv–xvi.

5. Joel D. Howell, "The Invention and Development of American Internal Medicine," *Journal of General Internal Medicine* 4 (1989): 127–133.

6. Magali Sarfatti Larson, *The Rise of Professionalism: A Sociological Analysis* (Berkeley: University of California Press, 1977); Andrew Abbott, *The System of Professions: An Essay on the Division of Expert Labor* (Chicago: University of Chicago Press, 1988).

7. Jeffrey Lionel Berlant, *Profession and Monopoly: A Study of Medicine in the United States and Great Britain* (Berkeley: University of California Press, 1975); Larson, *Rise of Professionalism.*

8. George Weisz, "Medical Directories and Medical Specialization in France, Britain, and the United States," *Bulletin of the History of Medicine* 71, no. 1 (1997): 23–68.

9. Sydney A. Halpern, *American Pediatrics: The Social Dynamics of Professionalism, 1880–1980* (Berkeley: University of California Press, 1988), 157.

10. Glenn Gritzer and Arnold Arluke, *The Making of Rehabilitation: A Political Economy of Medical Specialization, 1890–1980* (Berkeley: University of California Press, 1985), 7.

11. Samuel Haber, *Efficiency and Uplift: Scientific Management in the Progressive Era, 1890–1920* (Chicago: University of Chicago Press, 1964), 19; Judith A. Merkle, *Management and Ideology: The Legacy of the International Scientific Management Movement* (Berkeley: University of California Press, 1980), 81.

12. Adam Smith, *Selections from the Wealth of Nations* (1776; rpt., Arlington Heights, Ill.: AHM Publishing, 1957); Harry Braverman, *Labor and Monopoly Capital: The Degradation of Work in the Twentieth Century* (New York: Monthly Review Press, 1974).

13. Charles Gordon Heyd, "Relation of American Medical Association to Certification of Specialists," *Journal of the American Medical Association* 108, no. 13 (1937): 1017–1019.

14. George Rosen, "Changing Attitudes of the Medical Profession to Specialization," *Bulletin of the History of Medicine* 12 (1942): 343–354.

15. Eliot Freidson, "Review Essay: Health Factories, the New Industrial Sociology," *Social Problems* 14 (1967): 493–500.

16. Paul Starr, *The Social Transformation of American Medicine* (New York: Basic Books, 1982), 220–221.

17. Toby Gelfand, "The Origins of a Modern Concept of Medical Specialization: John Morgan's *Discourse* of 1765," *Bulletin of the History of Medicine* 50, no. 4 (1976): 511–535.

18. Worthington Hooker and James Kennedy, *Report of the Committee of Medical Ethics on Specialties* (Philadelphia: Collins, 1866), reprinted in Charles E. Rosenberg, ed., *The Origins of Specialization in American Medicine: An Anthology of Sources* (New York: Garland, 1989), 19–30.

19. Ashbel Woodward, "Specialism in Medicine" (1866), in Rosenberg, *Origins of Specialization in American Medicine,* 31–37.

20. William H. Welch, "The Interdependence of Medicine and Other Sciences of Nature" (1907), in J. McKeen Cattell, ed., *Science and Education,* vol. 2: *Medical Research and Education* (New York: Science Press, 1913), 143–164.

21. John L. Hildreth, "The General Practitioner and the Specialist," *Boston Medical and Surgical Journal* 155 (1906): 79–83.
22. Frederic A. Washburn, *The Massachusetts General Hospital: Its Development, 1900–1935* (Boston: Houghton Mifflin, 1939), 259.
23. Michael M. Davis, "Group Medicine," *American Journal of Public Health* 9 (1919): 358–362.
24. E. A. Codman, "The Product of a Hospital," *Surgery, Gynecology and Obstetrics* 18, no. 4 (1914): 491–496; "Davis, Michael Marks," in Martin Kaufman, Stuart Galishoff, and Todd L. Savitt, eds., *Dictionary of American Medical Biography* (Westport, Conn.: Greenwood Press, 1984), 186–187.
25. Michael M. Davis and Andrew R. Warner, *Dispensaries: Their Management and Development* (New York: Macmillan, 1918), 80.
26. Hugh Cabot, "Is Urology Entitled to Be Regarded as a Specialty?" *Transactions of the American Urological Association* 5 (1911): 1–20.
27. Hugh Cabot, *The Doctor's Bill* (New York: Columbia University Press, 1935), 64, 69.
28. Richard C. Cabot, *Training and Rewards of the Physician* (Philadelphia: J. B. Lippincott, 1918), 123.
29. Richard C. Cabot, "More Light on This Subject: Better Doctoring for Less Money," *American Magazine* 81 (1916): 43–44, 76–78, 81; Cabot, *Doctor's Bill,* 129.
30. Richard C. Cabot, "What Dispensary Work Should Stand For," *Modern Hospital* 7 (1916): 467–469.
31. Lewellys F. Barker, "On the Present Status of Therapy and Its Future," *Bulletin of the Johns Hopkins Hospital* 11 (1900): 149–156.
32. Lewellys F. Barker, "The Organization of the Laboratories in the Medical Clinic of the Johns Hopkins Hospital," *Bulletin of the Johns Hopkins Hospital* 18 (1907): 193–198.
33. Rosemary Stevens, "The Changing Idea of a Medical Specialty," *Transactions and Studies of the College of Physicians of Philadelphia* 2, no. 3 (1980): 159–177; Nicholas Jardine, "The Laboratory Revolution in Medicine as Rhetorical and Aesthetic Accomplishment," in Andrew Cunningham and Perry Williams, eds., *The Laboratory Revolution in Medicine* (Cambridge: Cambridge University Press, 1992), 304–323.
34. Barker, "On the Present Status of Therapy and Its Future," 149–156; Lewellys F. Barker, "Some Tendencies in Medical Education in the United States" (1911), in J. McKeen Cattell, ed., *Science and Education,* vol. 2: *Medical Research and Education* (New York: Science Press, 1913), 241–278.
35. Barker, "Some Tendencies in Medical Education in the United States," 241–278.
36. Lewellys F. Barker, "The Specialist and the General Practitioner: In Relation to Team-work in Medical Practice," *Journal of the American Medical Association* 78 (1922): 773–779.
37. Barker, "Specialist and the General Practitioner," 773–779.
38. Frederick Winslow Taylor, *The Principles of Scientific Management* (New York: Harper and Brothers, 1911), 125.
39. Quoted in Peter F. Drucker, *Innovation and Entrepreneurship: Practice and Principles* (New York: Harper and Row, 1985), 212.
40. Allen B. Kanavel, "The Standardized Hospital as a Medical Education Center," *Bulletin of the American College of Surgeons* 16, no. 4A (1932): 9–12.

41. Franklin H. Martin, *Fifty Years of Medicine and Surgery* (Chicago: Surgical Publishing Co. of Chicago, 1934).

42. Eugene H. Pool and Frederick W. Bancroft, "Systematization of a Surgical Service," *Journal of the American Medical Association* 69, no. 19 (1917): 1599–1603.

43. George Gray Ward, "Hospital Standardization and Its Application to the Organization of a Special Hospital," *American Journal of Obstetrics and Diseases of Women and Children* 78, no. 1 (1918): 65–78.

44. Duncan Neuhauser, *Coming of Age: A 50-Year History of the American College of Hospital Administrators and the Profession It Serves, 1933–1983* (Chicago: Pluribus Press, 1983), 173.

45. Maurice Leven, *The Incomes of Physicians: An Economic and Statistical Analysis* (Chicago: University of Chicago Press, 1932), 50, 59.

46 I. S. Falk, C. Rufus Rorem, and Martha D. Ring, *The Costs of Medical Care: A Summary of Investigations on the Economic Aspects of the Prevention and Care of Illness,* CCMC no. 27 (Chicago: University of Chicago Press, 1933), 212, 580, 386.

47. Falk, Rorem, and Ring, *Costs of Medical Care,* 386, 212.

48. Susan M. Reverby, *Ordered to Care: The Dilemma of American Nursing, 1850–1945* (Cambridge: Cambridge University Press, 1987); Joel D. Howell, *Technology in the Hospital: Transforming Patient Care in the Early Twentieth Century* (Baltimore: Johns Hopkins University Press, 1995).

49. Morris L. Cooke, "The Spirit and Social Significance of Scientific Management," *Journal of Political Economy* 21, no. 6 (1913): 481–493. Cooke claimed that scientific management could operationalize democracy as well as Christianity.

50. Morris Llewellyn Cooke, foreword, in Edward Eyre Hunt, ed., *Scientific Management since Taylor* (New York: McGraw-Hill, 1924), vii–ix.

51. Howard Berliner, "Medical Modes of Production," in Peter Wright and Andrew Treacher, eds., *The Problem of Medical Knowledge: Examining the Social Construction of Medicine* (Edinburgh: Edinburgh University Press, 1982), 162–173.

52. Lewellys F. Barker, "The Unveiling of the Cell," *Journal of the American Medical Association* 38 (1902): 577–582.

53. Carolyn Merchant, *The Death of Nature: Women, Ecology, and the Scientific Revolution* (San Francisco: HarperSanFrancisco, 1980), 177–186.

54. Merkle, *Management and Ideology.*

55. Camilla Stivers, *Bureau Men, Settlement Women: Constructing Public Administration in the Progressive Era* (Lawrence: University Press of Kansas, 2000), 70.

56. George Rosen, "The Efficiency Criterion in Medical Care, 1900–1920," *Bulletin of the History of Medicine* 50, no. 1 (1976): 28–44; Stephen J. Kunitz, "Efficiency and Reform in the Financing and Organization of American Medicine in the Progressive Era," *Bulletin of the History of Medicine* 55, no. 4 (1981): 497–515.

57. Edward T. Morman, intro., in Edward T. Morman, ed., *Efficiency, Scientific Management, and Hospital Standardization: An Anthology of Sources* (New York: Garland, 1989).

58. Rothstein, *American Medical Schools and the Practice of Medicine,* 175–176.

59. Steven C. Wheatley, *The Politics of Philanthropy: Abraham Flexner and Medical Education* (Madison: University of Wisconsin Press, 1988), xii.

60. G. Canby Robinson, *Adventures in Medical Education: A Personal Narrative of the Great Advance of American Medicine* (Cambridge: Harvard University Press, 1957), 107, 113.

61. Charles R. Bardeen, "Medical School Plants," *Proceedings of the Annual Congress of Medical Education, Medical Licensing, and Hospitals* (1930): 13–31; "Huge New York Hospital–Cornell Medical Center Opened," *Hospital Management* 34 (1932): 26–29.

62. Allan M. Brandt and David C. Sloane, "Of Beds and Benches: Building the Modern American Hospital," in Peter Galison and Emily Thompson, eds., *The Architecture of Science* (Cambridge: MIT Press, 1999), 281–305.

63. Falk, Rorem, and Ring, *Costs of Medical Care,* 316. Because these figures include all hospitals with interns and more than two hundred beds, they are higher than they would be for strictly academic hospitals.

64. Donald L. Madison, "Notes on the History of Group Practice: The Tradition of the Dispensary," *Medical Group Management Journal* (September–October 1990): 52–60, 86–91.

65. Lewellys F. Barker, "Group Diagnosis and Group Therapy," *Illinois Medical Journal* 39 (1921): 1–22.

66. Davis and Warner, *Dispensaries,* 350.

67. Harry H. Moore, *American Medicine and the People's Health* (New York: D. Appleton, 1927), 20.

68. Hugh Cabot, "Medicine—A Profession or a Trade," *Boston Medical and Surgical Journal* 173, no. 19 (1915): 685–688.

69. Michael M. Davis, *Hospital Administration: A Career, the Need of Trained Executives for a Billion Dollar Business, and How They May Be Trained* (New York: Rockefeller Foundation, 1929), 42.

70. Lewellys F. Barker, "Medicine and the Universities," *American Medicine* 4 (1902): 143–147.

71. Lewellys F. Barker, "Some Tendencies in Medical Education in the United States," *Maryland Medical Journal* (October 1911): 295–303, (November 1911): 311–324.

72. John D. Spelman, "What Is the Ideal Organization of the Medical Staff in Order to Promote Efficiency of the Professional Work of the Hospital?" *Transactions of the American Hospital Association* 30 (1928): 323–328.

73. Barton Cooke Hirst, "The Equipment, the Organization, and the Scope of Teaching in the Obstetric Department of a Modern Medical School," *American Journal of Obstetrics and Gynecology* 1 (1920): 128–130.

74. Lewellys F. Barker, *Time and the Physician* (New York: G. Putnam, 1942). Barker's colleague Franklin Mall is credited for first advocating a full-time system in the United States.

75. Letter from Ray Lyman Wilbur to Lewellys F. Barker, December 11, 1913, Ray Lyman Wilbur papers, Lane Medical Library Archives, Stanford University Medical Center.

76. Lewellys F. Barker, "The Future of Medicine in America," *New York State Journal of Medicine* 21 (1921): 189–194.

77. J. Whitridge Williams, "Dispensary Abuse and Certain Problems of Medical Practice," *Journal of the American Medical Association* 66, no. 25 (1916): 1902–1908.

78. Abraham Flexner, *Medical Education: A Comparative Study* (New York: Macmillan, 1925), 51.

79. George Dock, "Full-time Clinical Departments," *Southern Medical Journal* 15, no. 12 (1922): 1013–1020.

80. William Allen Pusey, "Some Tendencies in the Business of the Practice of Medicine," *Journal of the American Medical Association* 90, no. 23 (1928): 1897–1902.

81. Emmett Keating, "Wanted—A John Stuart Mill, within the Ranks of the Medical Profession," *Northwest Medical Bulletin,* Northwest Branch, Chicago Medical Society (April 1929): n.p., Ray Lyman Wilbur papers, Lane Medical Library Archives, Stanford University Medical Center.

82. Nathan B. Van Etten, "The Teaching Clinic," *Journal of the American Medical Association* 102, no. 14 (1934): 1160–1161.

83. Milton Friedman and Simon Kuznets, *Income from Independent Professional Practice* (New York: National Bureau of Economic Research, 1945).

84. Allon Peebles, *A Survey of Statistical Data on Medical Facilities in the United States* (Washington, D.C.: Committee on the Costs of Medical Care, 1929), 75.

85. Thomas S. Huddle and Jack Ende, "Osler's Clinical Clerkship: Origins and Interpretations," *Journal of the History of Medicine and Allied Sciences* 49, no. 4 (1994): 483–503.

86. William H. Welch, "The Relation of the Hospital to Medical Education and Research" (1907) and other papers, in Cattell, *Science and Education,* 2:183–194.

87. Lewellys F. Barker, "The Teaching of Clinical Medicine," in Association of American Medical Colleges, *Proceedings of the Twenty-sixth Annual Meeting,* Chicago, February 8, 1916, 43–57.

88. Lewellys F. Barker, "Osler as Chief of a Medical Clinic," *Johns Hopkins Medical Bulletin* 341 (1919): 189–193.

89. James B. Herrick, "The Educational Function of Hospitals and the Hospital," in Cattell, *Science and Education,* 2:388–394.

90. Harold L. Foss, "A Plan for the Systematic Instruction and Supervision of Internes and Resident Physicians," *Bulletin of the American College of Surgeons* 15 (1931): 29–32; Malcolm T. MacEachern, *Hospital Organization and Management* (Chicago: Physicians' Record Co., 1935).

91. Several papers in Morris J. Vogel, ed., *On the Administrative Frontier of Medicine: The First Ten Years of the American Hospital Association, 1899–1908* (New York: Garland, 1989).

92. James F. Gifford, *The Evolution of a Medical Center: A History of Medicine at Duke University to 1941* (Durham: Duke University Press, 1972), 123.

93. Michael J. Lepore, *Death of the Clinician: Requiem or Reveille?* (Springfield, Ill.: Charles C. Thomas, 1982), 229.

94. Rothstein, *American Medical Schools and the Practice of Medicine,* 134–137; Kenneth M. Ludmerer, *Time to Heal: American Medical Education from the Turn of the Century to the Era of Managed Care* (New York: Oxford University Press, 1999), 92.

95. George Rosen, *The Structure of American Medical Practice, 1875–1941* (Philadelphia: University of Pennsylvania Press, 1983), 85.

96. Davis, *Hospital Administration.*

97. Malcolm T. MacEachern, "Summary of the 1929 Hospital Standardization Survey Twelve Years in Retrospect," *Bulletin of the American College of Surgeons* 13, no. 4 (1929): 3–8.

98. John D. Spelman, "What Is the Ideal Organization of the Medical Staff in Order to

Promote Efficiency of the Professional Work of the Hospital?" *Transactions of the American Hospital Association* 31 (1928): 323–328.

99. Barker, *Time and the Physician,* 178–181.

100. George L. Jordan, "Presidential Address: The Impact of Specialization on Health Care," *Annals of Surgery* 201, no. 5 (1985): 537–544. The author continued: "The surgical operating team as we know it today, however, was still in the future."

101. Helen Clapesattle, *The Doctors Mayo* (Minneapolis: University of Minnesota Press, 1941), 392.

102. Frederick C. Holden, "An Inventory of Gynecological Clinics," *American Journal of Obstetrics and Diseases of Women and Children* 78 (1918): 93–107.

103. Loyal Davis, *A Surgeon's Odyssey* (Garden City, N.Y.: Doubleday, 1973), 159–161, 186.

104. Davis and Warner, *Dispensaries,* 19.

105. Michael M. Davis, *Clinics, Hospitals and Health Centers* (New York: Harper, 1927), 422.

106. Michael M. Davis, "Efficiency Tests of Out-patient Work," *Boston Medical and Surgical Journal* 166 (1912): 915–921, reprinted in Morman, *Efficiency, Scientific Management, and Hospital Standardization,* 173–179.

107. Moore, *American Medicine and the People's Health,* 320.

108. Louis S. Reed, *Midwives, Chiropodists, and Optometrists: Their Place in Medical Care,* CCMC no. 15 (Chicago: University of Chicago Press, 1932), 63–64.

109. B. P. Watson, "Can Our Methods of Obstetric Practice Be Improved?" *Bulletin of the New York Academy of Medicine* 6, no. 10 (1930): 647–663.

110. Jane Pacht Brickman, "Public Health, Midwives, and Nurses, 1880–1930," in Ellen Condliffe Lagemann, ed., *Nursing History: New Perspectives, New Possibilities* (New York: Teachers College Press, 1983), 65–88.

111. Edward A. Ayers, "Prenatal Diagnosis, the Major Need in Obstetrics," *American Journal of Surgery* 30, no. 1 (1916): 369–371.

112. Mary Ayres Burgess, *Nurses, Patients, and Pocketbooks* (New York: Committee on the Grading of Nursing Schools, 1928), 457.

113. Karen Buhler-Wilkerson, "False Dawn: The Rise and Decline of Public Health Nursing in America, 1900–1930," in Lagemann, *Nursing History,* 89–106.

114. Committee for the Study of Nursing Education, *Nursing and Nursing Education in the United States* (New York: Macmillan, 1923), 347–364.

115. C. Rufus Rorem, "Comparative Costs of Undergraduate and Graduate Nursing," *Proceedings of the Annual Congress of Medical Education and Licensing* (1933): 76–79.

116. National League of Nursing Education, *A Study on the Use of the Graduate Nurse for Bedside Nursing in the Hospital* (New York: The League, 1933), 61–62.

117. David Wagner, "The Proletarianization of Nursing in the United States, 1932–1946," *International Journal of Health Services* 10 (1980): 271–291; Barbara Melosh, *"The Physician's Hand": Work Culture and Conflict in American Nursing* (Philadelphia: Temple University Press, 1982); Susan Reverby, *Ordered to Care: The Dilemma of American Nursing, 1850–1945* (Cambridge: Cambridge University Press, 1987).

118. Robert L. Hanson, *Management Systems for Nursing Service Staffing* (Rockville, Md.: Aspen, 1983), 48.

119. Barbara Melosh, "More than 'The Physician's Hand': Skill and Authority in

Twentieth-Century Nursing," in Judith Walzer Leavitt, ed., *Women and Health in America* (Madison: University of Wisconsin Press, 1984), 482–496.

120. Robert L. Brannon, *Intensifying Care: The Hospital Industry, Professionalization, and the Reorganization of the Nursing Labor Process* (Amityville, N.Y.: Baywood, 1994).

121. Burgess, *Nurses, Patients, and Pocketbooks,* 482–496.

122. Ethel Johns and Blanche Pfefferkorn, *An Activity Analysis of Nursing* (New York: Committee on the Grading of Nursing Schools, 1934), 99.

123. Barker, "On the Present Status of Therapy and Its Future," 149–156.

124. Lewellys F. Barker, "On the Expansion of Nursing," *Johns Hopkins Nurses Alumnae Magazine* 8 (1909): 79–87.

125. Carolyn Conant Van Blarcom, *Obstetrical Nursing* (New York: Macmillan, 1925 and 1929).

126. Herbert Marion Stowe, "The Specially Trained Obstetric Nurse—Her Advantages and Field," *American Journal of Nursing* 10, no. 8 (1910): 550–554.

127. Carrie M. Hall, "Training the Obstetrical Nurse," *American Journal of Nursing* 27, no. 5 (1927): 373–379.

128. Burgess, *Nurses, Patients, and Pocketbooks,* 265.

129. Elizabeth Fee, "The Social History of the Hospital: From Charity Care to the Management of Medicine: A Review Essay," *Radical History Review* 28–30 (1984): 472–481.

Three   Dividing Labor, Industrializing Birth

1. Lewellys F. Barker, "Some Tendencies in Medical Education in the United States," *Maryland Medical Journal* (November 1911): 311–324.

2. Howard C. Taylor, "The Making of a Woman's Hospital," *Obstetrics and Gynecology* 31, no. 4 (1968): 566–574.

3. Barton Cooke Hirst, "The Equipment, the Organization, and the Scope of Teaching in the Obstetric Department of a Modern Medical School," *American Journal of Obstetrics and Gynecology* 1 (1920): 128–130.

4. Charles Edward Ziegler, "The Elimination of the Midwife," *Journal of the American Medical Association* 60, no. 1 (1913): 32–38.

5. Barbara Melosh, *"The Physician's Hand": Work Culture and Conflict in American Nursing* (Philadelphia: Temple University Press, 1982), 159.

6. R. A. Johnson and R. S. Siddall, "Is the Usual Method of Preparing Patients for Delivery Beneficial or Necessary?" *American Journal of Obstetrics and Gynecology* 4 (1922): 645–650.

7. R. W. Stearns, "Analgesics in the First Stage of Labor," *Northwest Medicine* 17 (1918): 71–74; Edward P. Davis, "The Non-Operative Treatment of Labor," *Therapeutic Gazette* 39 (1915): 622–627.

8. American Academy of Pediatrics and American College of Obstetricians and Gynecologists, *Guidelines for Perinatal Care,* 4th ed. (Elk Grove Village, Ill.: American Academy of Pediatrics; and Washington, D.C.: American College of Obstetricians and Gynecologists, 1997), 26–27.

9. Michael Nathanson, "Single-Room Maternity Care Seen as Way to Attract Patients, Cut Costs," *Modern Healthcare* 15, no. 7 (1985): 72, 74.

10. American Academy of Pediatrics and American College of Obstetricians and

Gynecologists, *Guidelines for Perinatal Care,* 3d ed. (Elk Grove Village, Ill.: American Academy of Pediatrics; and Washington, D.C.: American College of Obstetricians and Gynecologists, 1992), 13.

11. Carolyn Conant Van Blarcom, *Obstetrical Nursing* (New York: Macmillan, 1929), 272, 434.

12. Benjamin P. Watson, "Can Our Methods of Obstetric Practice Be Improved?" *Bulletin of the New York Academy of Medicine* 6, no. 10 (1930): 647–663.

13. Brooke M. Anspach, "The Drudgery of Obstetrics and Its Effect upon the Practice of the Art, with Some Suggestions for Relief," *American Journal of Obstetrics and Gynecology* 2 (1921): 245–248.

14. E. D. Plass, "The Increase in Hospital Deliveries," *American Journal of Obstetrics and Gynecology* 40, no. 4 (1940): 659–661.

15. Frederick C. Holden, "Obstetrics and Gynecology under Ideal Conditions in a General Hospital," *Journal of the American Medical Association* 67, no. 16 (1916): 1130–1131.

16. Henry Schwarz, "Teaching Obstetrics under Improved Conditions," *American Journal of Obstetrics and Diseases of Women and Children* 74, no. 6 (1916): 981–989.

17. Samuel A. Cosgrove, "Proper Training of Internes and Residents in Obstetrics through Arrangement of Services, Supervision of Work and Instruction," *Bulletin of the American College of Surgeons* 24, no. 3 (1939): 200–201.

18. American Hospital Association, *Manual on Obstetrical Practice in Hospitals* (Chicago: American Hospital Association, 1935); Herbert M. Little, "Essentials for an Efficient Obstetrical Service," *Bulletin of the American College of Surgeons* 9, no. 1 (1925): 81–85.

19. George Gray Ward, "Hospital Standardization and Its Application to the Organization of a Special Hospital," *American Journal of Obstetrics and Diseases of Women and Children* 78, no. 1 (1918): 65–78; Committee on Maternity Care of the Children's Welfare Federation and a Special Committee Appointed by the New York Obstetrical Society, "Standards for Maternity Care," *American Journal of Obstetrics and Gynecology* 20 (1930): 133–141.

20. Committee on Maternal Welfare, *Maternal Mortality in Philadelphia: 1931–1933* (Philadelphia: Philadelphia County Medical Society, 1934), 133.

21. Robert Latou Dickinson, "Standardization of Surgery: An Attack on the Problem," *Journal of the American Medical Association* 63, no. 9 (1914): 763–765; Robert Latou Dickinson, "Hospital Efficiency from the Standpoint of a Hospital Surgeon," *Boston Medical and Surgical Journal* 172, no. 21 (1915): 775–778.

22. Robert L. Dickinson, "The New 'Efficiency' Systems and Their Bearing on Gynecological Diagnosis," *American Journal of Obstetrics and Diseases of Women and Children* 70, no. 6 (1914): 865–884.

23. Ward, "Hospital Standardization," 65–78.

24. Judith Walzer Leavitt, *Brought to Bed: Childbearing in America, 1750 to 1950* (New York: Oxford University Press, 1986), 171; Richard W. Wertz and Dorothy C. Wertz, *Lying-in: A History of Childbirth in America* (New York: Free Press, 1977), 173.

25. Unsigned editorial note, *Obstetrical and Gynecological Survey* 1 (1946): 461–463. Nicholson J. Eastman and Emil Novak were joint editors.

26. Roslyn Lindheim, "Birthing Centers and Hospices: Reclaiming Birth and Death," *Annual Review of Public Health* 2 (1981): 1–29.

27. Quoted in "How to Plan the Labor-Delivery Suite," *Modern Hospital* 102, no. 1 (1964): 84–87, 154, 156.

28. "Maternity Center Designed for 'Assembly-line' Efficiency," *Hospitals, JAHA* 38 (1964): 73–74, 77.

29. Gladys Denny Schultz, "Cruelty in Maternity Wards," *Ladies' Home Journal* (May 1958): 44–45, 52–55.

30. Rudolf A. Clemen, *By-products in the Packing Industry* (Chicago: University of Chicago Press, 1927), 207–208.

31. Richard C. Norris, "The Use and Abuse of Pituitrin in Obstetrics," *American Journal of Obstetrics and Diseases of Women and Children* 71 (1915): 741–747; J. Hofbauer, "Forty Years of Postpituitary Extract in Obstetrics," *American Journal of Obstetrics and Gynecology* 69, no. 4 (1955): 822–825; Sidney R. Sogolow, "An Historical Review of the Use of Oxytocin Prior to Delivery," *Obstetrical and Gynecological Survey* 21 (1966): 155–172.

32. Bandler, "The Use of Pituitary Extract in Obstetric Practice," summarized in *Therapeutic Gazette* 39 (1915): 349–352.

33. J. C. Applegate, "Rational Obstetrics from the Teaching Viewpoint," *American Journal of Obstetrics and Gynecology* 7 (1924): 181–188. Comment by Daniel Longaker, discussion, 222–227.

34. J. K. Quigley, "Pituitrin in Obstetrics," *New York State Journal of Medicine* 13, no. 6 (1913): 317–324.

35. George M. Boyd, "Conservative Obstetrics: Some Lessons Learned in a Twenty-five Years' Service at the Philadelphia Lying-in Charity," *Bulletin of the Lying-in Hospital of the City of New York* 10, no. 4 (1916): 209–218.

36. Joseph J. Mundell, "The Present Status of Pituitary Extract in Labor," *Journal of the American Medical Association* 68, no. 22 (1917): 1601–1604.

37. B. P. Watson, "Pituitary Extract in Obstetrical Practice," *Canadian Medical Association Journal* 3, no. 9 (1913): 739–758; B. P. Watson, "Further Experience with Pituitary Extract in the Induction of Labor," *American Journal of Obstetrics and Gynecology* 4 (1922): 603–608. Obstetricians named a "sense of oppression" as an undesirable effect of pituitary extract, which can lead to interesting conjectures about doctor-patient relationships and dominance theories.

38. Charles B. Reed, "The Induction of Labor at Term: A Supplemental Report," *Surgery, Gynecology and Obstetrics* 27, no. 2 (1918): 163–168.

39. Charles B. Reed, "The Induction of Labor at Term," *American Journal of Obstetrics and Gynecology* 1 (1920): 24–33.

40. Nicholson J. Eastman, "Pituitary Extract in Uterine Inertia: Is It Justifiable?" *American Journal of Obstetrics and Gynecology* 53, no. 3 (1947): 432–441.

41. Howard C. Taylor, "Notes on Fifty Years of Progress in Gynecology," *American Journal of Surgery* 51, no. 1 (1941): 97–109.

42. John Harley Warner, *The Therapeutic Perspective: Medical Practice, Knowledge, and Identity in America, 1820–1885* (Cambridge: Harvard University Press, 1986), 12.

43. A. M. Mendenhall, "Teaching Undergraduate Obstetrics," *American Journal of Obstetrics and Gynecology* 3 (1922): 53–61. John Polak, in discussion, 86–88.

44. White House Conference on Child Health and Protection, Subcommittee on Obstetric Teaching and Education, *Obstetric Education* (New York: Century, 1932), 83. Secretary of the Interior and CCMC chairman Ray Lyman Wilbur served as overall chair of the conference.

45. Wertz and Wertz, *Lying-in,* 143.
46. Roy W. Mohler, "A Report of the Cesarean Sections Done at the Philadelphia Lying-in Pennsylvania Hospital," *American Journal of Obstetrics and Gynecology* 45, no. 3 (1943): 466–478. Years 1929–1942.
47. Ralph H. Pomeroy, "Shall We Cut and Reconstruct the Perineum for Every Primipara?" *American Journal of Obstetrics and Diseases of Women and Children* 78 (1918): 211–220.
48. Frances E. Kobrin, "The American Midwife Controversy: A Crisis of Professionalization," *Bulletin of the History of Medicine* 40, no. 4 (1966): 350–363; Wertz and Wertz, *Lying-in,* 141; Jessica Mitford, *The American Way of Birth* (New York: Penguin Books, 1992), 58; Mary M. Lay, *The Rhetoric of Midwifery: Gender, Knowledge, and Power* (New Brunswick: Rutgers University Press, 2000), 63.
49. Irvine Loudon, *Death in Childbirth: An International Study of Maternal Care and Maternal Mortality, 1800–1950* (Oxford: Clarendon, 1992), chaps. 19, 21.
50. Margot Edwards and Mary Waldorf, *Reclaiming Birth: History and Heroines of American Childbirth Reform* (Trumansburg, N.Y.: Crossing Press, 1984), 9; William Ray Arney, *Power and the Profession of Obstetrics* (Chicago: University of Chicago Press, 1982), 54.
51. Joseph B. DeLee, "The Prophylactic Forceps Operation," *American Journal of Obstetrics and Gynecology* 1 (1920): 34–44.
52. David A. Richardson, Mark I. Evans, and Luis A. Cibils, "Midforceps Delivery: A Critical Review," *American Journal of Obstetrics and Gynecology* 145, no. 5 (1983): 621–632. Year periods: 1931–1941, 1941–1946, 1946–1951.
53. Illinois Department of Public Health, *Services for Mothers and Infants in Illinois Hospitals: A Twenty-Five Year Summary, 1943–1967* (Illinois Department of Public Health, 1971).
54. Robert A. Hahn, *Sickness and Healing: An Anthropological Perspective* (New Haven: Yale University Press, 1995), 216–217.
55. Arthur H. Bill, "The Choice of Methods for Making Labor Easy," *American Journal of Obstetrics and Gynecology* 3 (1922): 65–71.
56. Pomeroy, "Shall We Cut and Reconstruct the Perineum for Every Primipara?" 211–220.
57. Bertha Van Hoosen, *Petticoat Surgeon* (Chicago: Pellegrini and Cudahy, 1947), 283.
58. Ian D. Graham, *Episiotomy: Challenging Obstetric Interventions* (Oxford: Blackwell Science, 1997).
59. Stephen B. Thacker and H. David Banta, "Benefits and Risks of Episiotomy: An Interpretative Review of the English-Language Literature, 1860–1980," *Obstetrical and Gynecological Survey* 38, no. 6 (1983): 322–338.
60. American Academy of Pediatrics and American College of Obstetricians and Gynecologists, *Guidelines for Perinatal Care* (Evanston, Ill.: American Academy of Pediatrics; and Washington, D.C.: American College of Obstetricians and Gynecologists, 1983), 65.
61. Lola Jean Kozak and Julie Dawson Weeks, "U.S. Trends in Obstetric Procedures, 1990–2000," *Birth* 29, no. 3 (2002): 157–161; U.S. Department of Health and Human Services, "National Hospital Discharge Survey: Annual Summary, 1994," *Vital and Health Statistics* 13, no. 128 (1997): 8.
62. Paul G. Schoon, "A Guest Editorial: Episiotomy: Yea or Nay," *Obstetrical and Gynecological Survey* 56, no. 11 (2001): 667–669.

63. G. Carroli, J. Balizan, and G. Stamp, in J. P. Neilson et al., eds., "Episiotomy Policies in Vaginal Births," *Pregnancy and Childbirth Module of the Cochrane Database of Systematic Reviews* (Oxford: Cochrane Collection, Issue 4, Update Software, 1997); M. Gabrielle Meyers-Helfgott and Andrew W. Helfgott, "Routine Use of Episiotomy in Modern Obstetrics: Should It Be Performed?" *Obstetrics and Gynecology Clinics of North America* 26, no. 2 (1999): 305–325.

64. Van Hoosen, *Petticoat Surgeon,* 282–283.

65. Regina Markell Morantz-Sanchez, *Sympathy and Science: Women Physicians in American Medicine* (New York: Oxford University Press, 1985), 222–231. Virginia G. Drachman, *Hospital with a Heart: Women Doctors and the Paradox of Separation at the New England Hospital, 1862–1969* (Ithaca: Cornell University Press, 1984), made a similar case.

66. Ornella Moscucci, *The Science of Woman: Gynaecology and Gender in England, 1800–1929* (Cambridge: Cambridge University Press, 1990).

67. Rudolph W. Holmes, "The Fads and Fancies of Obstetrics: A Comment on the Pseudoscientific Trend of Modern Obstetrics," *American Journal of Obstetrics and Gynecology* 2, no. 3 (1921): 225–237.

68. White House Conference on Child Health and Protection, *Obstetric Education,* 50.

69. Alfred C. Beck, "The Management of Normal Labor," *Journal of the American Medical Association* 99, no. 21 (1932): 1742–1744.

70. Magnus A. Tate, "A Method of Delivery in Normal Cases," *American Journal of Obstetrics and Gynecology* 3 (1922): 61–65.

71. Joseph B. DeLee, "Meddlesome Midwifery in Renaissance," *Journal of the American Medical Association* 67, no. 16 (1916): 1126–1129.

72. Arney, *Power and the Profession of Obstetrics,* 51.

73. Charles Edward Ziegler, "The Teaching of Obstetrics," *American Journal of Obstetrics and Diseases of Women and Children* 73 (1916): 50–66.

74. J. F. Moran, "The Endowment of Motherhood," *Journal of the American Medical Association* 64 (1915): 122.

75. Steven C. Wheatley, *The Politics of Philanthropy: Abraham Flexner and Medical Education* (Madison: University of Wisconsin Press, 1988), 14; Regina Markell Morantz-Sanchez, *Conduct Unbecoming a Woman: Medicine on Trial in Turn-of-the-Century Brooklyn* (New York: Oxford University Press, 1999), 78, 110.

76. J. Whitridge Williams, "A Criticism of Certain Tendencies in American Obstetrics," *New York State Journal of Medicine* 22, no. 11 (1922): 493–499.

77. William H. Morley, "Conduct of Labor during the Second Stage," *Physician and Surgeon* 18 (1906): 113–118.

78. *Dilatation* is the commonly accepted term. But Arthur Hertig, reproductive pathologist and chairman of the Pathology Department at Harvard Medical School, told its Medical Sciences class in 1965 that his department secretary had informed him that *dilatation* was unnecessarily complex and meant the same thing as *dilation* and that he would henceforth use the latter term. I also will henceforth use the term *dilation.*

79. James Robert Goodall, "A Plea for Prophylactic Intervention in the Second Stage of Labor," *Surgery, Gynecology and Obstetrics* 58, no. 5 (1934): 882–885.

80. L. M. Hellman and Harry Prystowsky, "The Duration of the Second Stage of Labor," *American Journal of Obstetrics and Gynecology* 63, no. 6 (1952): 1223–1233.

The authors noted that the two-hour rule appeared in the first edition (1903) of Williams's textbook and that DeLee terminated the argument by terminating most labors before two hours were up. The third stage is delivery of the placenta.

81. Charles Rosenberg, "The Practice of Medicine in New York City a Century Ago," *Bulletin of the History of Medicine* 41, no. 3 (1967): 223–253.

82. Elizabeth Fee, "The Social History of the Hospital: From Charity Care to the Management of Medicine: A Review Essay," *Radical History Review* 28–30 (1984): 472–481.

83. Keith Wailoo, *Drawing Blood: Technology and Disease Identity in Twentieth-Century America* (Baltimore: Johns Hopkins University Press, 1997), 111, 128–129.

84. Charles Edward Ziegler, "The Elimination of the Midwife," *Journal of the American Medical Association* 60, no. 1 (1913): 32–38; Charles Edward Ziegler, "How Can We Best Solve the Midwifery Problem," *American Journal of Public Health* 12 (1922): 405–413.

85. George W. Kosmak, "Prenatal Care and Maternity Welfare from the Standpoint of the Maternity Center without Hospital Connection," *New York State Journal of Medicine* 23, no. 8 (1923): 335–338.

86. U.S. Public Health Service, *Maternal Care in Michigan: A Study of Obstetric Practices,* bulletin no. 8, Sickness and Medical Care Series (Washington, D.C.: U.S. Public Health Service, 1938), 17–18.

87. Rosemary Stevens, *In Sickness and in Wealth: American Hospitals in the Twentieth Century* (New York: Basic Books, 1989), 105–107.

88. Selwyn D. Collins, "Variation in Hospitalization with Size of City, Family Income, and Other Environmental Factors," *Public Health Reports* 57, no. 44 (1942): 1635–1659.

89. Mendenhall, "Teaching Undergraduate Obstetrics," 53–61, 86–88.

90. U.S. Department of Labor, Children's Bureau, *The Promotion of the Welfare and Hygiene of Maternity and Infancy* (Washington, D.C.: U.S. Government Printing Office, 1926), 7.

91. George Clark Mosher, "Report of the Committee on Maternal Welfare of the American Association of Obstetricians, Gynecologists and Abdominal Surgeons, Cleveland Meeting, September, 1924," *American Journal of Obstetrics and Gynecology* 9 (1925): 269–276; Charles R. King, "The New York Maternal Mortality Study: A Conflict of Professionalization," *Bulletin of the History of Medicine* 65 (1991): 476–502.

92. Morris J. Vogel, *The Invention of the Modern Hospital: Boston, 1870–1930* (Chicago: University of Chicago Press, 1980), 116.

93. White House Conference on Child Health and Protection, "Prenatal and Maternal Care," *White House Conference 1930: Addresses and Abstracts of Committee Reports* (New York: Century, 1931), 76–77.

94. I. S. Falk, C. Rufus Rorem, and Martha D. Ring, *The Costs of Medical Care: A Summary of Investigations on the Economic Aspects of the Prevention and Care of Illness,* CCMC report no. 27 (Chicago: University of Chicago Press, 1933), 307.

95. James W. Markoe, "Obstetrical Technique for the General Practitioner," *Bulletin of the Lying-in Hospital of New York* 9 (1913–1914): 159–171.

96. American Gynecological Society, "Symposium: To What Extent Should Delivery Be Hastened or Assisted by Operative Interference?" *American Journal of Obstetrics and Gynecology* 2, no. 3 (1921): 297–307.

97. U.S. Public Health Service, *Maternal Care in Michigan,* 33. I took mid-career general practitioners as the most appropriate comparison group. Interestingly, the use of drugs for labor induction and acceleration was reversed.

98. Leavitt, *Brought to Bed,* 79–86.

99. U.S. Department of Labor, Children's Bureau, *Causal Factors in Infant Mortality,* Publication no. 142 (Washington, D.C.: U.S. Government Printing Office, 1925), 236.

100. Jennie C. Goddard, *Medical and Nursing Services for the Maternal Cases of the National Health Survey,* Public Health Bulletin no. 264 (Washington, D.C.: U.S. Government Printing Office, 1941), 45. Figures estimated from graph.

101. Committee on Maternal Welfare, *Maternal Mortality in Philadelphia,* 75.

102. Roy W. Mohler, "A Report of the Cesarean Sections Done at the Philadelphia Lying-in Pennsylvania Hospital," *American Journal of Obstetrics and Gynecology* 45, no. 3 (1943): 466–478. Data were from 1932–1937; the rates lowered in the following decade.

103. George Clark Mosher, "Ten Years of Painless Childbirth," *American Journal of Obstetrics and Gynecology* 3, no. 2 (1922): 142–149.

104. Edward Reynolds, "Primary Operations for Obstetrical Debility," *Surgery, Gynecology, and Obstetrics* 4 (1907): 306–318; Barbara Ehrenreich and Deirdre English, *For Her Own Good: 150 Years of the Experts' Advice to Women* (Garden City, N.Y.: Doubleday, 1978), 93.

105. Franklin S. Newell, "The Effect of Overcivilization on Maternity," *American Journal of the Medical Sciences* 136 (1908): 532–541.

106. Donald G. Tollefson and Aaron M. Webb, "Uterine Inertia in the First Stage of Labor," *Western Journal of Surgery, Obstetrics and Gynecology* 45, no. 3 (1937): 156–167.

107. Judith Walzer Leavitt, "Joseph B. DeLee and the Practice of Preventive Obstetrics," *American Journal of Public Health* 78, no. 10 (1988): 1353–1360.

108. DeLee, quoted in William Danforth, "Contemporary Titans: Joseph Bolivar DeLee and John Whitridge Williams," *American Journal of Obstetrics and Gynecology* 120, no. 5 (1974): 577–588.

109. Joseph B. DeLee, "Obstetrics versus Midwifery," *Journal of the American Medical Association* 103, no. 5 (1934): 307–311.

110. Morris Fishbein, *Joseph Bolivar DeLee: Crusading Obstetrician* (New York: E. P. Dutton, 1949), 98, 167.

111. J. Whitridge Williams, "Dispensary Abuse and Certain Problems of Medical Practice," *Journal of the American Medical Association* 66, no. 25 (1916): 1901–1908; Alan M. Chesney, *The Johns Hopkins Hospital and the Johns Hopkins University School of Medicine: A Chronicle* (Baltimore: Johns Hopkins Press, 1963), 139.

112. Ziegler, "Teaching of Obstetrics," 50–66.

113. Harold Speert, *Obstetrics and Gynecology in America* (Chicago: American College of Obstetricians and Gynecologists, 1980), 14.

114. Joseph B. DeLee and Fred Lyman Adair, "University of Chicago Division of Biological Sciences Department of Obstetrics and Gynecology and the Chicago Lying-in Hospital and Dispensary," *Methods and Problems of Medical Education* (New York: Rockefeller Foundation, 1931), 149–162.

115. DeLee and Adair, "University of Chicago Division of Biological Sciences," 149–162.

116. Sylvester J. Goodman, "Recent Progress in Obstetrics—A Review," *American Journal of Surgery* 30, no. 11 (1916): 371–377. It is not clear whether the author was referring to obstetricians or general practitioners.

117. Holmes, "Fads and Fancies of Obstetrics," 225–237.

118. American Gynecological Society, "Symposium: To What Extent Should Delivery Be Hastened or Assisted by Operative Interference?" *American Journal of Obstetrics and Gynecology* 2, no. 3 (1921): 297–307.

119. New York Obstetrical Society, "Symposium on Operative Delivery vs. Spontaneous Delivery," *American Journal of Obstetrics and Gynecology* 1, no. 9 (1921): 986–1000; Vern L. Bullough, "Irving W. Potter and Podalic Version: A Buffalo Case Study," in Lilli Sentz, ed., *Medical History in Buffalo, 1846–1996* (Buffalo: State University of New York at Buffalo, 1996), 233–246.

120. Charles A. Gordon, "The Conduct of Labor and the Management of Obstetric Emergencies," *American Journal of Obstetrics and Gynecology* 13 (1927): 501–506.

121. White House Conference on Child Health and Protection, *Report of Subcommittee on Factors and Causes of Fetal, Newborn, and Maternal Morbidity and Mortality* (New York: D. Appleton-Century, 1933), 231.

122. Robert L. De Normandie, "Cesarean Section in Massachusetts in 1939," *New England Journal of Medicine* 224, no. 23 (1941): 963–971.

123. White House Conference on Child Health and Protection, *Factors and Causes of Fetal, Newborn, and Maternal Morbidity and Mortality,* 222, 233.

124. George W. Kosmak, "The Training of Medical Students in Obstetrics," *Proceedings of the Annual Congress of Medical Education* (1936): 15–18.

125. White House Conference on Child Health and Protection, *Factors and Causes of Fetal, Newborn and Maternal Morbidity and Mortality,* 242.

126. Frederick C. Irving, "Maternal Mortality at the Boston Lying-in Hospital in 1933, 1934, and 1935," *New England Journal of Medicine* 217, no. 18 (1937): 693–695.

127. Rosemary Stevens, *American Medicine and the Public Interest* (Berkeley: University of California Press, 1998), 86.

128. Rosemary Stevens, "The Curious Career of Internal Medicine: Functional Ambivalence, Social Success," in Russell C. Maulitz and Diana E. Long, eds., *Grand Rounds: One Hundred Years of Internal Medicine* (Philadelphia: University of Pennsylvania Press, 1988), 339–364.

129. J. Whitridge Williams, "The Abuse of Caesearean Section," *Surgery, Gynecology, and Obstetrics* 25 (1917): 194–201.

130. White House Conference on Child Health and Protection, *Factors and Causes of Fetal, Newborn and Morbidity and Mortality,* 211.

131. Mendenhall, "Teaching Undergraduate Obstetrics," 53–61, discussion 86–88.

132. Michael M. Davis and Mary C. Jarrett, *A Health Inventory of New York City* (New York: Welfare Council of New York City, 1929), 89. Maternal mortality was to join the general decline in mortality rates in the mid-1930s.

133. James E. Davis, "Pathology of the Reproductive Cycle Based upon Over Half a Million Obstetric Deliveries in Detroit," *American Journal of Obstetrics and Gynecology* 27 (1934): 457–465.

134. Julius Levy, "Maternal Mortality and Mortality in the First Month of Life in Relation to Attendant at Birth," *American Journal of Public Health* 13, no. 1 (1923): 88–95.

135. New York Academy of Medicine, *Maternal Mortality in New York City: A Study of All Puerperal Deaths, 1930–1932* (New York: Commonwealth Fund, 1933), 180–182.

136. American Gynecological Society, "Symposium: To What Extent Should Delivery Be Hastened or Assisted by Operative Interference?" 297–307.

137. J. Whitridge Williams, "Medical Education and the Midwife Problem in the United States," *Journal of the American Medical Association* 58, no. 1 (1912): 1–7.

Four   Committee on the Costs of Medical Care

1. Roger M. Battistella and David B. Smith, "Control of Health Services," in Roger M. Battistella and Thomas G. Rundall, eds., *Health Care Policy in a Changing Environment* (Berkeley: McCutchan, 1978), 194–252; Stephen J. Kunitz, "Efficiency and Reform in the Financing and Organization of American Medicine in the Progressive Era," *Bulletin of the History of Medicine* 55 (1981): 497–515. I use CCMC reports and writings of its leaders and staff to identify goals and concepts of "the committee" and identify separately the views of the dissenting minority. As Parks noted, the work was "primarily directed by the executive committee and the research staff, not by the general committee." Douglas R. Parks, *Expert Inquiry and Health Care Reform in New Era America: Herbert Hoover, Ray Lyman Wilbur, and the Travails of the Disinterested Experts* (Ann Arbor, Mich.: UMI Dissertation Services, 1994), 222.

2. Letter from Paul Kellogg and Haven Emerson to Ray Lyman Wilbur, April 22, 1924, Ray Lyman Wilbur papers, Lane Medical Library Archives, Stanford University Medical Center, hereafter called "Wilbur papers." They wrote Michael Davis, Louis I. Dublin, Lee K. Frankel, C.-E. A. Winslow, Homer Folks, Linsley Williams, W. S. Rankin, Mrs. William K. Draper, Hugh Cabot, Richard Cabot, and Robert L. Dickinson, among others.

3. C.-E. A. Winslow, "Public Health at the Crossroads," *American Journal of Public Health* 16, no. 11 (1926): 1075–1085.

4. Harry H. Moore, *American Medicine and the People's Health* (New York: D. Appleton, 1927), vii.

5. I. S. Falk, "Some Lessons from the Fifty Years since the CCMC Final Report, 1932," *Journal of Public Health Policy* 4, no. 2 (1983): 135–161.

6. Committee on the Costs of Medical Care, *The Five-Year Program of the Committee on the Costs of Medical Care,* report no. 1 (Washington, D.C.: CCMC, 1928).

7. Harry H. Moore, *American Medicine and the People's Health.*

8. "Report of the Committee of Five Submitted to the Conference on the Economic Factors Affecting the Organization of Medicine," May 17, 1927, Washington, D.C., Wilbur papers.

9. "Minutes of a Meeting of the Committee on the Cost of Medical Care," May 18, 1927, Washington, D.C., Wilbur papers. Following a lengthy discussion on the implications of different names for the committee, an *s* was added to *cost* in 1930.

10. Daniel M. Fox, *Health Policies, Health Politics: The British and American Experience, 1911–1965* (Princeton: Princeton University Press, 1986), 46.

11. Richard L. McCormick, "Evaluating the Progressives," in Leon Fink, ed., *Major*

Problems in the Gilded Age and the Progressive Era (Lexington, Mass.: D. C. Heath, 1993), 315–329; Glenn Porter, *The Rise of Big Business, 1860–1910* (New York: Thomas Y. Crowell, 1973), 3–6.

12. David W. Noble, *The Paradox of Progressive Thought* (Minneapolis: University of Minnesota Press, 1958), 163–171; James Weinstein, *The Corporate Ideal in the Liberal State, 1900–1918* (Boston: Beacon Press, 1968), x.

13. J. B. Bury, *The Idea of Progress: An Inquiry into Its Origin and Growth* (New York: Dover, 1932), 220–221.

14. Alfred P. Sloan, *My Years with General Motors* (New York: Doubleday, 1963), xv, 248.

15. Carolyn Merchant, *The Death of Nature: Women, Ecology, and the Scientific Revolution* (San Francisco: HarperSanFrancisco, 1980), 179–185.

16. Guy Alchon, *The Invisible Hand of Planning: Capitalism, Social Science, and the State in the 1920s* (Princeton: Princeton University Press, 1985), 131; Daniel T. Rogers, "In Search of Progressivism," *Reviews in American History* 10 (1982): 113–132; David F. Noble, *America by Design: Science, Technology, and the Rise of Corporate Capitalism* (Oxford: Oxford University Press, 1977).

17. Clarke A. Chambers, *Paul U. Kellogg and the SURVEY: Voices for Social Justice and Social Welfare* (Minneapolis: University of Minnesota Press, 1971), 108.

18. S. E. Berki, "Book Review," *Medical Care* 18, no. 8 (1980): 878–879.

19. Walton H. Hamilton, "Organization, Economic," in Edwin R. A. Seligman, ed., *Encyclopaedia of the Social Sciences* (New York: Macmillan, 1937), 8:484–490; Walton H. Hamilton, "Competition," in Edwin R. A. Seligman, ed., *Encyclopaedia of the Social Sciences* (New York: Macmillan, 1937), 3:141–147; Allan G. Gruchy, "The Concept of National Planning in Institutional Economics," *Southern Economic Journal* 6, no. 2 (1939): 121–144.

20. William Appleman Williams, *The Contours of American History* (Chicago: Quadrangle Books, 1961); Ellis W. Hawley, "Introduction: Secretary Hoover and the Changing Framework of New Era Historiography," in Ellis W. Hawley, ed., *Herbert Hoover as Secretary of Commerce: Studies in New Era Thought and Practice* (Iowa City: University of Iowa Press, 1981), 1–16.

21. Ellis W. Hawley, "Secretary Hoover and the Bituminous Coal Problem, 1921–1928," *Business History Review* 42 (1968): 247–270.

22. Edward Eyre Hunt, intro., in Edward Eyre Hunt, ed., *Scientific Management since Taylor* (New York: McGraw-Hill, 1924), xi–xv; Herbert Hoover, foreword, in President's Research Committee on Social Trends, *Recent Social Trends in the United States,* vol. 1 (New York: McGraw-Hill, 1933).

23. Ray Lyman Wilbur and Arthur Mastick Hyde, *The Hoover Policies* (New York: Charles Scribner's Sons, 1937); Barry D. Karl, "Presidential Planning and Social Science Research: Mr. Hoover's Experts," *Perspectives in American History* 3 (1969): 347–409; Ellis W. Hawley, "Herbert Hoover and Modern American History: Sixty Years After," in Mark M. Dodge, ed., *Herbert Hoover and the Historians* (West Branch, Iowa: Herbert Hoover Presidential Library Association, 1989), 1–38; Murray N. Rothbard, "Herbert Hoover and the Myth of Laissez-Faire," in Ronald Radosh and Murray N. Rothbard, eds., *A New History of Leviathan* (New York: E. P. Dutton, 1972), 111–145.

24. Note from M.M.D. [presumably Michael M. Davis] to E.R.E. [Edwin R. Embree, director of the Julius Rosenwald Fund], internal routing slip, June 18, 1932, Michael

Marks Davis papers, Historical Collection, New York Academy of Medicine Library, hereafter called "Davis papers."

25. Guy Alchon, "Mary Van Kleek and Scientific Management," in Daniel Nelson, ed., *A Mental Revolution: Scientific Management since Taylor* (Columbus: Ohio State University Press, 1992), 102–129; Steven C. Wheatley, *The Politics of Philanthropy* (Madison: University of Wisconsin Press, 1988), 114.

26. Fox, *Health Policies, Health Politics,* 47–48.

27. Moore, *American Medicine and the People's Health,* 13, 65, 318.

28. Walton H. Hamilton, "The Problem of Bituminous Coal," *American Labor Legislation Review* 16 (1926): 217–229.

29. Lucy Sprague Mitchell, *Two Lives: The Story of Wesley Clair Mitchell and Myself* (New York: Simon and Schuster, 1953), 396.

30. President's Research Committee on Social Trends, "Review of Findings," in *Recent Social Trends* lvi. Lucy Sprague Mitchell attributed the unsigned introduction to Wesley Mitchell (*Two Lives,* 367).

31. Ray Lyman Wilbur, "The Trouble with Doctors," as told to Frank J. Taylor of the *Post,* draft copy sent for approval, n.d., Wilbur papers.

32. "Conference on the Economic Factors Affecting the Organization of Medicine," Wilbur papers.

33. Michael M. Davis and C. Rufus Rorem, *The Crisis in Hospital Finance and Other Studies in Hospital Economics* (Chicago: University of Chicago Press, 1932).

34. Haven Emerson, C. Rufus Rorem, and Louis S. Reed, "The Problem of Medical Care: A Statement and Analysis of the Deficiencies of the Present Economic Organization of Medicine," part of a Confidential Report to the Executive Committee, November 23, 1931, 25, Countway Library of Medicine Historical Collection, Boston.

35. CCMC, *Five-Year Program,* 10–11.

36. I. S. Falk, C. Rufus Rorem, and Martha D. Ring, *The Costs of Medical Care: A Summary of Investigations on the Economic Aspects of the Prevention and Care of Illness,* CCMC report no. 27 (Chicago: University of Chicago Press, 1933), 384–387.

37. Paul Starr, *The Social Transformation of American Medicine* (New York: Basic Books, 1982), 199, 264–265.

38. Rosemary Stevens, *In Sickness and in Wealth: American Hospitals in the Twentieth Century* (New York: Basic Books, 1989), 135.

39. Alan Derickson, "'Health for Three-Thirds of the Nation,' Public Health Advocacy of Universal Access to Medical Care in the United States," *American Journal of Public Health* 92, no. 2 (2002): 180–190.

40. Forrest A. Walker, "Americanism versus Sovietism: A Study of the Reaction to the Committee on the Costs of Medical Care," *Bulletin of the History of Medicine* 53, no. 4 (1979): 489–504.

41. Steven A. Schroeder, "Group Practice Recommendations of the Committee on the Costs of Medical Care," *Milbank Memorial Fund Quarterly* 56, no. 2 (1978): 169–186.

42. Daniel M. Fox, "From Reform to Relativism: A History of Economists and Health Care," *Milbank Memorial Fund Quarterly* 57, no. 3 (1979): 297–336.

43. Davis and Rorem, *Crisis in Hospital Finance,* 173.

44. Roger I. Lee, Lewis Webster Jones, and Barbara Jones, *The Fundamentals of Good Medical Care,* report no. 22 (Chicago: University of Chicago Press, 1933), 111.

45. C. Rufus Rorem, *Capital Investment in Hospitals,* report no. 7 (Washington, D.C.: CCMC, 1930), 10.
46. Davis and Rorem, *Crisis in Hospital Finance,* 103.
47. Martin Bulmer, "Knowledge for the Public Good: The Emergence of Social Sciences and Social Reform in Late-Nineteenth- and Early-Twentieth-Century America, 1880–1940," in David L. Featherman and Maris A. Vinovskis, eds., *Social Science and Policy-Making: A Search for Relevance in the Twentieth Century* (Ann Arbor: University of Michigan Press, 2001), 16–39.
48. Camilla Stivers, *Bureau Men, Settlement Women: Constructing Public Administration in the Progressive Era* (Lawrence: University Press of Kansas, 2000), 70.
49. C. Rufus Rorem, *The Public's Investment in Hospitals* (Chicago: University of Chicago Press, 1930).
50. C.-E. A. Winslow, "The Business of Medicine," *Yale Review* 21 (1931): 318–329.
51. Douglas R. Parks, *Expert Inquiry and Health Care Reform in New Era America: Herbert Hoover, Ray Lyman Wilbur, and the Travails of the Disinterested Experts* (Ann Arbor, Mich.: UMI Dissertation Services, 1994).
52. Haven Emerson and Gertrude E. Sturges, "Method of Making a Community Diagnosis," *Method of Survey, Part 11* (Cleveland: Cleveland Hospital and Health Survey, 1920), 1003.
53. Haven Emerson, Louis I. Reed, and C. Rufus Rorem, "Some Tentative Conclusions and Recommendations Based upon the Work of the Committee on the Costs of Medical Care," part of a Confidential Report to the Executive Committee, November 23, 1931, 3, Davis papers.
54. Michael M. Davis, *Hospital Administration: A Career. The Need of Trained Executives for a Billion Dollar Business and How They May Be Trained* (New York: Rockefeller Foundation, 1929), 4.
55. Committee on the Costs of Medical Care, *Medical Care for the American People,* final report (Chicago: University of Chicago Press, 1932), 28.
56. Julius Rosenwald, "Hospitals from a Business Man's Point of View," *Transactions of the American Hospital Association* 32 (1930): 106–111.
57. CCMC, *Medical Care for the American People,* 28.
58. Bureau of Medical Economics, *An Introduction to Medical Economics* (Chicago: American Medical Association, 1935), 16–17, 21–23.
59. R. G. Leland, "Prepayment Plans for Hospital Care," *Journal of the American Medical Association* 100 (1933): 870–873.
60. Bureau of Medical Economics, *Medical Economics,* 21–22.
61. Walton Hamilton, "Statement," in CCMC, *Medical Care for the American People,* 189–200.
62. Davis and Rorem, *Crisis in Hospital Finance,* 69.
63. Dorothy Ross, *The Origins of American Social Science* (Cambridge: Cambridge University Press, 1991), 378–382, 410–412.
64. Falk, Rorem, and Ring, *Costs of Medical Care,* 324.
65. Niles Carpenter, *Hospital Service for Patients of Moderate Means* (Washington, D.C.: CCMC, 1930), 45; Rorem, *Public's Investment in Hospitals,* 208–209.
66. Davis and Rorem, *Crisis in Hospital Finance,* 5–6.
67. Rorem, *Capital Investment in Hospitals,* 37.
68. C. Rufus Rorem, "Some Economic Issues in Hospital Management," *Bulletin* of the Taylor Society for the Advancement of Management, February 1932, reprinted in

C. Rufus Rorem, *A Quest for Certainty: Essays on Health Care Economics, 1930–1970* (Ann Arbor, Mich.: Health Administration Press, 1982), 19–27.

69. Michael M. Davis, "Group Medicine," *American Journal of Public Health* 9 (1919): 358–362.

70. Lewellys F. Barker, "Group Diagnosis and Group Therapy," *Illinois Medical Journal* 39 (1921): 1–9.

71. Lewellys F. Barker, "The Specialist and the General Practitioner in Relation to Team-Work in Medical Practice," *Journal of the American Medical Association* 78 (1922): 773–779.

72. Haven Emerson, C. Rufus Rorem, and Louis S. Reed, "The Problem of Medical Care: A Statement and Analysis of the Deficiencies of the Present Economic Organization of Medicine," part of a Confidential Report to the Executive Committee, November 23, 1931, 25, Countway Library of Medicine Historical Collection, Boston.

73. Haven Emerson, "Society and Medicine" (1936), in *Selected Papers of Haven Emerson* (Battle Creek, Mich.: W. K. Kellogg Foundation, 1949), 343–352.

74. Lewellys F. Barker, Harry H. Moore, and Watson Davis, "Can We Afford to Be Sick?" University of Chicago Press, Economics Series Presentation no. 17, radio broadcast, 1933.

75. C. Rufus Rorem, *Private Group Clinics,* report no. 8 (Washington, D.C.: CCMC, 1931), 11, 20, 26, 36, 47, 59, 71.

76. Rorem, *Private Group Clinics,* 19.

77. Lee, Jones, and Jones, *Fundamentals of Good Medical Care.* Calculated from data on 295.

78. Falk, Rorem, and Ring, *Costs of Medical Care,* 387–388.

79. Edward A. Filene, "Autocare versus Medical Care," *Journal of the American Medical Association* 93 (1929): 1247–1249.

80. Letter to Dr. Winslow from Evans Clark, September 1, 1931, Wilbur papers.

81. CCMC, *Medical Care for the American People,* 109–110, 120.

82. "Seven Major Questions," discussion paper for the Executive Committee meeting, April 12 and 13, 1931, 22–28, Wilbur papers.

83. Harry H. Moore, "Health and Medical Practice," in the President's Research Committee on Social Trends, *Recent Social Trends in the United States* (New York: McGraw-Hill, 1934), 1061–1113.

84. Lewis Webster Jones and Barbara Jones, "Medicine: Economic Organization," in Edwin R. A. Seligman, *Encyclopaedia of the Social Sciences* (New York: Macmillan, 1933), 9: 292–301.

85. David A. Pearson, "The Concept of Regionalized Personal Health Services in the United States, 1920–1955," in Ernest W. Saward, ed., *The Regionalization of Personal Health Services* (New York: Prodist, 1976), 3–51. Kerr White in discussion, 56.

86. Committee on the Costs of Medical Care, "Minority Report Number One," *Medical Care for the American People,* CCMC final report (Chicago: University of Chicago Press, 1932), 173.

87. Alphonse M. Schwitalla, "Basic Considerations in Minority Report of Committee on the Costs of Medical Care," *Journal of the American Medical Association* 100, no. 12 (1933): 863–867.

88. CCMC, "Minority Report Number One," 175.

89. C. Rufus Rorem, "Developments in Group Medical Practice," *American Journal of Public Health* 48, no. 8 (1958): 983–986.

90. James C. Robinson, "Physician-Hospital Integration and the Economic Theory of the Firm," *Medical Care Research and Review* 54, no. 1 (1997): 3–24.

91. CCMC, *Medical Care for the American People,* 112–113.

92. Paul Starr, *The Social Transformation of American Medicine* (New York: Basic Books, 1982), 161; Charles E. Rosenberg, *The Care of Strangers: The Rise of America's Hospital System* (New York: Basic Books, 1987), 238.

93. S. S. Goldwater, "The Hospital and the Surgeon," *Modern Hospital* 7 (1916): 371–377, in Edward T. Morman, ed., *Efficiency, Scientific Management, and Hospital Standardization: An Anthology of Sources* (New York: Garland, 1989), 252–258.

94. Lewellys F. Barker, "The Development of the Science of Diagnosis," *Journal of the South Carolina Medical Association* 12 (1916): 278–284.

95. Michael M. Davis and Edward Hartshorn, "A Self-Supporting Eye Clinic for Working People," *Archives of Ophthalmology* 43 (1914): 643–646.

96. Andrew R. Warner, "The Evening Pay Clinic," *Modern Hospital* 11 (1918): 143–145.

97. Lowell T. Coggeshall, "The Chicago Plan," in "Symposium on the Compensation of Faculties of Clinical Departments," *Journal of Medical Education* 31, no. 7 (1956): 476–481.

98. Michael M. Davis, *The Cornell Clinic, 1921–1924: Medical Service on a Self-Supporting Basis for Persons of Moderate Means* (New York: United Hospital Fund, 1925), 13, 36.

99. Michael Davis, *Hospitals and Dispensaries: Part 10* (Cleveland: Cleveland Hospital Council, 1920), 870.

100. Michael M. Davis and Andrew R. Warner, *Dispensaries: Their Management and Development* (New York: Macmillan, 1918), 330.

101. Ralph E. Pumphrey, "Michael M. Davis and the Development of the Health Care Movement, 1900–1928," *Societas* 2 (1972): 27–41.

102. Carpenter, *Patients of Moderate Means,* 21–25.

103. Davis and Rorem, *Crisis in Hospital Finance,* 175.

104. Ellen C. Potter, "Developing Standards of Accounting and Administration," *Modern Hospital* 26 (1926): 389–394.

105. Rosenwald, "Business Man's Point of View."

106. Stewart R. Roberts, "Comparison of Medical and Hospital Costs for Individuals in Moderate Circumstances," *Bulletin of the American College of Surgeons* 13, no. 4 (1929): 24–25.

107. CCMC, *Five-Year Program,* 13.

108. Carpenter, *Patients of Moderate Means,* 25, 44–45.

109. Davis and Rorem, *Crisis in Hospital Finance,* 129.

110. C. Rufus Rorem, "Accounting as a Science," *Journal of Accountancy* 48, no. 2 (1929): 87–98; C. Rufus Rorem, "Social Control through Accounts," *Accounting Review* 3, no. 3 (1928): 261–268.

111. Emerson, Rorem, and Reed, "Problem of Medical Care," 28.

112. Davis and Rorem, *Crisis in Hospital Finance,* 170.

113. Michael M. Davis, "Methods and Technical Problems of the Committee on the Costs of Medical Care," *American Statistical Association Journal* 28 (1933): 92–97.

114. Everett A. Johnson, Montague Brown, and Richard L. Johnson, *The Economic Era*

of Health Care: A Revolution in Organized Delivery Systems (San Francisco: Jossey-Bass, 1996), x.

115. Ray Lyman Wilbur, "Address of President Ray Lyman Wilbur," *Journal of the American Medical Association* 82, no. 24 (1924): 1968–1969.

Five Regional Health Planning

1. Thomas K. McCraw, *Prophets of Regulation* (Cambridge: Harvard University Press, 1984), 110.

2. David W. Noble, *The Progressive Mind, 1890–1917* (Chicago: Rand McNally, 1970), 152.

3. "Theodore Roosevelt on the New Nationalism," in Leon Fink, ed., *Major Problems in the Gilded Age and the Progressive Era* (Lexington, Mass.: D. C. Heath, 1993), 345–346; John Milton Cooper, "The New Nationalism versus the New Freedom," in Fink, *Major Problems in the Gilded Age,* 352–363.

4. Guy Alchon, *The Invisible Hand of Planning: Capitalism, Social Science, and the State in the 1920s* (Princeton: Princeton University Press, 1985), 10, 46, 67.

5. Samuel Haber, *Efficiency and Uplift: Scientific Management in the Progressive Era, 1890–1920* (Chicago: University of Chicago Press, 1964), 156–158.

6. Ellis W. Hawley, *The Great War and the Search for a Modern Order: A History of the American People and Their Institutions, 1917–1933* (New York: St. Martin's, 1979), 120, 201, 213.

7. William G. Scott, *Chester I. Barnard and the Guardians of the Managerial State* (Lawrence: University Press of Kansas, 1992), 5; David W. Eakins, "The Origins of Corporate Liberal Policy Research, 1916–1922: The Political-Economic Expert and the Decline of Public Debate," in Jerry Israel, ed., *Building the Organizational Society* (New York: Free Press, 1972), 163–179, 288–291; David F. Noble, *America by Design: Science, Technology, and the Rise of Corporate Capitalism* (Oxford: Oxford University Press, 1977), 61–65.

8. Allan G. Gruchy, "The Concept of National Planning in Institutional Economics," *Southern Economic Journal* 6, no. 2 (1939): 121–144; Wesley C. Mitchell, "The Social Sciences and National Planning" (1935), reprinted in Findlay Mackenzie, ed., *Planned Society: Yesterday, Today, Tomorrow* (New York: Prentice-Hall, 1937), 108–127; Wesley Clair Mitchell, "Intelligence and the Guidance of Economic Evolution," *Scientific Monthly* 43 (1936): 450–465.

9. Howard W. Odum and Harry Estill Moore, *American Regionalism: A Cultural-Historical Approach to National Integration* (New York: Henry Holt, 1938), 256. Authors were quoting L. S. Lorwin, "The Problem of Economic Planning," The Hague, World Economic Congress, 1931.

10. Eli Ginzberg, "The Many Meanings of Regionalization in Health," in Eli Ginzburg [*sic*], ed., *Regionalization and Health Policy* (Washington, D.C.: U.S. Department of Health, Education, and Welfare, 1977), 1–6; Daniel M. Fox, *Health Policies, Health Politics: The British and American Experience, 1911–1965* (Princeton: Princeton University Press, 1986), xi; Kevin Grumbach and Thomas Bodenheimer, "The Organization of Health Care," *JAMA* 273, no. 2 (1995): 160–167.

11. Abraham Flexner, *Medical Education in the United States and Canada* (New York: Carnegie Foundation for the Advancement of Teaching, 1910).

12. Philadelphia County Medical Society, Committee on Hospital Efficiency, *Reports* (1914), reprinted in Edward T. Morman, ed., *Efficiency, Scientific Management, and Hospital Standardization: An Anthology of Sources* (New York: Garland, 1989), 207–217.

13. Great Britain Ministry of Health, Consultative Council on Medical and Allied Services, *Interim Report on the Future Provision of Medical and Allied Services* (London: His Majesty's Stationery Office, 1920); David A. Pearson, "The Concept of Regionalized Personal Health Services in the United States, 1920–1955," in Ernest W. Saward, ed., *The Regionalization of Personal Health Services* (New York: Prodist, 1976), 3–51.

14. C. E. A. Winslow, "Public Health at the Crossroads," *American Journal of Public Health* 16, no. 11 (1926): 1075–1085.

15. Michael Davis, "Community Planning," in *Hospitals and Dispensaries: Part 10* (Cleveland: Cleveland Hospital Council, 1920), 966–972.

16. Haven Emerson and Gertrude E. Sturges, "Method of Making a Community Diagnosis," *Method of Survey: Part 11* (Cleveland: Cleveland Hospital Council, 1920), 1003–1017.

17. Davis, "Community Planning," 966–972; Michael M. Davis, "The Cleveland Hospital and Health Survey," *Modern Hospital* 15, no. 4 (1920): 306–307.

18. I. S. Falk, C. Rufus Rorem, and Martha D. Ring, *The Costs of Medical Care,* CCMC no. 27 (Chicago: University of Chicago Press, 1933), 344, 431, 589.

19. Joseph E. Garland, *An Experiment in Medicine: The First Twenty Years of the Pratt Clinic and the New England Center Hospital of Boston* (Cambridge: Riverside Press, 1960), 35, 81.

20. "Parran on Health and Hospitals in the Near Future," *Hospitals* 18, no. 8 (1944): 41.

21. C. Rufus Rorem, "Areawide Planning Is Here to Stay" (1964), in *A Quest for Certainty: Essays on Health Care Economics, 1930–1970* (Ann Arbor, Mich.: Health Administration Press, 1982), 163–168.

22. Kerr L. White, "Life and Death and Medicine," in *Life and Death and Medicine* (San Francisco: W. H. Freeman, 1973), 3–13.

23. Roger M. Battistella and Thomas P. Weil, "Comprehensive Health Care Planning," *New York State Journal of Medicine* 69, no. 17 (1969): 2350–2370; W. Shonick, *Elements of Planning for Area-Wide Personal Health Services* (St. Louis: C. V. Mosby, 1976), 77; Herbert Harvey Hyman, *Health Planning: A Systematic Approach* (Rockville, Md.: Aspen, 1982), 90.

24. E. Richard Weinerman, "The Regional Concept," from "Regionalization of Medical Services," in *Annual of the Western Branch* [of the American Public Health Association] (1949), reprinted in Committee on Medical Care Teaching of the Association of Teachers of Preventive Medicine, ed., *Readings in Medical Care* (Chapel Hill: University of North Carolina Press, 1958), 350–356.

25. Gary W. Shannon and G. E. Alan Dever, *Health Care Delivery: Spatial Perspectives* (New York: McGraw-Hill, 1974), 4–6, 10–14; Leslie Mayhew, *Urban Hospital Location* (London: Allen and Unwin, 1986).

26. Brian J. L. Berry, Edgar C. Conkling, and D. Michael Ray, *The Geography of Economic Systems* (Englewood Cliffs, N.J.: Prentice-Hall, 1976), 8.

27. John Friedmann, intro., "Regional Development and Planning," *Journal of the American Institute of Planners* 30, no. 2 (1964): 82–83.

28. John Friedmann, "Cities in Social Transformation," in John Friedmann and William Alonso, eds., *Regional Development and Planning: A Reader* (Cambridge, Mass.: MIT Press, 1964), 343–360; Jos. G. M. Hilhorst, *Regional Planning: A Systems Approach* (Rotterdam: Rotterdam University Press, 1971).

29. For a more detailed comparison of planning and managed competition, see Barbara Bridgman Perkins, "Re-Forming Medical Delivery Systems: Economic Organization and Dynamics of Regional Planning and Managed Competition," *Social Science and Medicine* 48, no. 2 (1999): 241–251.

30. Avedis Donabedian, "Models for Organizing the Delivery of Personal Health Services and Criteria for Evaluating Them," *Milbank Memorial Fund Quarterly* 50, no. 4, pt. 2 (1972): 103–154.

31. George P. Schultz, "The Logic of Health Care Facility Planning," *Socio-Economic Planning Sciences* 4 (1970): 383–393; George P. Schultz, "Facility Patterns for a Regional Health Care System" (MS, Regional Science Research Institute, Philadelphia, 1969); Thomas M. Stanback, "Regionalization of Professional Services: Private Sector Analogue," in Ginzburg [*sic*], ed., *Regionalization and Health Policy* 7–14; Gerald F. Pyle, *Applied Medical Geography* (Washington, D.C.: V. H. Winston and Sons, 1979).

32. Melinda S. Meade and Robert J. Earickson, *Medical Geography,* 2d ed. (New York: Guilford Press, 2000), 358.

33. C. Rufus Rorem, "Preface to the Reprint Edition," *Private Group Clinics* (New York: Milbank Memorial Fund, 1971), v–xi.

34. ALPHA Center for Health Planning, *A Guide for Improving Health System Capacity through Multi-Institutional Cooperation* (Bethesda, Md.: ALPHA Center for Health Planning, 1979).

35. U.S. Department of Health, Education, and Welfare, "National Health Priorities," *Papers on the National Health Guidelines: Conditions for Change in the Health Care System* (Hyattsville, Md.: Health Resources Administration, 1977), v.

36. Thomas C. Cochran, *The American Business System: A Historical Perspective, 1900–1955* (New York: Harper and Row, 1957), 34.

37. James O. Hepner, "Multihospital Systems: An Overview," in James O. Hepner, ed., *Health Planning for Emerging Multihospital Systems* (St. Louis: C. V. Mosby, 1978), 3–10; National Center for Health Services Research, *National Conference Monograph: Evaluating the Performance of Multi-Institutional Systems* (Hyattsville, Md.: National Center for Health Services Research, 1982).

38. U.S. House of Representatives, Committee on Interstate and Foreign Commerce, *A Discursive Dictionary of Health Care* (Washington, D.C.: U.S. Government Printing Office, 1976).

39. S. E. Berki, *Hospital Economics* (Lexington, Mass.: D. C. Heath, 1972), 115.

40. C. Rufus Rorem, *Capital Investment in Hospitals: The Place of "Fixed Charges" in Hospital Financing and Costs,* CCMC no. 7 (Washington, D.C.: CCMC, 1930), 32, 37; Elliott H. Pennell, Joseph W. Mountin, and Kay Pearson, "Business Census of Hospitals, 1935," *Public Health Reports,* supp. no. 154 (1939); Haven Emerson, *The Hospital Survey for New York* (New York: United Hospital Fund, 1937), 1:161, 167, 171–172; Duncan Neuhauser, "Hospital Size and Structure," in *Hospital Size and Efficiency* (Chicago: University of Chicago Graduate School of Business, 1966), 11–17.

41. Howard Larkin, "Finance: Old and Poor: Small Rurals on Financial Edge," *Hospitals* (November 20, 1988): 32, 34.

42. Sara McLafferty, "The Geographical Restructuring of Urban Hospitals: Spatial Dimensions of Corporate Strategy," *Social Science and Medicine* 23, no. 10 (1986): 1079–1086.

43. Roice D. Luke, Yasar A. Oxcan, and Peter C. Olden, "Local Markets and Systems: Hospital Consolidations in Metropolitan Areas," *HSR: Health Services Research* 30, no. 4 (1995): 555–575; Paul B. Ginsburg, "The Dynamics of Market-Level Change," *Journal of Health Politics, Policy and Law* 22, no. 2 (1997): 363–382; David Dranove and William D. White, *How Hospitals Survived: Competition and the American Hospital* (Washington, D.C.: AEI Press, 1999), 51–52.

44. Steven R. Hollis, "Strategic and Economic Factors in the Hospital Conversion Process," *Health Affairs* 16, no. 2 (1997): 131–143.

45. Stephen M. Shortell et al., *Remaking Health Care in America: The Evolution of Organized Delivery Systems* (San Francisco: Jossey-Bass, 2000), 25.

46. Everett A. Johnson, Montague Brown, and Richard L. Johnson, *The Economic Era of Health Care: A Revolution in Organized Delivery Systems* (San Francisco: Jossey-Bass, 1996), 38.

47. *New York Times,* December 21, 1938; Walton H. Hamilton and Horace R. Hansen, *The Labor-Health Venture and the Law* (New York: American Labor Health Association, 1959).

48. *New York Times,* August 1, 1938.

49. Walton H. Hamilton, "Competition," in Edwin R. A. Seligman, ed., *Encyclopaedia of the Social Sciences* (New York: Macmillan, 1937), 3:141–147. Hamilton was not particularly distinguishing regulated competition from regulated monopoly, however. He identified the "new industrial revolution" as "organized competition within and between great industries."

50. Rickey Hendricks, *A Model for National Health Care: The History of Kaiser Permanente* (New Brunswick: Rutgers University Press, 1993), 207.

51. Warren Winkelstein, "Is There an Alternative to the Comprehensive Approach to Health Care?" in *Papers on the National Health Guidelines,* 59–64; National Council on Health Planning and Development, *Productivity and Health* (Hyattsville, Md.: National Council on Health Planning and Development, 1980), 17–18.

52. John E. Kralewski and Roice D. Luke, "The Group Practice of Medicine: Some Implications for Health Planning," in *Papers on the National Health Guidelines: The Priorities of Section 1502* (Rockville, Md.: Health Services Administration, 1977), 45–55.

53. Paul M. Ellwood, "Models for Organizing Health Services and Implications of Legislative Proposals," *Milbank Memorial Fund Quarterly* 50, no. 4, pt. 2 (1972): 73–101.

54. Alain C. Enthoven, *Health Plan: The Only Practical Solution to the Soaring Cost of Medical Care* (Reading, Mass.: Addison-Wesley, 1980).

55. White House Domestic Policy Council, *The President's Health Security Plan* (New York: Times Books, 1993).

56. John D. Wilkerson, Kelly J. Devers, and Ruth S. Given, "The Emerging Competitive Managed Care Marketplace," in John D. Wilkerson, Kelly J. Devers, and Ruth S. Given, *Competitive Managed Care: The Emerging Health Care System* (San Francisco: Jossey-Bass, 1997), 3–29.

57. Samuel Levey et al., *The Rise of a University Teaching Hospital: A Leadership Perspective: The University of Iowa Hospitals and Clinics* (Chicago: Health Administration Press, 1996), 99–110. Unlike many other revenue-generating faculty practice plans, Iowa did not initially target private patients primarily but, instead, contracted with state government to provide clinical services for indigent patients residing throughout the state. I frequently use the University of Iowa as an example for the expedient reason that its leaders left a legacy of published books on its development.

58. Viscount Dawson, "Medicine and the Public Welfare," *Medical Care* 2, no. 4 (1942): 322–336. Ray Lyman Wilbur in invited comments.

59. Thomas Parran, *Statement before the Senate Subcommittee on Wartime Health and Education (July 12, 1944)* (Washington, D.C.: U.S. Government Printing Office, 1944), 1774–1791.

60. U.S. Senate, Subcommittee on Wartime Health and Education, *Interim Report from the Committee on Education and Labor* (Washington, D.C.: U.S. Government Printing Office, 1945), 14–15.

61. Joseph W. Mountin, Elliott H. Pennell, and Vane M. Hoge, *Health Service Areas: Requirements for General Hospitals and Health Centers,* Public Health Bulletin no. 292 (Washington, D.C.: U.S. Government Printing Office, 1945); Commission on Hospital Care, *Hospital Care in the United States* (New York: Commission on Hospital Care, 1947).

62. Subcommittee on Medical Care, "The Quality of Medical Care in a National Health Program," *American Journal of Public Health* 39, no. 7 (1949): 898–924.

63. "Symposium on the Compensation of Faculties of Clinical Departments," *Journal of Medical Education* 31, no. 7 (1956): 476–492.

64. John E. Deitrick and Robert C. Berson, *Medical Schools in the United States at Mid-Century* (New York: McGraw-Hill, 1953), 153–154.

65. "Report of the [AMA] Council on Medical Service: Private Practice by Medical School Faculty Members," in Augustus J. Carroll, *A Study of Medical College Costs* (Evanston, Ill.: Association of American Medical Colleges, 1958), 116–120.

66. E. Richard Weinerman, "Organization and Quality of Service in a National Health Program," *Yale Journal of Biology and Medicine* 44, no. 1 (1971): 133–152; E. Richard Weinerman, "Medical Schools and the Quality of Medical Care: A Survey of Recent Trends," *New England Journal of Medicine* 239, no. 22 (1948): 810–817; E. Richard Weinerman, "The Response of the University Medical Center to Social Demands," *Journal of Medical Education* 45, no. 11 (1970): 69–78.

67. Marie Callender, "Personal Health Services—as Defined and Organized by E. Richard Weinerman, M.D.," *Yale Journal of Biology and Medicine* 44, no. 1 (1971): 164–171.

68. E. Richard Weinerman, "Organization and Quality of Service in a National Health Program," *Yale Journal of Biology and Medicine* 44, no. 1 (1971): 133–152.

69. E. Richard Weinerman, "The Quality of Medical Care," in "Medical Care for Americans," *Annals of the American Academy of Political and Social Science* 273 (1951): 185–191.

70. E. Richard Weinerman, "Problems and Perspectives of Group Practice," *Bulletin of the New York Academy of Medicine* 44, no. 11 (1968): 1423–1434.

71. National Council on Health Planning and Development, *Productivity and Health.*

72. Stephen J. Williams and Paul R. Torrens, eds., *Introduction to Health Services* (New York: John Wiley, 1980), 330.

73. Gerald Katz, Abby Mitchell, and Elaine Markezin, intro., in Gerald Katz, Abby Mitchell, and Elaine Markezin, eds., *Ambulatory Care and Regionalization in Multi-Institutional Health Systems* (Rockville, Md.: Aspen, 1982), 3–8.

74. John H. Knowles, "Medical School, Teaching Hospital, and Social Responsibility," in John H. Knowles, ed., *The Teaching Hospital* (Cambridge: Harvard University Press, 1966), 84–145; John S. Millis, *A Rational Public Policy for Medical Education and Its Financing* (New York: National Fund for Medical Education, 1971), 96, 117.

75. Committee on Medical Schools and the AAMC in Relation to Training for Family Practice, "Planning for Comprehensive and Continuing Care of Patients through Education," *Journal of Medical Education* 43, no. 6 (1968): 751–759.

76. William C. Keettel, *A History of the Department of Obstetrics and Gynecology: The University of Iowa, 1848–1980* (Iowa City: University of Iowa Press, 1981), 109–111; Samuel Levey et al., *Rise of a University Teaching Hospital*, 245, 288, 342, 351.

77. John R. Evans, "Organizational Patterns for New Responsibilities," *Journal of Medical Education* 45, no. 12 (1970): 988–999.

78. Kenneth M. Ludmerer, *Time to Heal: American Medical Education from the Turn of the Century to the Era of Managed Care* (New York: Oxford University Press, 1999), 166–167.

79. R. Glenn Hubbard, *Medical School Financing and Research* (Washington, D.C.: American Enterprise Institute for Public Policy Research, 1998), table 1. This figure had grown from 6 percent in 1960 and 1965.

80. Edmund D. Pellegrino, "The Regionalization of Academic Medicine: The Metamorphosis of a Concept," *Journal of Medical Education* 48, no. 2 (1973): 119–133.

81. Charles Perrow, "Markets, Hierarchies and Hegemony" (1981), in Thomas K. McCraw, ed., *The Essential Alfred Chandler: Essays Toward a Historical Theory of Big Business* (Boston: Harvard Business School Press, 1988), 432–447.

82. Robert Earickson, *The Spatial Behavior of Hospital Patients* (Chicago: University of Chicago Department of Geography Research Paper no. 124, 1970).

83. Pellegrino, "Regionalization of Academic Medicine," 119–133.

84. Harold S. Luft, John P. Bunker, and Alain C. Enthoven, "Should Operations Be Regionalized? The Empirical Relation between Surgical Volume and Mortality," *New England Journal of Medicine* 301, no. 25 (1979): 1364–1369.

85. Association of American Medical Colleges, *AAMC Data Book* (Washington, D.C.: Association of American Medical Colleges, 2000), table G9.

86. Thomas C. Ricketts et al., *Geographic Methods for Health Services Research* (Lanham, Md.: University Press of America, 1994), 195.

87. Jerome H. Grossman, "Conference Summary: Vertical Integration and the Future of Academic Health Centers," in *Vertical Integration in Health Care: Implications for Medical Education and Practice* (Orlando: American Medical Association Conference, 1986), 203–216.

88. William L. Dowling, "Strategic Alliances as a Structure for Integrated Delivery Systems," in Arnold D. Kaluzny, Howard S. Zuckerman, and Thomas C. Ricketts, eds., *Partners for the Dance: Forming Strategic Alliances in Health Care* (Ann Arbor, Mich.: Health Administration Press, 1995), 139–175; Douglas A. Conrad and

Stephen M. Shortell, "Integrated Health Systems: Promise and Performance," *Frontiers of Health Services Management* 13, no. 1 (1996): 3–40.

89. W. Richard Scott et al., *Institutional Change and Healthcare Organizations: From Professional Dominance to Managed Care* (Chicago: University of Chicago Press, 2000), 265.

90. Kelly J. Devers et al., "Implementing Organized Delivery Systems: An Integration Scorecard," *Health Care Management Review* 19, no. 3 (1994): 7–20.

91. Roice D. Luke, "Spatial Competition and Cooperation in Local Hospital Markets," *Medical Care Review* 48, no. 2 (1991): 207–237; Roice D. Luke, "Local Hospital Systems: Forerunners of Regional Systems?" *Frontiers of Health Services Management* 9, no. 2 (1992): 3–51.

92. Sam J. W. Romeo, "Faculty Practice Plans," in William F. Minogue, ed., *Managing in an Academic Health Care Environment* (Tampa: American College of Physician Executives, 1992), 21–27; Mark C. Rogers, Ralph Snyderman, and Elizabeth L. Rogers, "Sounding Board: Cultural and Organizational Implications of Academic Managed-Care Networks," *New England Journal of Medicine* 331, no. 20 (1994): 1374–1377.

93. James D. Bentley et al., "Faculty Practice Plans: The Organization and Characteristics of Academic Medical Practice," *Academic Medicine* 66, no. 8 (1991): 433–439; Walter A. Zelman, *The Changing Health Care Marketplace: Private Ventures, Public Interests* (San Francisco: Jossey-Bass, 1996), 284–286; Lawrence D. Devoe, "Facing the Next Millennium of Managed Health Care: Can Academic Maternal-Fetal Medicine Programs Survive?" *Seminars in Perinatology* 21, no. 6 (1997): 472–478.

94. Ralph Snyderman, "Model for a 21st Century Academic Health System," in *Conference: The Academic Health Center in the 21st Century,* <http://cfm.mc.duke.edu/chair/pcc/public/ahc/duke.htm>, accessed 9/3/01, 1996.

95. David Blumenthal and Gregg S. Meyer, "Academic Health Centers in a Changing Environment," *Health Affairs* 15, no. 2 (1996): 200–215.

96. James C. Robinson, "Academic Medical Centers and the Economics of Innovation in Health Care," in Henry J. Aaron, ed., *The Future of Academic Medical Centers* (Washington, D.C.: Brookings Institution Press, 2001), 49–74.

97. W. K. Kellogg Foundation, *Hospital Resources and Needs: Report of the Michigan Hospital Survey* (Battle Creek, Mich.: W. K. Kellogg Foundation, 1946); Frank G. Dickinson and Charles E. Bradley, *Medical Service Areas: Population, Square Miles and Primary Centers* (Chicago: American Medical Association, 1951).

98. Vicente Navarro, *National and Regional Health Planning in Sweden* (Rockville, Md.: U.S. Department of Health, Education, and Welfare, 1974); R. G. Bevan and A. H. Spencer, "Models of Resource Policy of Regional Health Authorities," in M. Clarke, ed., *Planning and Analysis in Health Care Systems* (London: Pion, 1984), 90–118.

99. Robert E. Dickinson, *City and Region: A Geographical Interpretation* (London: Routledge and Kegan Paul, 1964), 212; Neil Smith, "Deindustrialization and Regionalization: Class Alliance and Class Struggle," *Papers of the Regional Science Association* 54 (1984): 113–128.

100. ALPHA Center for Health Planning, *Guide for Improving Health System Capacity,* 26–27.

101. Philip N. Reeves and Russell C. Coile, *Introduction to Health Planning* (Arlington, Va.: Information Resources Press, 1989), 190.

102. David D. Rutstein, *Blueprint for Medical Care* (Cambridge, Mass.: MIT Press, 1974); Robert H. Ebert, ed., *The Financing of Medical Schools in an Era of Health Care Reform* (New York: Josiah Macy Jr. Foundation, 1995), 16.

103. Donald C. Harrison, John J. Hutton, and J. Randolph Hilliard, "Funding for the Colleges of Medicine: Integrated Delivery Systems to the Rescue," *Transactions of the American Clinical and Climatological Association* 107 (1995): 238–248; John E. Billi et al., "Potential Effects of Managed Care on Specialty Practice at a University Medical Center," *New England Journal of Medicine* 333, no. 15 (1995): 979–983.

104. David D. Rutstein, "At the Turn of the Next Century," in John H. Knowles, ed., *Hospitals, Doctors, and the Public Interest* (Cambridge: Harvard University Press, 1965), 293–317.

105. Reeves and Coile, *Introduction to Health Planning,* 129.

106. Karen Davis, "Regionalization and National Health Insurance," in Ginzburg [*sic*], *Regionalization and Health Policy,* 178–187.

107. Health Policy Advisory Center, "Medical Empires: Who Controls?" *Health PAC Bulletin* 6 (November–December 1968).

108. Richard Kronick et al., "The Marketplace in Health Care Reform: The Demographic Limitations of Managed Competition," *New England Journal of Medicine* 328, no. 2 (1993): 148–152.

109. Stephen M. Shortell and Kathleen E. Hull, "The New Organization of the Health Care Delivery System," in Stuart H. Altman and Uwe E. Reinhardt, eds., *Strategic Choices for a Changing Health Care System* (Chicago: Health Administration Press, 1996), 102–148.

110. Herbert E. Klarman, "Planning for Facilities," in Ginzburg [*sic*], *Regionalization and Health Policy,* 25–36; Louis Tannen, "Health Planning as a Regulatory Strategy: A Discussion of its History and Current Uses," *International Journal of Health Services* 10, no. 1 (1980): 115–132.

111. Arthur Young and Co., *Methods for Setting Priorities in Areawide Health Care Planning* (Washington, D.C.: U.S. Department of Health, Education, and Welfare, 1978); Booz-Allen and Hamilton, *Financial Analysis Workbook* (San Francisco: Western Center for Health Planning, n.d. [1979?]); Institute for Health Planning, *Improving Operations Management: Lessons from Multihospital Systems* (Hyattsville, Md.: Prepared for Bureau of Health Planning, 1982), 16; Victor G. Rodwin, *The Health Planning Predicament: France, Quebec, England, and the United States* (Berkeley: University of California Press, 1984).

112. Henrik L. Blum, *Expanding Health Care Horizons: From a General Systems Concept of Health to a National Health Policy* (Oakland, Calif.: Third Party Associates, 1978), 69, 92. Presaging managed competition, Blum also advised that it would be preferable to have more than one integrated system per region in order to offer consumer choice.

113. Many chapters in Alan Sheldon, Frank Baker, and Curtis P. McLaughlin, eds., *Systems and Medical Care* (Cambridge, Mass.: MIT Press, 1970).

114. Leahmae McCoy, "The Medical School as Coordinator of Health Services," *Journal of Medical Education* 46 (1971): 134–141.

115. William T. Butler, "Academic Medicine's Season of Accountability and Social Responsibility," *Academic Medicine* 67, no. 2 (1992): 68–73.

116. Michael R. Pollard, "Fostering Competition in Health Care," in Arthur Levin, ed., *Regulating Health Care: The Struggle for Control* (New York: Academy of Political

Science, 1980), 158–167; U.S. Department of Health and Human Services, *Research on Competition in the Financing and Delivery of Health Services: Future Research Needs* (Hyattsville, Md.: National Center for Health Services Research, 1982).

117. James A. Morone, *The Democratic Wish: Popular Participation and the Limits of American Government* (New York: Basic Books, 1990), 265–285.

118. J. Randall Evans, *Linkages between Planning, Regulation, and Rate Setting in New Jersey: The Case of a Perinatal Care Center Designation* (Boston: Harvard Center for Community Health and Medical Care, 1978), 79.

119. Paul J. Feldstein, "The Political Environment of Regulation," in Levin, *Regulating Health Care,* 6–20.

120. Bruce Spitz, "Community Control in a World of Regional Delivery Systems," *Journal of Health Politics, Policy and Law* 22, no. 4 (1997): 1021–1050.

121. Robert G. Evans, "Going for the Gold: The Redistributive Agenda behind Market-based Health Care Reform," *Journal of Health Politics, Policy and Law* 22, no. 2 (1997): 427–465.

122. Western Center for Health Planning, *Coalition Building with Major Purchasers: The Golden Empire Experience* (San Francisco: Western Center for Health Planning, 1981).

123. Meade and Earickson, *Medical Geography,* 368–369.

124. Evan M. Melhado, "Competition versus Regulation in American Health Policy," in Evan M. Melhado, Walter Fineberg, and Harold M. Swartz, eds., *Money, Power, and Health Care* (Ann Arbor, Mich.: Health Administration Press, 1988), 15–101.

125. Enthoven, *Health Plan,* 42.

126. U.S. General Accounting Office, *Health Care Alliances: Issues Relating to Geographic Boundaries* (Washington, D.C.: U.S. General Accounting Office, 1994), 6.

127. Thomas P. Weil, "Close to a Bull's Eye—A Concurring Opinion," *Health Care Management Review* 20, no. 2 (1995): 35–44.

128. Jeremiah Hurley, Stephen Birch, and John Eyles, "Geographically-Decentralized Planning and Management in Health Care: Some Informational Issues and Their Implications for Efficiency," *Social Science and Medicine* 41, no. 1 (1995): 3–11; Organisation for Economic Co-operation and Development, *Health Care Reform: The Will to Change* (Paris: Organisation for Economic Co-operation and Development, 1996), 14, 38.

129. Chris Ham, Judith Smith, and John Temple, *Hubs, Spokes and Policy Cycles* (London: King's Fund, 1998), 16–17.

130. Weinerman, "Quality of Medical Care," 185–191; Garland, *Experiment in Medicine,* 84.

Six Perinatal Regionalization

1. Joyce A. Martin et al., "Births: Final Data for 2000," *National Vital Statistics Reports* 50, no. 5 (2002): table 1; Warren H. Pearse, "Doctors and Patients in Obstetrics and Gynecology: The Next 15 Years," *American Journal of Obstetrics and Gynecology* 125, no. 3 (1976): 361–367; American College of Obstetricians and Gynecologists (ACOG), "Comparison of ACOG Fellowship with AMA Physician Data," Tab A, *Manpower Planning in Obstetrics and Gynecology;* Manpower data set sent every Health Systems Agency, various dates. ACOG figures are not entirely consistent from year to year; in addition, ACOG fellow figures are considerably lower

in earlier years than the number of physicians identifying themselves to the AMA as specialists in obstetrics and gynecology.

2. Quoted in "Doctors, Hospitals, and the Declining Birthrate," *Contemporary Ob/Gyn* 2, no. 4 (1973): 30–32, 37–39.

3. American Medical Association, *Areawide Planning: Report of the First National Conference on Areawide Health Facilities Planning* (Chicago: American Medical Association, 1965), 82, 100–112.

4. Duncan E. Reid, "To Everything There Is a Season," *Obstetrics and Gynecology* 30, no. 2 (1967): 269–280.

5. American College of Obstetricians and Gynecologists, Committee on Maternal Health, *National Study of Maternity Care: Survey of Obstetric Practice and Associated Services in Hospitals in the United States* (Chicago: American College of Obstetricians and Gynecologists, 1970), 7.

6. American Medical Association House of Delegates, "Recommendations on White House Conference on Children" and "Centralized Community or Regionalized Perinatal Intensive Care," in American Medical Association Committee on Maternal and Child Care, *Action Guide for Maternal and Child Care Committees* (Chicago: American Medical Association, 1974), 71, 73; H. Belton P. Meyer, "Regional Care for Mothers and Their Infants," *Clinics in Perinatology* 7, no. 1 (1980): 205–221.

7. Committee on Perinatal Health, *Toward Improving the Outcome of Pregnancy* (White Plains, N.Y.: National Foundation-March of Dimes, 1976).

8. L. Joseph Butterfield, "Organization of Regional Perinatal Programs," *Seminars in Perinatology* 1, no. 3 (1977): 217–233; L. Joseph Butterfield, "Historical Perspectives of Neonatal Transport," *Pediatric Clinics of North America* 40, no. 2 (1993): 221–239. The two sources differ on the quantity of reports issued.

9. U.S. Department of Health, Education, and Welfare, *National Guidelines for Health Planning* (Washington, D.C.: U.S. Department of Health, Education, and Welfare, 1978), 7–8.

10. Areawide and Local Planning for Health Action, *ALPHA Regional Plan for Obstetric and Pediatric Hospital Services* (Syracuse, N.Y.: Areawide and Local Planning for Health Action, 1975); Medical Service Consultants, *Criteria and Standards Monograph for Review of Obstetrics/Gynecology Inpatient Services* (Arlington, Va.: Medical Service Consultants, n.d. [1976?]).

11. David E. Gagnon and Sherry Allison-Cooke, "Adaptations to Perinatal Regionalization," in Robert A. Knuppel and Joan E. Drukker, eds., *High-Risk Pregnancy: A Team Approach* (Philadelphia: W. B. Saunders, 1993), 47–61.

12. March of Dimes Birth Defects Foundation, *Toward Improving the Outcome of Pregnancy: The 90s and Beyond* (Wilkes-Barre, Pa.: March of Dimes Birth Defects Foundation, 1993).

13. American Academy of Pediatrics and American College of Obstetricians and Gynecologists, *Guidelines for Perinatal Care,* 4th ed. (Elk Grove Village, Ill.: American Academy of Pediatrics, and Washington, D.C.: American College of Obstetricians and Gynecologists, 1997), xvii.

14. American Academy of Pediatrics and American College of Obstetricians and Gynecologists, *Guidelines for Perinatal Care* (Evanston, Ill.: American Academy of Pediatrics, and Washington, D.C.: American College of Obstetricians and Gynecologists, 1983), 1.

15. Gary Pettett, Sally Sewell, and Gerald B. Merenstein, "Regionalization and Transport in Perinatal Care," in Gerald B. Merenstein and Sandra L. Gardner, eds., *Handbook of Neonatal Intensive Care,* 4th ed. (St. Louis: Mosby, 1998), 30–45.

16. American College of Obstetricians and Gynecologists, *National Study of Maternity Care: Survey of Obstetric Practice and Associated Services in Hospitals in the United States* (Chicago: American College of Obstetricians and Gynecologists, 1970).

17. Massachusetts Department of Public Health, "New Regulations for Newborn Services," *New England Journal of Medicine* 286, no. 25 (1972): 1363–1364.

18. American Academy of Pediatrics and American College of Obstetricians and Gynecologists, *Guidelines for Perinatal Care* (1983 ed.), 37.

19. National Perinatal Information Center, *A Study of the Impact of Recent Developments in the Health Care Environment on Perinatal Regionalization* (Providence, R.I.: National Perinatal Information Center, n.d. [1988?]), 2–13.

20. Association of American Medical Colleges, *AAMC Data Book* (Washington, D.C.: Association of American Medical Colleges, 1996), table G9, data for 1993.

21. Mark W. Tomlinson et al., "Change in Health Care Delivery: A Threat to Academic Obstetrics," *American Journal of Obstetrics and Gynecology* 173, no. 5 (1995): 1614–1616.

22. March of Dimes Birth Defects Foundation, *Toward Improving the Outcome of Pregnancy: The 90s and Beyond,* 34, 103.

23. Earl Siegel et al., "A Controlled Evaluation of Rural Regional Perinatal Care: Impact on Mortality and Morbidity," *American Journal of Public Health* 75, no. 3 (1985): 246–253; Marie C. McCormick, Sam Shapiro, and Barbara H. Starfield, "The Regionalization of Perinatal Services: Summary of the Evaluation of a National Demonstration Program," *JAMA* 253, no. 6 (1985): 799–804.

24. March of Dimes Birth Defects Foundation, *Toward Improving the Outcome of Pregnancy: The 90s and Beyond,* ix, 1.

25. J. Randall Evans, *Linkages between Planning, Regulation and Rate Setting in New Jersey: The Case of a Perinatal Care Center Designation* (Boston: Harvard Center for Community Health and Medical Care, 1978), 70, 79, 99.

26. Lucy Candib, "Obstetrics in Family Practice: A Personal and Political Perspective," *Journal of Family Practice* 3, no. 4 (1976): 391–396.

27. American Academy of Pediatrics and American College of Obstetricians and Gynecologists, *Guidelines for Perinatal Care,* 2d ed. (Elk Grove Village, Ill.: American Academy of Pediatrics; and Washington, D.C.: American College of Obstetricians and Gynecologists, 1988), 61.

28. Calvin J. Hobel, "Better Perinatal Health," *Lancet* 1, no. 8158 (1980): 31–33.

29. National Perinatal Information Center, *The Perinatal Partnership: An Approach to Organizing Care in the 1990's* (Providence, R.I.: National Perinatal Information Center, n.d. [1989?]), 7.

30. Douglas K. Richardson et al., "Perinatal Regionalization versus Hospital Competition: The Hartford Example," *Pediatrics* 96, no. 3 (1995): 417–423.

31. Irwin R. Merkatz and Kenneth G. Johnson, "Regionalization of Perinatal Care for the United States," *Clinics in Perinatology* 3, no. 2 (1976): 271–276.

32. Calvin J. Hobel, "Risk Assessment in Perinatal Medicine," *Clinical Obstetrics and Gynecology* 21, no. 2 (1978): 287–295.

33. U.S. Congress, Office of Technology Assessment, *Neonatal Intensive Care for Low Birthweight Infants* (Washington, D.C.: Office of Technology Assessment, 1987).

34. James D. Bentley et al., "Faculty Practice Plans: The Organization and Characteristics of Academic Medical Practice," *Academic Medicine* 66, no. 8 (1991): 433–439.

35. California Office of Statewide Planning and Development, *Aggregate Financial Data for California: Reports Ending 6/30/91 to 6/29/92* (Sacramento: Office of Statewide Planning and Development, 1993), table 8.3.

36. Peter P. Budetti et al., *A Study of the Perinatal Care Resources of Hospitals in Alameda and Contra Costa Counties, California* (San Francisco: Institute for Health Policy Studies, 1982).

37. U.S. Department of Health and Human Services, *Vital Statistics of the United States 1988,* vol. 2: *Mortality Part B* (Hyattsville, Md.: Department of Health and Human Services, 1990); Coalition to Fight Infant Mortality, *The Report of the Community Investigation of Alameda County's High Infant Mortality Rate* (Oakland, Calif.: Coalition to Fight Infant Mortality, n.d. [1980?]); California State Department of Consumer Affairs, *Pregnant Women and Newborn Infants in California: A Deepening Crisis in Health Care* (Sacramento, Calif.: Department of Consumer Affairs, 1982).

38. Murray Milner, *Unequal Care: A Case Study of Interorganizational Relations in Health Care* (New York: Columbia University Press, 1980).

39. Arthur W. Jones and Francesca K. Thomas, *Report of the Hospital Survey for New York* (New York: United Hospital Fund, 1938), 3:932, 943.

40. L. E. Weeks, ed., *C. RUFUS ROREM in First Person: An Oral History* (Chicago: American Hospital Association, 1983).

41. E. H. L. Corwin, *Infant and Maternal Care in New York City: A Study of Hospital Facilities* (New York: Columbia University Press, 1952), 64, 102, 104, 135.

42. John D. Thompson and Robert B. Fetter, "The Economics of the Maternity Service," *Yale Journal of Biology and Medicine* 36, no. 1 (1963): 91–103.

43. Hospital Review and Planning Council of Southern New York, *Guidelines and Recommendations for the Planning and Use of Obstetrical Facilities in Southern New York* (New York: Hospital Review and Planning Council of Southern New York, 1966), i; C. Rufus Rorem and Marvin D. Roth, "Need Every Hospital Offer an Obstetric Service?" *Hospitals* 40, no. 24 (1966): 50–52, 126.

44. American College of Obstetricians and Gynecologists, *Standards for Obstetric-Gynecologic Services* (Chicago: American College of Obstetricians and Gynecologists, 1974), 17.

45. Committee on Perinatal Health, *Toward Improving the Outcome of Pregnancy,* 2, 22.

46. Health, Education, and Welfare, *National Guidelines for Health Planning,* 51–52.

47. Daniel F. O'Keeffe and Jay Mayes, "Managed Obstetrical Care," *Clinical Obstetrics and Gynecology* 40, no. 2 (1997): 414–419.

48. Robinson C. Trowbridge, "Services, Revenue, Occupancy Increased by OB Merger," *Hospital Topics* 44, no. 10 (1966): 105; Irwin Goldberg and C. R. Youngquist, "Two Hospitals, One Obstetric Service," *Hospitals* 40, no. 24 (1966): 53–56.

49. American College of Obstetricians and Gynecologists, *National Needs in Obstetrics and Gynecology: 1971* (Chicago: American College of Obstetricians and Gynecologists, 1971).

50. Ross Laboratories, *Regionalization of Perinatal Care* (Columbus, Ohio: Ross Laboratories, 1974), 39–40.

51. "Doctors, Hospitals, and the Declining Birthrate," *Contemporary Ob/Gyn* 2, no. 4 (1973): 30–32, 37–39.

52. Boston University Center for Health Planning, *Consolidation of Maternity Services* (Boston: Boston University Center for Health Planning, 1977), 1.

53. Health Planning Council for Greater Boston, *Appropriateness Review Report: Maternity Services* (Boston: Health Planning Council for Greater Boston, 1981), viii–4.

54. Nancy M. Kane, "The Financial Health of Academic Medical Centers: An Elusive Subject," in Henry J. Aaron, ed., *The Future of Academic Medical Centers* (Washington, D.C.: Brookings Institution Press, 2001), 13–47. Quote seems to be editor's summary of Kane's comments.

55. American College of Obstetricians and Gynecologists, *National Study of Maternity Care,* 5.

56. Leonard J. Nelson and Janet M. Bronstein, "Medical Malpractice and Access to Obstetrical Care in Alabama," *Alabama Medicine* 60, no. 12 (1991): 14–23. Twenty-two percent of the obstetrics services closed.

57. California Office of Statewide Health Planning and Development, *Licensed Services and Utilization Profiles: Annual Report of Hospitals, 1990* (Sacramento, Calif.: Office of Statewide Health Planning and Development, 1991). Calculated from data provided.

58. American College of Obstetricians and Gynecologists, *National Study of Maternity Care;* Association of American Medical Colleges, *AAMC Data Book* (1996). Figures cited are reported by different sources and are not strictly comparable.

59. Robert Wood Johnson Foundation, *Special Report: Regionalized Perinatal Services* (Princeton, N.J.: Robert Wood Johnson Foundation, 1978), 5.

60. Ronald L. Williams, *Vital Record Data for Use in the Planning of Perinatal Health Services* (Sacramento: California Department of Health Services, 1980), 40.

61. Douglas K. Richardson et al., "Birth Weight and Illness Severity: Independent Predictors of Neonatal Mortality," *Pediatrics* 91, no. 5 (1993): 969–975.

62. U.S. Congress, Office of Technology Assessment, *The Quality of Medical Care: Information for Consumers* (Washington, D.C.: Office of Technology Assessment, 1988), 167–172.

63. More evidence for this conclusion is provided in Barbara Bridgman Perkins, "Rethinking Perinatal Policy: History and Evaluation of Minimum Volume and Level-of-Care Standards," *Journal of Public Health Policy* 14, no. 3 (1993): 299–319.

64. American Academy of Pediatrics and American College of Obstetricians and Gynecologists, *Guidelines for Perinatal Care* (1983 ed.), 1.

65. Metropolitan Council of the Twin Cities Area, *Consumer's Guide to Hospital Specialty Services: Twin Cities Metropolitan Area, 1984* (St. Paul, Minn.: Metropolitan Council of the Twin Cities Area, 1984).

66. National Perinatal Information Center, *Perinatal Partnership,* 8.

67. Ciaran S. Phibbs et al., "The Effects of Patient Volume and Level of Care at the Hospital of Birth on Neonatal Mortality," *JAMA* 276, no. 13 (1996): 1054–1059.

68. Marie C. McCormick and Douglas K. Richardson, "Access to Neonatal Intensive Care," *Future of Children: Low Birth Weight* 5, no. 1 (1995): 162–175.

69. Boston University Center for Health Planning, *Consolidation of Maternity Services;* Executive Programs in Health Policy and Management, *Planning Peri-Natal Services in Lewiston (A)* (Boston: Harvard School of Public Health, n.d. [late 1970s]).

70. John D. Thompson and Robert B. Fetter, "The Economics of the Maternity Service," *Yale Journal of Biology and Medicine* 36, no. 1 (1963): 91–103.

71. Teh-Wei Hu, "Hospital Costs and Pricing Behavior: The Maternity Ward," *Inquiry* 8, no. 4 (1971): 19–26; Ronald L. Williams, "Using CHFC [California Health Facilities Commission] Data to Understand the Variation in Hospital Maternity Costs," paper presented at the Second Annual Symposium Utilizing Commission Data in Health Planning, 1979.

72. Herman A. Hein and Norma N. Fergusun, "The Cost of Maternity Care in Rural Hospitals," *JAMA* 240, no. 19 (1978): 2051–2052; David Baron, "The Economics of Hospital Obstetrics Care," *Journal of Economics and Business* 30 (1977–1978): 98–107. The five studies used different ways of measuring cost.

73. Douglas Richardson, Arnold Rosoff, and Joseph P. McMenamin, "Referral Practices and Health Care Costs: The Dilemma of High Risk Obstetrics," *Journal of Legal Medicine* 6, no. 4 (1985): 427–464.

74. Gary W. Shannon and G. E. Alan Dever, *Health Care Delivery: Spatial Perspectives* (New York: McGraw-Hill, 1974), 18.

75. Cited in Frederick D. Mott and Milton I. Roemer, *Rural Health and Medical Care* (New York: McGraw-Hill, 1948), 499.

76. Commission on Hospital Care, *Hospital Care in the United States* (New York: Commonwealth Fund, 1947).

77. Special Study Committee, "Obstetrics in Northern Alameda County," sec. II-B (Joint BACHP [Bay Area Comprehensive Health Planning Council] / ACCHPC [Alameda County Comprehensive Health Planning Council], 1976), 29, 32.

78. Committee on Maternal and Child Care, *Action Guide for Maternal and Child Care Committees,* 1.

79. East Bay Perinatal Project, *East Bay Regional Perinatal Plan* (Berkeley: East Bay Perinatal Project, 1980).

80. American Academy of Pediatrics and American College of Obstetricians and Gynecologists, *Guidelines for Perinatal Care* (1983 ed.), 6.

81. National Perinatal Information Center, *Perinatal Partnership,* 8, 11.

82. March of Dimes Birth Defects Foundation, *Toward Improving the Outcome of Pregnancy: The 90s and Beyond,* 19–21, 93–95.

83. Robert J. Sokol, "Joint University and Private Hospital Models," *American Journal of Perinatology* 6 supp. (1989): 24–27.

84. O'Keeffe and Mayes, "Managed Obstetrical Care," 414–419.

85. Kenneth Krieg, "Obstetrics/Gynecology Network Development," *Clinical Obstetrics and Gynecology* 40, no. 2 (1997): 446–452.

86. National Perinatal Information Center, *Perinatal Partnership,* 6.

87. Keith P. Russell, Sprague H. Gardiner, and Ervin E. Nichols, "A Conceptual Model for Regionalization and Consolidation of Obstetric-Gynecologic Services," *American Journal of Obstetrics and Gynecology* 121, no. 6 (1975): 756–762; Herman A. Hein, "The Status and Future of Small Maternity Services in Iowa," *JAMA* 255, no. 14 (1985): 1899–1903; Roger A. Rosenblatt et al., "Outcomes of Regionalized Perinatal Care in Washington State," *Western Journal of Medicine* 149, no. 1 (1988): 98–102.

88. California Medical Association, *Goals for Regionalized Perinatal Care* (California Medical Association, n.d. [1976?]).

89. Gary S. Berger, Dennis B. Gillings, and Earl E. Siegel, "The Evaluation of Regionalized Perinatal Health Care Programs," *American Journal of Obstetrics and Gynecology* 125, no. 7 (1976): 924–932.

90. R. R. Nugent, K. B. Surles, and J. L. Rhyne, *Perinatal Regionalization and Concomitant Changes in Perinatal Mortality Rates: North Carolina, the Decade of the Seventies* (Division of Health Services, 1981). Level III utilization was up from 21 percent in 1969–1973, and level I was down from 35 percent.

91. Paul G. Tomich and Craig L. Anderson, "Analysis of a Maternal Transport Service within a Perinatal Region," *American Journal of Perinatology* 7, no. 1 (1990): 13–17; John M. Thorp et al., "Establishing Maternal-Fetal Medicine Consultative Services in Western North Carolina (Perinatal Region 1)," *North Carolina Medical Journal* 51, no. 6 (1990): 266–267; M. Karen Campbell et al., "Is Perinatal Care in Southwestern Ontario Regionalized?" *CMAJ: Canadian Medical Association Journal* 144, no. 3 (1991): 305–312; Susan Borker et al., "Interhospital Referral of High-Risk Newborns in a Rural Regional Perinatal Program," *Journal of Perinatology* 10, no. 2 (1990): 156–163; Leandro Cordero and Frederick Zuspan, "Very Low–Birth Weight Infants: Five Years Experience of a Regional Perinatal Program," *OHIO Medicine* 84, no. 12 (1988): 976–978; William F. Powers, Patricia D. Hegwood, and Young S. Kim, "Perinatal Regionalization as Measured by Antenatal Referral," *Obstetrics and Gynecology* 71, no. 3, pt. 1 (1988): 375–379; Jennifer A. Mayfield et al., "The Relation of Obstetrical Volume and Nursery Level to Perinatal Mortality," *American Journal of Public Health* 80, no. 7 (1990): 819–823; Herman A. Hein and S. S. Lathrop, "The Changing Pattern of Neonatal Mortality in a Regionalized System of Perinatal Care," *American Journal of Diseases of Children* 140 (1986): 989–993; L. Joseph Butterfield, "Newborn Country USA," *Clinics in Perinatology* 3, no. 2 (1976): 281–295; Watson A. Bowes, "A Review of Perinatal Mortality in Colorado, 1971 to 1978, and Its Relationship to the Regionalization of Perinatal Services," *American Journal of Obstetrics and Gynecology* 141, no. 8 (1981): 1045–1052; Thomas A. Hulsey et al., "Regionalized Perinatal Care in South Carolina," *Journal of the South Carolina Medical Association* 85, no. 8 (1989): 357–384; Congress of the United States, Office of Technology Assessment, *Neonatal Intensive Care for Low Birthweight Infants: Costs and Effectiveness* (Washington, D.C.: Office of Technology Assessment, 1987); Nugent, Surles, and Rhyne, *Perinatal Regionalization and Concomitant Changes in Perinatal Mortality Rates;* Nigel Paneth et al., "The Choice of Place of Delivery: Effect of Hospital Level on Mortality in All Singleton Births in New York City," *American Journal of Diseases of Children* 141, no. 1 (1987): 60–64; Alan D. Stiles et al., "Characteristics of Neonatal Intensive Care Unit Patients in North Carolina: A Cross-Sectional Survey," *Pediatrics* 87, no. 6 (1991): 904–908; August L. Jung and Nan Sherman Streeter, "Total Population Estimate of Newborn Special-Care Bed Needs," *Pediatrics* 75, no. 6 (1985): 993–996; Linda F. Samson, "Predicting the Marginal Cost of Direct Nursing Care for Newborns," *Journal of Nursing Administration* 21, no. 3 (1991): 42–47.

92. Sanjeev Mehta et al., "Differential Markers for Regionalization," *Journal of Perinatology* 20 (2000): 366–372.

93. Herman A. Hein, "Evaluation of a Rural Perinatal Care System," *Pediatrics* 66 (1980): 540–546.

94. Same set of notes as ratios of hospitals in level I, II, and III (note 91), plus Richard R. Nugent, "Perinatal Regionalization in North Carolina, 1967–1979: Services, Programs, Referral Patterns, and Perinatal Mortality Rate Declines for Very Low Birthweight Infants," *North Carolina Medical Journal* 43, no. 7 (1982): 513–515; Ronald L. Williams and Roger Wroblewski, *1984–1988 Maternal and Child Health Data Base: Descriptive Narrative* (Santa Barbara, Calif.: Community and Organization Research Institute, 1991); Sharon L. Dooley, Sally A. Freels, and Bernard J. Turnock, "Quality Assessment of Perinatal Regionalization by Multivariate Analysis: Illinois, 1991–1993," *Obstetrics and Gynecology* 89, no. 2 (1997): 193–198; John D. Yeast et al., "Changing Patterns in Regionalization of Perinatal Care and the Impact on Neonatal Mortality," *American Journal of Obstetrics and Gynecology* 178, no. 1, pt. 1 (1998): 131–135.

95. Susan E. Gerber, Deborah G. Dobrez, and Peter P. Budetti, "Managed Care and Perinatal Regionalization in Washington State," *Obstetrics and Gynecology* 98, no. 1 (2001): 139–143.

96. Michelle M. Bode et al., "Perinatal Regionalization and Neonatal Mortality in North Carolina, 1968–1994," *American Journal of Obstetrics and Gynecology* 184, no. 6 (2001): 1302–1307.

97. Mike Janko, Data and Information Business Group, American Hospital Association, Chicago, personal communication, February 12, 1997. AHA statistics for 1995: Hospitals self-identifying as level I: 1614 units, 829,162 births; level II: 1093 units and 1,442,189 births; level III: 358 units and 1,022,863 births. In addition, 863 hospitals with bassinets collectively reported 612,024 births, and 1691 births were reported by hospitals with no bassinets. Twenty-one percent of total U.S. hospital births occurred in hospitals reporting level I units; adding to this the hospitals reporting bassinets and births but not reporting levels, the total is 37 percent. A different way of defining levels by their services and staffing capacity judged that 45 percent of births in 1988 occurred in level I, 23 percent in level II, and 32 percent in level III hospitals. Rachel M. Schwartz et al., "Use of High-Technology Care among Women with High-Risk Pregnancies in the United States," *Maternal and Child Health Journal* 4, no. 1 (2000): 7–18.

98. Ronald L. Williams et al., *1982–86 Maternal and Child Health Data Base* (Santa Barbara, Calif., Community and Organization Research Institute, 1990). Calculated from data provided. Levels of care designated by the California Maternal and Child Health Branch. In 1986, 74 percent of level IIIs were located in subcounty health facility planning areas with higher than the state mean expected perinatal mortality rate and with more than one thousand births, but, of the level IIs, 85 percent were located in areas below the mean expected perinatal mortality rate.

99. David C. Goodman et al., "Are Neonatal Intensive Care Resources Located According to Need? Regional Variation in Neonatologists, Beds, and Low Birth Weight Newborns," *Pediatrics* 108, no. 2 (2001): 426–431.

100. Institute of Medicine, National Research Council, *Research Issues in the Assessment of Birth Settings* (Washington, D.C.: National Academy Press, 1982).

101. Comprehensive Health Planning Association of Imperial, Riverside, and San Diego Counties, *Report of the High Risk Maternal and Newborn Study* (San Diego: Comprehensive Health Planning Association of Imperial, Riverside, and San Diego Counties, 1973). Calculated from data provided.

102. Paul R. Swyer and James W. Goodwin, eds., *Regional Services in Reproductive Medi-*

cine (Joint Committee of the Society of Obstetricians and Gynaecologists of Canada and the Canadian Paediatric Society, n.d. [1973?]).

103. John Stallworthy, "The Development of a Regional Maternity Service," *American Journal of Obstetrics and Gynecology* 109, no. 2 (1971): 285–291.

104. "Comments of the British Paediatric Association on the Proposal for Minimum Standards in Neonatal Care," in *South Western Regional Perinatal Survey, 1980–1982,* vol. 1: *The Report with Appendices* (Bristol: British Paediatric Association, n.d.), app. L.

105. Miranda Mugford and John Stilwell, "Maternity Services: How Well Have They Done and Could They Do Better?" in A. Harrison and J. Gretton, eds., *Health Care UK 1986* (Cambridge: Burlington Press, 1986), 53–64.

106. South East Thames Regional Health Authority, *Strategies and Guidelines for the Development of Obstetric Services* (Croydon: South East Thames Regional Health Authority, 1978), 8, 12.

107. North West Thames Regional Health Authority, *Report of Regional Working Party on Obstetric and Neonatal Services* (London: North West Thames Regional Health Authority, 1980), 28; North West Thames Regional Health Authority, Regional Working Party on Obsteric [*sic*] and Neonatal Services, *Report of Obstetricians* (London: North West Thames Regional Health Authority, 1980), 3, 14–17, 41, 51, 56–57; North West Thames Regional Health Authority, *Regional Strategy: Towards a Strategy for Maternity and Neo-natal Services* (London: North West Thames Regional Health Authority, 1984).

108. Alison MacFarlane et al., *Birth Counts: Statistics of Pregnancy and Childbirth,* vol. 2: *Tables* (London: Stationery Office, 2000), 455.

109. "What Future for Small Obstetric Units?" *Lancet* 2, no. 8452 (1985): 423–424.

110. Christine Hogg, *Centering Excellence? National and Regional Health Services in London* (London: King's Fund, 1992), 51.

111. Lindsay A. Thompson, David C. Goodman, and George A. Little, "Is More Neonatal Intensive Care Always Better? Insights from a Cross-national Comparison of Reproductive Care," *Pediatrics* 109, no. 6 (2002): 1036–1043.

Seven   Competing for the Birth Market

1. Howard C. Taylor, ed., *The Recruitment of Talent for a Medical Specialty* (St. Louis: C. V. Mosby, 1961), 52–53, 130, 141, 158. Taylor also attributed his specialty's poor showing in the competition for research funding to its "talent" problem. The term was a euphemism for the fact that the majority of ob-gyn residents came from the bottom third of their medical school classes.

2. Harold A. Kaminetzky, "The Effects of Litigation on Perinatal Practice," *Perinatal Practice and Malpractice Symposium* (New York: Academy Professional Information Services, 1984), 43–46.

3. W. Benson Harer, "Gender Bias in Health Care Services Valuations," *Obstetrics and Gynecology* 87, no. 3 (1996): 453–454.

4. Robert P. Lorenz, Robert J. Sokol, and Lawrence Chik, "Survey of Maternal-Fetal Medicine Subspecialists: Professional Activities, Job Setting, and Satisfaction," *Obstetrics and Gynecology* 74, no. 6 (1989): 962–966.

5. Robert C. Mendenhall, *Obstetrics/Gynecology Practice Study Report* (Hyattsville, Md.: U.S. Department of Health, Education, and Welfare, 1977); Ira M. Rutkow, "Ob-

stetric and Gynecologic Operations in the United States, 1979 to 1984," *Obstetrics and Gynecology* 67, no. 6 (1986): 755–759. Workload studies found that three-quarters of ob-gyn patient encounters entailed no problem or only a minimal one.

6. Geraldine McCord, "Enlargening the Market for Perinatal Procedures," in "Reconsidering the 'Market Model' in Obstetrics: Part II," *Birth* 12, no. 1 (1985): 40.

7. David A. Grimes, "Declining Surgical Case-Load of the Obstetrician-Gynecologist," *Obstetrics and Gynecology* 67, no. 6 (1986): 760–762.

8. Center for Health Policy Research, *Socioeconomic Characteristics of Medical Practice, 1986* (Chicago: American Medical Association, 1986), tables 11, 18.

9. U.S. Department of Health and Human Services, National Center for Health Statistics, *Vital and Health Statistics: National Hospital Discharge Survey: Annual Summary, 1994* 13, no. 128 (1997): table E. These data exclude procedures performed on newborn infants. Cardiac catheterization was number two.

10. U.S. Department of Health and Human Services, National Center for Health Statistics, *Vital and Health Statistics: National Ambulatory Medical Care Survey: 1993 Summary* 13, no. 136 (1998): tables C, D.

11. Peter Cherouny and Colleen Nadolski, "Underreimbursement of Obstetric and Gynecologic Invasive Services by the Resource-based Relative Value Scale," *Obstetrics and Gynecology* 87, no. 3 (1996): 328–331.

12. Ervin E. Nichols, "The Status of Obstetrics," in *The Roles of Family Practice, Internal Medicine, Obstetrics and Gynecology and Pediatrics in Providing Primary Care,* 73d Ross Conference on Pediatric Research (Columbus, Ohio: Ross Laboratories, 1977), 29–32.

13. Alan Guttmacher Institute, *Blessed Events and the Bottom Line: Financing Maternity Care in the United States* (New York: Alan Guttmacher Institute, 1987), 34; James W. Fossett et al., "Medicaid in the Inner City: The Case of Maternity Care in Chicago," *Milbank Quarterly* 68, no. 1 (1990): 111–141.

14. Edmond J. Graves, "Expected Principal Source of Payment for Hospital Discharges: United States, 1990," *Advance Data* 220 (1992). Private health insurance covered 54 percent of pregnant women in 1990.

15. Guttmacher Institute, *Blessed Events and the Bottom Line,* 46.

16. Walter L. Larimore and Barry S. Sapolsky, "Maternity Care in Family Medicine: Economics and Malpractice," *Journal of Family Practice* 40, no. 2 (1995): 153–160.

17. Task Force on Quality Health Care, *Quality Assurance in Obstetrics and Gynecology* (Washington, D.C.: American College of Obstetricians and Gynecologists, n.d. [1981?]), 37–41.

18. Barry D. Weiss, "Special Series: Hospital Privileges for Family Physicians," *Family Medicine* 25, no. 9 (1993): 562.

19. Jane Krieger, "Family Practice Privileges: An Update," *Family Medicine* 25, no. 9 (1993): 568–569.

20. William MacMillan Rodney, "Letters from the Front: Testimony on Behalf of OB Privileges for Family Physicians," *Family Medicine* 25, no. 9 (1993): 563–565.

21. Walter L. Larimore and James L. Reynolds, "Family Practice Maternity Care in America: Ruminations on Reproducing an Endangered Species—Family Physicians Who Deliver Babies," *Journal of the American Board of Family Practice* 7, no. 6 (1994): 478–488.

22. Thomas C. Rosenthal, David M. Holden, and Willow Woodward, "Primary Care

Obstetrics in Rural Western New York: A Multi-Center Case Review," *New York State Journal of Medicine* 90, no. 11 (1990): 537–540; Mark E. Deutchman, DeAnna Sills, and Pamela D. Connor, "Perinatal Outcomes: A Comparison between Family Physicians and Obstetricians," *Journal of the American Board of Family Practice* 8, no. 6 (1995): 440–447; William J. Hueston et al., "Practice Variations between Family Physicians and Obstetricians in the Management of Low-Risk Pregnancies," *Journal of Family Practice* 40, no. 4 (1995): 345–351.

23. American Academy of Family Physicians, *Facts about Family Practice* (Leawood, Kans.: American Academy of Family Physicians, 2000), tables 63–69.

24. Joseph E. Scherger et al., "Teaching Family-Centered Perinatal Care in Family Medicine, Part 1," *Family Medicine* 24, no. 4 (1992): 288–298; Walter L. Larimore, "Family-Centered Birthing: A Niche for Family Physicians," *American Family Physician* 47 (1993): 1365–1366.

25. H. Belton P. Meyer, "Regional Care for Mothers and Their Infants," *Clinics in Perinatology* 7, no. 1 (1980): 205–221.

26. Interprofessional Task Force on Health Care of Women and Children, *Joint Position Statement on the Development of Family-Centered Maternity/Newborn Care in Hospitals* (Chicago: Interprofessional Task Force on Health Care of Women and Children, 1978), 7.

27. Lewin and Associates, *Competition among Health Practitioners: The Influence of the Medical Profession on the Health Manpower Market,* vol. 2: *The Childbearing Center Case Study* (Washington, D.C.: Lewin and Associates, 1981), 9–10.

28. Howard C. Taylor, "Objectives and Principles in the Training of the Obstetrician-Gynecologist: Training for Surgical Virtuosity and Versatility or for Public Service," *American Journal of Surgery* 110, no. 1 (1965): 35–42.

29. Duncan E. Reid, "To Everything There Is a Season," *Obstetrics and Gynecology* 30, no. 2 (1967): 269–280.

30. American College of Obstetricians and Gynecologists, "National Needs in Obstetrics and Gynecology—1971" (Chicago: American College of Obstetricians and Gynecologists, 1971).

31. R. Clay Burchell et al., "Collaborative Practice in Obstetrics/Gynecology: Implications for Cost, Quality, and Productivity," *American Journal of Obstetrics and Gynecology* 144, no. 6 (1982): 621–625.

32. Phyllis A. Langton, "Obstetricians' Resistance to Independent, Private Practice by Nurse-Midwives in Washington, D.C., Hospitals," *Women and Health* 22, no. 1 (1994): 27–48.

33. Judith Pence Rooks, *Midwifery and Childbirth in America* (Philadelphia: Temple University Press, 1997), 196, 210. Rooks cited ACOG's 1995 *Guidelines for Implementing Collaborative Practice.*

34. Sara Rosenbaum, "Nurse Midwives and Care of the Poor," in Judith Rooks and J. Eugene Haas, eds., *Nurse-Midwifery in America* (Washington, D.C.: American College of Nurse Midwives Foundation, 1986), 54–56; Lawrence D. Platt et al., "Nurse-Midwifery in a Large Teaching Hospital," *Obstetrics and Gynecology* 66, no. 6 (1985): 816–820.

35. Cynthia P. Dickinson, Debra J. Jackson, and William H. Swartz, "Making the Alternative Mainstream: Maintaining a Family-Centered Focus in a Large Freestanding Birth Center for Low-Income Women," *Journal of Nurse-Midwifery* 39, no. 2

(1994): 112–118; Thomas J. Garite et al., "Development and Experience of a University-Based, Freestanding Birthing Center," *Obstetrics and Gynecology* 86, no. 3 (1995): 411–416.

36. Langton, "Obstetricians' Resistance to Independent Private Practice," 27–48.

37. Sandra Howell-White, *Birth Alternatives: How Women Select Childbirth Care* (Westport, Conn.: Greenwood Press, 1999), 124.

38. Deanne R. Williams, "Credentialing Certified Nurse-Midwives," *Journal of Nurse-Midwifery* 39, no. 4 (1994): 258–264.

39. Frances Mayes et al., "A Retrospective Comparison of Certified Nurse-Midwife and Physician Management of Low Risk Births," *Journal of Nurse-Midwifery* 32, no. 4 (1987): 216–221.

40. Julian N. Robinson et al., "Predictors of Episiotomy Use at First Spontaneous Vaginal Delivery," *Obstetrics and Gynecology* 96, no. 2 (2000): 214–218.

41. Roger A. Rosenblatt et al., "Interspecialty Differences in the Obstetric Care of Low-Risk Women," *American Journal of Public Health* 87, no. 3 (1997): 344–351.

42. Rooks, *Midwifery and Childbirth in America,* chaps. 10 and 11.

43. Murray Enkin et al., "Effective Care in Pregnancy and Childbirth: A Synopsis," *Birth* 28, no. 1 (2001): 41–51.

44. Charles Krauthammer, "A Lack of Maternal Instinct," *Manchester Guardian Weekly,* June 2, 1996, 16.

45. J. D. Kleinke, *Bleeding Edge: The Business of Health Care in the New Century* (Gaithersburg, Md.: Aspen, 1998), 251.

46. Committee on Assessing Alternative Birth Settings, *Research Issues in the Assessment of Birth Settings* (Washington, D.C.: National Academy Press, 1982).

47. Shirley Mayer, in U.S. House of Representatives, Committee on Interstate and Foreign Commerce, "Maternal and Child Health Care Act—1976" (Washington, D.C.: U.S. Government Printing Office, 1976).

48. Gigliola Baruffi et al., "A Study of Pregnancy Outcomes in a Maternity Center and a Tertiary Care Hospital," *American Journal of Public Health* 74, no. 9 (1984): 973–978; Anne Scupholme et al., "A Birth Center Affiliated with the Tertiary Care Center: Comparison of Outcome," *Obstetrics and Gynecology* 67, no. 4 (1986): 598–603; Leah L. Albers and Vern L. Katz, "Birth Setting for Low-Risk Pregnancies: An Analysis of the Current Literature," *Journal of Nurse-Midwifery* 36, no. 4 (1991): 215–220.

49. Ricki Rusting, "Safe Passage? Study Fuels Debate over Safety of Birth Centers," *Scientific American* 262 (1990): 36.

50. John L. Kiely et al., "Fetal Death during Labor: An Epidemiologic Indicator of Level of Obstetrical Care," *American Journal of Obstetrics and Gynecology* 153, no. 7 (1985): 721–727.

51. Elizabeth Feldman and Marsha Hurst, "Outcomes and Procedures in Low Risk Birth: A Comparison of Hospital and Birth Center Settings," *Birth* 14, no. 1 (1987): 18–24.

52. Judith P. Rooks, Norman L. Weatherby, and Eunice K. M. Ernst, "The National Birth Center Study: Part II—Intrapartum and Immediate Postpartum and Neonatal Care," *Journal of Nurse-Midwifery* 37, no. 5 (1992): 301–330.

53. Women's Institute for Childbearing Policy, *Childbearing Policy within a National Health Program: An Evolving Consensus for New Directions* (Roxbury, Vt.: Women's Institute for Childbearing Policy, 1994), 38–39.

54. Kathleen F. Miller, "Birth of a Business," *Puget Sound Business Journal* (November 3–9, 2000): 37.

55. Alice Allgaier, "Alternative Birth Centers Offer Family-Centered Care," *Hospitals* 52, no. 24 (1978): 97–112; Dorma Kohler, Danny N. Bellenger, and Gordon E. Whyte, "The Role of Birthing Centers in Hospital Marketing," *Health Care Management Review* 15, no. 3 (1990): 71–77.

56. Kathe B. Dobbs and Kirkwood K. Shy, "Alternative Birth Rooms and Birth Options," *Obstetrics and Gynecology* 58, no. 5 (1981): 626–630.

57. American Academy of Pediatrics and American College of Obstetricians and Gynecologists, *Guidelines for Perinatal Care* (Evanston, Ill.: American Academy of Pediatrics; and Washington, D.C.: American College of Obstetricians and Gynecologists, 1983), 59.

58. Pamela S. Eakins and Gary A. Richwald, *Free-Standing Birth Centers in California: Structure, Cost, Medical Outcome and Issues* (Stanford: Stanford University Institute for Research on Women and Gender, 1986), 36.

59. Patricia Benner and Judith Wrubel, *The Primacy of Caring* (Menlo Park, Calif.: Addison-Wesley, 1989), 400.

60. Dorothy C. Wertz and Pamela S. Eakins, "A Note on the Future of American Birth," in Pamela S. Eakins, ed., *The American Way of Birth* (Philadelphia: Temple University Press, 1986), 331–337.

61. Lola Jean Kozak and Julie Dawson Weeks, "U.S. Trends in Obstetric Procedures, 1990–2000," *Birth* 29, no. 3 (2002): 157–161.

62. Colin Francome and Peter J. Huntingford, "Births by Caesarean Section in the United States of America and in Britain," *Journal of Biosocial Science* 12 (1980): 353–362.

63. Jean Comaroff, "Conflicting Paradigms of Pregnancy: Managing Ambiguity in Ante-Natal Encounters," in Alan Davis and Gordon Horobin, eds., *Medical Encounters: The Experience of Illness and Treatment* (New York: St. Martins, 1977), 115–134; Hilary Graham and Ann Oakley, "Competing Ideologies of Reproduction: Medical and Maternal Perspectives on Pregnancy," in Helen Roberts, ed., *Women, Health and Reproduction* (London: Routledge and Kegan Paul, 1981), 50–74; Robbie E. Davis-Floyd, *Birth as an American Rite of Passage* (Berkeley: University of California Press, 1992), chaps. 2 and 4.

64. Pamela S. Summey and Marsha Hurst, "Ob/Gyn on the Rise; The Evolution of Professional Ideology in the Twentieth Century—Part II," *Women and Health* 11, no. 2 (1986): 103–122.

65. Barbara K. Rothman, quoted in Judith Ann Carveth, "Conceptual Models in Nurse-Midwifery," *Journal of Nurse-Midwifery* 32, no. 1 (1987): 20–25.

66. Wayne R. Cohen, "Influence of the Duration of Second Stage Labor on Perinatal Out-come and Puerperal Morbidity," *Obstetrics and Gynecology* 49, no. 3 (1977): 266–269.

67. J. Selwyn Crawford, "The Stages and Phases of Labour: An Outworn Nomenclature That Invites Hazard," *Lancet* 2, no. 8344 (1983): 271–272; J. Selwyn Crawford, "The Phases and Stages of Labour," *British Journal of Hospital Medicine* 34, no. 1 (1985): 32–36.

68. Michelle Harrison, *A Woman in Residence* (Harmondsworth, U.K.: Penguin, 1982), 227.

69. Carol Sakala, "Midwifery Care and Out-of-Hospital Birth Settings: How Do They Reduce Unnecessary Cesarean Section Births?" *Social Science and Medicine* 37, no. 10 (1993): 1233–1250.

70. American Hospital Association Resource Center, *Examples of Monitoring and Evaluation in Obstetrics and Gynecology* (Chicago: American Hospital Association 1988), 18.

71. Richard W. Walker, "Obstetrical Risk Management: Establishing Documents of Defense," *Texas Medicine* 86 (June 1990): 32–38.

72. Barbara Bridgman Perkins, "Intensity, Stratification, and Risk in Perinatal Care: Redefining Problems and Restructuring Levels," *Women and Health* 21, no. 1 (1994): 17–31. I am not charging a lack of "objectivity" but pointing out that systemic structure as well as our positions in it shape the perceptions of us all.

73. Cited in Mary M. Lay, *The Rhetoric of Midwifery: Gender, Knowledge, and Power* (New Brunswick: Rutgers University Press, 2000), 87, 90.

74. Jimmie W. Westberg, Dayton Clark, and Gilbert A. Webb, "An Evaluation of High Risk Maternity Care in a Community Hospital," *American Journal of Obstetrics and Gynecology* 116, no. 4 (1973): 557–563.

75. Walter L. Larimore and Matthew K. Cline, "Keeping Normal Labor Normal," *Primary Care* 27, no. 1 (2000): 221–236.

76. Frederick M. Ettner, "Hospital Technology Breeds Pathology," *Women and Health* 2, no. 2 (1977): 17–23.

77. Bonnie B. O'Connor, "The Home Birth Movement in the United States," *Journal of Medicine and Philosophy* 18 (1993): 147–174.

78. Carol Shepherd McClain, "Perceived Risk and Choice of Childbirth Service," *Social Science and Medicine* 17, no. 23 (1983): 1857–1865.

79. Thomas H. Strong, *Expecting Trouble: The Myth of Prenatal Care in America* (New York: New York University Press, 2000), 129.

80. *New York Times,* November 13, 1988, front page.

81. Daniel F. O'Keeffe and Jay Mayes, "Managed Obstetrical Care," *Clinical Obstetrics and Gynecology* 40, no. 2 (1997): 414–419.

82. K. K. Barker, "A Ship upon a Stormy Sea: The Medicalization of Pregnancy," *Social Science and Medicine* 47, no. 8 (1998): 1067–1076.

83. Kathryn Strother Ratcliff, "Health Technologies for Women: Whose Health? Whose Technology?" in Katherine Strother Ratcliff et al., eds., *Healing Technology: Feminist Perspectives* (Ann Arbor: University of Michigan Press, 1989), 173–198.

84. Jan Williams, "The Controlling Power of Childbirth in Britain," in Hilary Marland and Anne Marie Rafferty, eds., *Midwives, Society and Childbirth: Debates and Controversies in the Modern Period* (London: Routledge, 1997), 232–247.

85. Karen D. Bonar, Andrew M. Kaunitz, and Luis Sanchez-Ramos, "The Effect of Obstetric Resident Gender on Forceps Delivery Rate," *American Journal of Obstetrics and Gynecology* 182, no. 5 (2000): 1050–1051.

86. Carol S. Weisman, *Women's Health Care: Activist Traditions and Institutional Change* (Baltimore: Johns Hopkins University Press, 1998), 146.

87. Catherine Kohler Riessman and Constance A. Nathanson, "The Management of Reproduction: Social Construction of Risk and Responsibility," in Linda H. Aiken and David Mechanic, eds., *Applications of Social Science to Clinical Medicine and Health Policy* (New Brunswick: Rutgers University Press, 1986), 251–281.

88. Joann Kovacich, "The Medical Profession and the Medicalization of Society," in

Frank N. Magill, ed., *Survey of Social Science: Sociology Series* (Pasadena, Calif.: Salem Press, 1994), 1159–1165.

89. U.S. Department of Health and Human Services, *Vital and Health Statistics: Trends in Hospital Utilization: United States, 1988–92* 13, no. 124 (1996): table 28. In 1980: 1.26 million procedures, 64.7 percent of all male newborns; in 1992: 1.17 million procedures, 60.7 percent of male newborns.

90. *American Journal of Public Health* 88, no. 2 (1998): 171.

91. Lewis F. McLean et al., "The Present-Day Safety of Cesarean Section," *American Journal of Obstetrics and Gynecology* 60, no. 4 (1950): 860–865; Madeleine M. Donnelly, "Cesarean Sections: A Five-year Statewide Survey in Iowa, 1949–53," *Obstetrics and Gynecology* 7, no. 4 (1956): 412–417.

92. Robert H. Fagan, "Maternal and Infant Mortality," *Western Journal of Surgery* 59 (1951): 324–329.

93. Sally C. Curtin and Lola Jean Kozak, "Decline in U.S. Cesarean Delivery Rate Appears to Stall," *Birth* 25, no. 4 (1998): 259–262.

94. John T. Queenan, "Editorial: The C/S Rate: Out of Sight, but Not Out of Mind," *Contemporary Ob/Gyn* 28, no. 4 (1986): 7–8; Public Citizen Health Research Group, *Unnecessary Cesarean Sections: How to Cure a National Epidemic* (Washington, D.C.: Public Citizen Health Research Group, 1989).

95. Kozak and Weeks, "U.S. Trends in Obstetric Practice," 157–161.

96. U.S. General Accounting Office, *A Review of Research Literature and Federal Involvement Relating to Selected Obstetric Practices* (Washington, D.C.: General Accounting Office, 1979), 70.

97. U.S. Department of Health and Human Services, *Cesarean Childbirth: Report of a Consensus Development Conference* (Bethesda, Md.: National Institutes of Health, 1981), 23.

98. James K. Quigley, "A Ten-Year Study of Cesarean Section in Rochester and Monroe County, 1937 to 1946," *American Journal of Obstetrics and Gynecology* 58, no. 1 (1949): 41–53; R. Gordon Douglas and Robert Landesman, "Recent Trends in Cesarean Section," *American Journal of Obstetrics and Gynecology* 59, no. 1 (1950): 96–107.

99. Warren H. Pearse, "To Section or Not to Section," *American Journal of Public Health* 73, no. 8 (1983): 843–844.

100. Benjamin P. Sachs, "Is the Rising Rate of Cesarean Sections a Result of More Defensive Medicine?" in Committee to Study Medical Professional Liability and the Delivery of Obstetrical Care, *Medical Professional Liability and the Delivery of Obstetrical Care* (Washington, D.C.: National Academy Press, 1989), 2:27–40.

101. Helen I. Marieskind, *An Evaluation of Caesarean Section in the United States* (Washington, D.C.: U.S. Department of Health, Education, and Welfare, 1979), 3.

102. George B. Feldman and Jennie A. Freiman, "Prophylactic Cesarean Section at Term?" *New England Journal of Medicine* 312, no. 19 (1985): 1264–1267.

103. Warren H. Pearse, "Professional Liability: Epidemiology and Demography," *Clinical Obstetrics and Gynecology* 31, no. 1 (1988): 148–152.

104. Opinion Research Corporation, *Professional Liability and its Effects: Report of a 1987 Survey of ACOG's Membership* (Washington, D.C.: American College of Obstetricians and Gynecologists, 1988). Calculated from data in tables 26, 32.

105. Laura-Mae Baldwin et al., "Defensive Medicine and Obstetrics," *JAMA* 274, no. 20

(1995): 1606–1610; Lisa Dubay, Robert Kaestner, and Timothy Waidmann, "The Impact of Malpractice Fears on Cesarean Section Rates," *Journal of Health Economics* 18, no. 4 (1999): 491–522.

106. Roger A. Rosenblatt and Barbara Detering, "Changing Patterns of Obstetric Practice in Washington State: The Impact of Tort Reform," *Family Medicine* 20, no. 2 (1988): 101–107.

107. Dana Hughes et al., "Obstetrical Care for Low-Income Women: The Effects of Medical Malpractice on Community Health Centers," in Committee to Study Medical Professional Liability and the Delivery of Obstetrical Care, *Medical Professional Liability,* 2:59–77.

108. David A. Richardson, Mark I. Evans, and Luis A. Cibils, "Midforceps Delivery: A Critical Review," *American Journal of Obstetrics and Gynecology* 145, no. 5 (1983): 621–632.

109. Russell E. Mardon, Kimberly D. Shafer, and Scott A. Hinton, "Cesarean Deliveries in Florida: Current Trends and Related Factors," *Journal of Florida Medical Association* 84, no. 5 (1997): 310–315.

110. Haider H. Shamsi, Roy H. Petrie, and Charles M. Steer, "Changing Obstetric Practices and Amelioration of Perinatal Outcome in a University Hospital," *American Journal of Obstetrics and Gynecology* 133, no. 8 (1979): 855–858.

111. Paul J. Placek and Selma M. Taffel, "Recent Patterns in Cesarean Delivery in the United States," *Obstetrics and Gynecology Clinics of North America* 15, no. 4 (1988): 607–627.

112. Community and Organization Research Institute, "1970–1977 California Vital Record Data for HSA 11 by Hospital of Birth" (MS, Community and Organization Research Institute, Santa Barbara, n.d.); Community and Organization Research Institute, *1984–1988 Maternal and Child Health Data Base: Statistical Appendix* (Santa Barbara, Calif.: Community and Organization Research Institute, 1991), 360, 370.

113. "Rates of Cesarean Delivery—United States, 1993," *Morbidity and Mortality Weekly Report* 44, no. 15 (1995): 303–307.

114. American College of Obstetricians and Gynecologists, *Standards for Obstetric-Gynecologic Services,* 5th ed. (Washington, D.C.: American College of Obstetricians and Gynecologists, 1982), 23.

115. American Academy of Pediatrics and American College of Obstetricians and Gynecologists, *Guidelines for Perinatal Care,* 2d ed. (Elk Grove Village, Ill.: American Academy of Pediatrics; and Washington, D.C.: American College of Obstetricians and Gynecologists, 1988), 71.

116. Michael S. Kinsella et al., "Cesarean Section Urgency-Use Clinical Definitions," *BMJ* 323, no. 7318 (2001): 931.

117. U.S. Department of Health and Human Services, National Center for Health Services Research, *Who Receives Cesareans: Patient and Hospital Characteristics* (Rockville, Md.: National Center for Health Services Research, 1984).

118. Albert Haverkamp in U.S. Senate, Committee on Human Resources, *Obstetrical Practices in the United States, 1978* (Washington, D.C.: U.S. Government Printing Office, 1978), 58–59.

119. David A. Miller and Richard H. Paul, "Cesarean Section for Fetal Distress," in Bruce L. Flamm and Edward J. Quilligan, eds., *Cesarean Section: Guidelines for Appropriate Utilization* (New York: Springer-Verlag, 1995), 95–114.

120. Paul J. Placek and Selma M. Taffel, "Trends in Cesarean Section Rates for the United States, 1970–78," *Public Health Reports* 95, no. 6 (1980): 540–548.

121. New York State Department of Health, *Cesarean Childbirth in New York State* (New York State Department of Health, 1987), fig. 19.

122. Randall S. Stafford, "Cesarean Section Use and Source of Payment: An Analysis of California Hospital Discharge Abstracts," *American Journal of Public Health* 80, no. 3 (1990): 313–315.

123. S. B. Thacker and D. F. Stroup, "Continuous Electronic Fetal Heart Monitoring during Labor," in J. P. Neilson et al., eds., *Pregnancy and Childbirth Module of the Cochrane Database of Systematic Reviews* (Oxford: Cochrane Collaboration, Issue 4, Update Software, updated September 1, 1997).

124. Bruce L. Flamm, intro., in Flamm and Quilligan, eds., *Cesarean Section,* xv–xvi.

125. A. Dale Tussing and Martha A. Wojtowycz, "The Cesarean Decision in New York State, 1986: Economic and Non-Economic Aspects," *Medical Care* 30, no. 6 (1992): 529–540; Laura B. Gardner, "Economic Considerations in Cesarean Section Use," in Flamm and Quilligan, eds., *Cesarean Section,* 173–190.

126. Jonathan Gruber and Maria Owings, *Physician Financial Incentives and Cesarean Section Delivery* (Cambridge, Mass.: National Bureau of Economic Research, 1994). Actual number of births might have been more to the point than fertility rates.

127. Center for Health Policy Research, *Socioeconomic Characteristics of Medical Practice, 1983* (Chicago: American Medical Association, 1983), table 39; Center for Health Policy Research, *Socioeconomic Characteristics of Medical Practice, 1989* (Chicago: American Medical Association, 1989), table 42; Center for Health Policy Research, *Physician Socioeconomic Statistics, 1999–2000* (Chicago: American Medical Association, 1999), table 36.

128. Eugene M. Lewit and Alan C. Monheit, "Expenditures on Health Care for Children and Pregnant Women," *Future of Children* 2, no. 2 (1992): 95–114.

129. Mary T. Koska, "Reducing Cesareans—A $1 Million Trade-off," *Hospitals* 63, no. 5 (1989): 26.

130. Joanne Zorn Heilbrunn and Rolla Edward Park, *Variations in the Use of Cesarean Sections: Literature Synthesis* (Santa Monica, Calif.: RAND, 1995).

131. Tracy Vanner and Jason Gardosi, "Intrapartum Assessment of Uterine Activity," *Bailliere's Clinical Obstetrics and Gynaecology* 10, no. 2 (1996): 243–257; James A. Thorp, "Epidural Analgesia during Labor," *Clinical Obstetrics and Gynecology* 42, no. 4 (1999): 785–801; Arthur S. Maslow and Amy L. Sweeny, "Elective Induction of Labor as a Risk Factor for Cesarean Delivery among Low-Risk Women at Term," *Obstetrics and Gynecology* 95, no. 6, pt. 1 (2000): 917–922.

132. Jeffrey P. Phelan, "Cesarean Delivery: A Medical-Legal Perspective," in Flamm and Quilligan, eds., *Cesarean Section,* 163–171.

133. Carol Sakala, "Medically Unnecessary Cesarean Section Births: Introduction to a Symposium," *Social Science and Medicine* 37, no. 10 (1993): 1177–1198.

134. Colin Francome and Wendy Savage, "Cesarean Section in Britain and the United States, 12% or 24%: Is Either the Right Rate?" *Social Science and Medicine* 37, no. 10 (1993): 1199–1218; J. F. A. Murphy, "The Relentless Rise in Caesarean Sections," *Irish Medical Journal* 94, no. 7 (2001): 196.

135. Committee on Perinatal Health, *Toward Improving the Outcome of Pregnancy* (White Plains, N.Y.: Committee on Perinatal Health, 1976), 2.

Eight　Capital Intensive Medicine

1. Samuel Levey et al., *The Rise of a University Teaching Hospital: A Leadership Perspective: The University of Iowa Hospitals and Clinics* (Chicago: Health Administration Press, 1996), 295–296.

2. Robert G. Petersdorf, "The Evolution of Departments of Medicine," *New England Journal of Medicine* 303, no. 9 (1980): 489–496; Leighton E. Cluff, "Economic Incentives of Faculty Practice," *JAMA* 250, no. 21 (1983): 2931–2934.

3. Julie Fairman, "Economically Practical and Critically Necessary? The Development of Intensive Care at Chestnut Hill Hospital," *Bulletin of the History of Medicine* 74, no. 1 (2000): 80–106.

4. Lee Anderson, *Internal Medicine and the Structures of Modern Medical Science: The University of Iowa, 1870–1990* (Ames: Iowa State University Press, 1996), 112, 157–183.

5. Philip Jacobs and Thomas W. Noseworthy, "National Estimates of Intensive Care Utilization and Costs: Canada and the United States," *Critical Care Medicine* 18, no. 11 (1990): 1282–1286.

6. Richard H. Aubrey and John C. Pennington, "Identification and Evaluation of High-Risk Pregnancy: The Perinatal Concept," *Clinical Obstetrics and Gynecology* 16, no. 1 (1973): 3–27.

7. Mary T. Koska, "High-Tech Specialties Generate Top Dollars," *Hospitals,* October 20, 1988, 72–73.

8. Lynne Cunningham and Charles Koch, *Involving Physicians in Product Line Marketing* (Chicago: Pluribus Press, 1987), 109–113; Steven G. Hillestad and Eric N. Berkowitz, *Health Care Marketing Plans: From Strategy to Action,* 2d ed. (Gaithersburg, Md.: Aspen, 1991), 154–156.

9. U.S. Department of Health, Education, and Welfare, *Trends Affecting the U.S. Health Care System,* Health Information and Planning Series no. 1 (Rockville, Md.: U.S. Department of Health, Education, and Welfare, 1976), 322; Lis Dragsted and Jesper Qvist, "Epidemiology of Intensive Care," *International Journal of Technology Assessment in Health Care* 8, no. 3 (1992): 395–407.

10. Louise Russell, *Technology in Hospitals: Medical Advances and Their Diffusion* (Washington, D.C.: Brookings Institution, 1979), 55–57.

11. Jeffrey P. Baker, *The Machine in the Nursery: Incubator Technology and the Origins of Newborn Intensive Care* (Baltimore: Johns Hopkins University Press, 1996), 114–122.

12. Murdina MacFarquhar Desmond, *Newborn Medicine and Society: European Background and American Practice (1750–1975)* (Austin, Tex.: Eakin Press, 1998), 225–226.

13. H. Belton P. Meyer, "Regional Care for Mothers and Their Infants," *Clinics in Perinatology* 7, no. 1 (1980): 205–221.

14. Committee on Maternal and Child Health Care, *AMA National Conference on Infant Mortality, San Francisco, 1966* (Chicago: American Medical Association, 1967).

15. U.S. Congress, *Neonatal Intensive Care for Low Birthweight Infants: Costs and Effectiveness* (Washington, D.C.: Office of Technology Assessment, 1987), 12; American Hospital Association, *Survey of Obstetric and Newborn Services—1989* (Chicago: American Hospital Association, 1990), table 2b; Rachel M. Schwartz, "Supply and Demand for Neonatal Intensive Care: Trends and Implications," *Journal of*

Perinatology 16, no. 6 (1996): 483–489. Different sources provide different figures. One of the larger differences is the enumeration of 429 level III NICUs on a combined list from National Perinatal Information Center and Ross Laboratories in 1991 (Rita G. Harper et al., "Limitation of Private Attending Physicians' Neonatal Intensive Care Privileges in Level III Institutions throughout the United States," *Pediatrics* 94, no. 2 [1994]: 190–193).

16. Stanford Erickson, "Infant I.C.U.s Save Lives—But Too Many Units May Add Cost and Hamper Growth," *Modern Hospital* 115, no. 4 (1970): 80–84.

17. Louis Gluck et al., "Neonatal Intensive Care in Community Hospitals and Remote Areas," *Clinics in Perinatology* 3, no. 2 (1976): 297–306.

18. Michael B. Resnick et al., "Prospective Pricing System for Tertiary Neonatal Intensive Care," *Pediatrics* 78, no. 5 (1986): 820–828.

19. Morris Cohen, "Management of the Neonatal Intensive Care Unit and Neonatal Service," in W. J. Sibbald and T. Massaro, eds., *The Business of Critical Care: A Textbook for Clinicians Who Manage Special Care Units* (Armonk, N.Y.: Futura, 1996), 377–401; Thomas Chiu and Lana Brennan, "University Neonatal Centers and Level II Centers Compatibility," *Journal of the Florida Medical Association* 79, no. 7 (1992): 464–468.

20. Kevin Grumbach, "Specialists, Technology, and Newborns—Too Much of a Good Thing," *New England Journal of Medicine* 346, no. 20 (2002): 1574–1575.

21. Sheldon B. Korones, *High-Risk Newborn Infants: The Basis for Intensive Nursing Care* (St. Louis: C. V. Mosby, 1972), 223–233.

22. Peter A. M. Auld, "Training and Staffing in the Neonatal Intensive Care Unit," *Clinics in Perinatology* 7, no. 1 (1980): 155–158.

23. Julie Fairman and Joan E. Lynaugh, *Critical Care Nursing: A History* (Philadelphia: University of Pennsylvania Press, 1998), 17.

24. Doris J. Biester, "Changing Role of the Nurse as a Member of the Perinatal Intensive Care Team," in Silvio Aladjem and Audrey K. Brown, eds., *Perinatal Intensive Care* (St. Louis: C. V. Mosby, 1977), 42–48; Lois Tschetter and Dianna Spies Sorenson, "Educational Preparation for the Neonatal Nurse Clinician/Practitioner: From Past to Future," *Journal of Perinatal and Neonatal Nursing* 5, no. 3 (1991): 61–69.

25. Qtd. in Mitzi L. Duxbury, "Personnel and Staffing Needs for Perinatal Programs," *Seminars in Perinatology* 1, no. 3 (1977): 267–277.

26. Alba Mitchell-DiCenso et al., "A Controlled Trial of Nurse Practitioners in Neonatal Intensive Care," *Pediatrics* 98, no. 6, pt. 1 (1996): 1143–1148; Marjorie Schulman, Katherine R. Lucchese, and Ann C. Sullivan, "Transition from Housestaff to Nonphysicians as Neonatal Intensive Care Providers: Cost, Impact on Revenue, and Quality of Care," *American Journal of Perinatology* 12, no. 6 (1995): 442–446.

27. Michele C. Walsh-Sukys, "Persistent Pulmonary Hypertension of the Newborn," *Clinics in Perinatology* 20, no. 1 (1993): 127–143.

28. K. Rais-Bahrami and Billie L. Short, "The Current Status of Neonatal Extracorporeal Membrane Oxygenation," *Seminars in Perinatology* 24, no. 6 (2000): 406–417.

29. Robert H. Bartlett et al., "Extracorporeal Circulation in Neonatal Respiratory Failure: A Prospective Randomized Study," *Pediatrics* 76, no. 4 (1985): 479–487.

30. Jen-Tien Wung and L. Stanley James, "Optimizing Conventional Respiratory Support," in Robert M. Arensman and J. Devn Cornish, eds., *Extracorporeal Life Support* (Boston: Blackwell Scientific, 1993), 51–67.

31. Robert E. Schumacher and Stephen Baumgart, "Extracorporeal Membrane Oxygenation 2001: The Odyssey Continues," *Clinics in Perinatology* 28, no. 3 (2001): 629–653.

32. Yves W. Brans et al., "Newer Technologies and the Neonate," ed. intro., *Clinics in Perinatology* 18, no. 3 (1991): vii and whole special issue.

33. Shoo K. Lee, "Neonatal Intensive Care," in Benjamin P. Sachs et al., eds., *Reproductive Health Care for Women and Babies* (New York: Oxford University Press, 1995), 420–430.

34. Kwang-Sun Lee et al., "Neonatal Mortality: An Analysis of the Recent Improvement in the United States," *American Journal of Public Health* 70, no. 1 (1980): 15–21; Ronald L. Williams and Peter M. Chen, "Identifying the Sources of the Recent Decline in Perinatal Mortality Rates in California," *New England Journal of Medicine* 306, no. 4 (1982): 207–214.

35. John C. Sinclair et al., "Evaluation of Neonatal-Intensive-Care Programs," *New England Journal of Medicine* 305, no. 9 (1981): 489–494.

36. William A. Silverman, "Preface," *Birth and the Family Journal* 7, no. 4 (1980): 213.

37. Peter P. Budetti and Peggy McManus, "Assessing the Effectiveness of Neonatal Intensive Care," *Medical Care* 20, no. 10 (1982): 1027–1039.

38. U.S. Congress, *The Implications of Cost-Effectiveness Analysis of Medical Technology: Case Study #10: The Costs and Effectiveness of Neonatal Intensive Care* (Washington, D.C.: Office of Technology Assessment, 1981).

39. U.S. Congress, *Health Technology Case Study 38: Neonatal Intensive Care for Low Birthweight Infants: Costs and Effectiveness* (Washington, D.C.: Office of Technology Assessment, 1987).

40. Ronald L. Williams and Roger Wroblewski, *1984–1988 Maternal and Child Health Data Base: Descriptive Narrative* (Santa Barbara, Calif.: Community and Organization Research Institute, 1991).

41. W. H. Kitchen et al., "A Longitudinal Study of Very Low-Birthweight Infants. I: Study Design and Mortality Rates," *Developmental Medicine and Child Neurology* 20 (1978): 605–618. See Barbara Bridgman Perkins, "Rethinking Perinatal Policy: History and Evaluation of Minimum Volume and Level-of-Care Standards," *Journal of Public Health Policy* 14, no. 3 (1993): 299–319, for more extensive data supporting this conclusion.

42. Thomas E. Cone, *History of the Care and Feeding of the Premature Infant* (Boston: Little, Brown, 1985), 51.

43. Julius H. Hess and Evelyn C. Lundeen, *The Premature Infant: Medical and Nursing Care,* 2d ed. (Philadelphia: J. B. Lippincott, 1949), 339.

44. U.S. Department of Health Education and Welfare, *Comparison of Neonatal Mortality From Two Cohort Studies: United States, January–March 1950 and 1960* (Rockville, Md.: National Center for Health Statistics, 1972).

45. James W. Buehler et al., "Birth Weight–Specific Infant Mortality, United States, 1960 and 1980," *Public Health Reports* 102, no. 2 (1987): 151–161.

46. William A. Silverman, *Where's the Evidence? Controversies in Modern Medicine* (Oxford: Oxford University Press, 1998), 10; Ronald J. Ozminkowski, Paul M. Wortman, and Dietrich W. Roloff, "Evaluating the Effectiveness of Neonatal Intensive Care: What Can the Literature Tell Us?" *American Journal of Perinatology* 4, no. 4 (1987): 339–347; Jon E. Tyson, "Use of Unproven Therapies in Clinical Practice and Re-

search: How Can We Better Serve Our Patients and Their Families?" *Seminars in Perinatology* 19, no. 2 (1995): 98–111.

47. Russell S. Kirby, "A Parable Wrapped in an Enigma: Population-Based Assessments of Outcomes among High-Risk Neonates Are Even Less Achievable in the Age of Clinical Informatics," *Archives of Pediatrics and Adolescent Medicine* 153, no. 8 (1999): 789–792.

48. Sue Halpern, "Miracle Baby," *Ms.* (September 1989): 56–60, 62, 64.

49. Lucky Jain and D. Vidyasagar, "Iatrogenic Disorders in Modern Neonatology," *Clinics in Perinatology* 16, no. 1 (1989): 255–273.

50. Sinclair et al., "Evaluation of Neonatal-Intensive-Care Programs," 489–494.

51. California Health and Welfare Agency, *Licensed Services and Utilization Profiles: Annual Report of Hospitals* (Sacramento: Office of Statewide Health Planning and Development, multiple years). Calculated figure in the 1990 report incorrect, as verified by telephone, March 15, 1993.

52. California Health and Welfare Agency, *Annual Report of Hospitals, 1995,* disk version (Sacramento: Office of Statewide Health Planning and Development, 1996).

53. National Perinatal Information Center, *The Perinatal Center Directory* (Providence, R.I.: National Perinatal Information Center, 1987), 71. These enumerations do not correct for infants admitted to more than one NICU.

54. Lindsay A. Thompson, David C. Goodman, and George A. Little, "Is More Neonatal Intensive Care Always Better? Insights from a Cross-National Comparison of Reproductive Care," *Pediatrics* 109, no. 6 (2002): 1036–1043.

55. Boston University Center for Health Planning, *A Review of Planning Methods and Criteria for Neonatal Intensive Care Units,* vol. 1: *Planning Methods* (Boston: Boston University Center for Health Planning, n.d. [1980?]), table 22.

56. Joyce A. Martin et al., "Births: Final Data for 2000," *National Vital Statistics Reports* 50, no. 5 (2002): table 44 and other reports in this series.

57. Martin et al., "Births: Final Data for 2000," 18.

58. Sanjeev Mehta et al., "Differential Markers for Regionalization," *Journal of Perinatology* 20 (2000): 366–372.

59. Murdina M. Desmond, Arnold J. Rudolph, and Phuangnoi Phitaksphraiwan, "The Transitional Care Nursery," *Pediatric Clinics of North America* 13, no. 3 (1966): 651–668.

60. Ciaran S. Phibbs, Ronald L. Williams, and Roderic H. Phibbs, "Newborn Risk Factors and Costs of Neonatal Intensive Care," *Pediatrics* 68, no. 3 (1981): 313–321.

61. John A. F. Zupancic and Douglas K. Richardson, "Characterization of the Triage Process in Neonatal Intensive Care," *Pediatrics* 102, no. 6 (1998): 1432–1436.

62. Sonya M. Stevens et al., "Estimating Neonatal Mortality Risk: An Analysis of Clinicians' Judgements," *Pediatrics* 93, no. 6 (1994): 945–950.

63. Paula A. Braveman et al., "Differences in Hospital Resource Allocation among Sick Newborns According to Insurance Coverage," *JAMA* 266, no. 23 (1991): 3300–3308.

64. Yves W. Brans et al., eds., "Innovative Planning of Perinatal Centers," special issue of *Clinics in Perinatology* 10, no. 1 (1983).

65. Bruce M. Thogmartin, "Major Architectural Considerations in Programming Perinatal Care Facilities," *Clinics in Perinatology* 3, no. 2 (1976): 337–347; Kathleen Bajo, "Equipment Costs: The Neonatal Care Unit and the Modern Obstetric Unit," *Clinics in Perinatology* 10, no. 1 (1983): 175–187; Robert Wood Johnson Foundation,

Special Report: The Perinatal Program: What Has Been Learned (Princeton: Robert Wood Johnson Foundation, 1985).

66. William N. Spellacy, "Survival of Departments of Obstetrics and Gynecology: Ten Points for Association of Professors of Gynecology and Obstetrics Action in the 1980s," *American Journal of Obstetrics and Gynecology* 144, no. 6 (1982): 626–629.

67. Robin Scott MacStravic, "Product-Line Administration in Hospitals," *Health Care Management Review* 11, no. 2 (1986): 35–43; James X. Reynolds, "Using DRGs for Competitive Positioning and Practical Business Planning," *Health Care Management Review* 11, no. 3 (1986): 37–55. The reproductive endocrinology subspecialty and its in-vitro fertilization procedures also became a highly successful product line.

68. Robert J. Gray, "Marketing for Success through Product-Line Development," *Topics in Health Care Financing* 14, no. 3 (1988): 76–83.

69. Levey et al., *Rise of a University Teaching Hospital,* 342.

70. Warren H. Pearse and Kathleen G. Poole, "Current Trends in Obstetric and Gynecologic Academic Faculty Manpower," *Obstetrics and Gynecology* 86, no. 6 (1995): 1018–1020.

71. Society of Perinatal Obstetricians, *1995–1996 Directory of Fellowship Programs in Maternal-Fetal Medicine* (Washington, D.C.: Society of Perinatal Obstetricians, 1995).

72. R. Clay Burchell et al., "Collaborative Practice in Obstetrics/Gynecology: Implications for Cost, Quality, and Productivity," *American Journal of Obstetrics and Gynecology* 144, no. 6 (1982): 621–625.

73. Robert A. Knuppel and Joan E. Drukker, *High-Risk Pregnancy: A Team Approach* (Philadelphia: W. B. Saunders, 1993), 4; American College of Nurse-Midwives, American College of Obstetricians and Gynecologists, and Nurses Association of the American College of Obstetricians and Gynecologists, "Joint Statement on Maternity Care" (1971) and "Supplementary Statement" (1975) (Washington, D.C., and Chicago).

74. National Perinatal Information Center, *Perinatal Center Directory,* 71.

75. Madeleine H. Shearer, "Maternity Patients' Advocates in the 1990s: Changing Debaters and New Debaters," *International Journal of Technology Assessment in Health Care* 7, no. 4 (1991): 519–529.

76. Dianne Hales and Timothy R. B. Johnson, *Intensive Caring: New Hope for High-Risk Pregnancy* (New York: Crown, 1990), 50.

77. Jorge D. Blanco, "The Private Practice Model," *American Journal of Perinatology* 6, supp. (1989): 17–20.

78. David B. Schwartz, "The Hospital's Perspective," *American Journal of Perinatology* 6, supp. (1989): 3–11.

79. Lawrence D. Devoe, "Facing the Next Millennium of Managed Health Care: Can Academic Maternal-Fetal Medicine Programs Survive?" *Seminars in Perinatology* 21, no. 6 (1997): 472–478.

80. Edward H. Hon, "Biophysical Intrapartal Fetal Monitoring," *Clinics in Perinatology* 1, no. 1 (1974): 149–159; Richard H. Paul, "Electronic Fetal Monitoring and Later Outcome: A Thirty-Year Overview," *Journal of Perinatology* 14, no. 5 (1994): 393–395.

81. Barbara Ehrenreich, "Birth Is Their Business," *Seven Days,* May 5, 1979, 26–27; Stephen B. Thacker, "The Impact of Technology Assessment and Medical Malpractice on the Diffusion of Medical Technologies: The Case of Electronic Fetal Moni-

toring," in Committee to Study Medical Professional Liability and the Delivery of Obstetrical Care, *Medical Professional Liability and the Delivery of Obstetrical Care* (Washington, D.C.: Institute of Medicine, 1989), 2:9–26; H. David Banta and Stephen B. Thacker, "Historical Controversy in Health Technology Assessment: The Case of Electronic Fetal Monitoring," *Obstetrical and Gynecological Survey* 56, no. 11 (2001): 707–719.

82. Judith R. Kunisch, "Electronic Fetal Monitors: Marketing Forces and the Resulting Controversy," in Kathryn Strother Ratcliff et al., eds., *Healing Technology: Feminist Perspectives* (Ann Arbor: University of Michigan Press, 1989), 41–60.

83. Margarete Sandelowski, *Devices and Desires: Gender, Technology, and American Nursing* (Chapel Hill: University of North Carolina Press, 2000), 149–175.

84. Thomas H. Strong and Richard H. Paul, "Intrapartum Uterine Activity: Evaluation of an Intrauterine Pressure Transducer," *Obstetrics and Gynecology* 73, no. 3, pt. 1 (1989): 432–434.

85. Edward J. Quilligan, "Perinatology as a Subspecialty," *Clinics in Perinatology* 1, no. 1 (1974): 47–51.

86. William C. Mabie and Baha M. Sibai, "Treatment in an Obstetric Intensive Care Unit," *American Journal of Obstetrics and Gynecology* 162, no. 1 (1990): 1–4.

87. Lawrence D. Devoe et al., "Monitoring Intrauterine Pressure during Active Labor: A Prospective Comparison of Two Methods," *Journal of Reproductive Medicine* 34, no. 10 (1989): 811–814.

88. Haider H. Shamsi, Roy H. Petrie, and Charles M. Steer, "Changing Obstetric Practices and Amelioration of Perinatal Outcome in a University Hospital," *American Journal of Obstetrics and Gynecology* 133, no. 8 (1979): 855–858.

89. Harvey A. Gabert and Morton A. Stenchever, "Electronic Fetal Monitoring as a Routine Practice in an Obstetric Service: A Progress Report," *American Journal of Obstetrics and Gynecology* 118, no. 4 (1974): 534–537.

90. Douglas Richardson, Arnold Rosoff, and Joseph P. McMenamin, "Referral Practices and Health Care Costs: The Dilemma of High Risk Obstetrics," *Journal of Legal Medicine* 6, no. 4 (1985): 427–464.

91. Thacker, "Impact of Technology Assessment and Medical Malpractice on the Diffusion of Medical Technologies," 2:9–26.

92. Paul J. Placek et al., "Electronic Fetal Monitoring in Relation to Cesarean Section Delivery, for Live Births and Stillbirths in the U.S., 1980," *Public Health Reports* 99, no. 2 (1984): 173–183; Stephanie J. Ventura et al., "Births: Final Data for 1998," *National Vital Statistics Reports* 48, no. 3 (2000): table 27 and other years in this series.

93. Charles B. Gassner and William J. Ledger, "The Relationship of Hospital-Acquired Maternal Infection to Invasive Intrapartum Monitoring Techniques," *American Journal of Obstetrics and Gynecology* 126, no. 1 (1976): 33–37.

94. Leah L. Albers and Cara J. Krulewitch, "Electronic Fetal Monitoring in the United States in the 1980s," *Obstetrics and Gynecology* 82, no. 1 (1993): 8–10.

95. U.S. Senate, Committee on Human Resources, *Obstetrical Practices in the United States, 1978* (Washington, D.C.: U.S. Government Printing Office, April 17, 1978), 61.

96. Edward J. Quilligan and Richard H. Paul, "Fetal Monitoring: Is It Worth It?" *Obstetrics and Gynecology* 45, no. 1 (1975): 96–100.

97. Miriam D. Orleans and Albert D. Haverkamp, "Birth: Electronic Fetal Monitoring," in Stanley Joel Reiser and Michael Anbar, eds., *The Machine at the Bedside: Strate-*

gies for Using Technology in Patient Care (Cambridge: Cambridge University Press, 1984), 303–306.

98. A. Dale Tussing and Martha A. Wojtowycz, "Malpractice, Defensive Medicine, and Obstetric Behavior," *Medical Care* 35, no. 2 (1997): 172–191.

99. Barry S. Schifrin, "The ABCs of Electronic Fetal Monitoring," *Journal of Perinatology* 14, no. 5 (1994): 396–402.

100. Barry S. Schifrin, "Medicolegal Ramifications of Electronic Fetal Monitoring during Labor," *Clinics in Perinatology* 22, no. 4 (1995): 837–854.

101. David A. Grimes, "Technology Follies: The Uncritical Acceptance of Medical Innovation," *JAMA* 269, no. 23 (1993): 3030–3033.

102. Ken L. Bassett, Nitya Iyer, and Arminee Kazanjian, "Defensive Medicine during Hospital Obstetrical Care: A By-product of the Technological Age," *Social Science and Medicine* 51, no. 4 (2000): 523–537.

103. Ann Oakley, *Women Confined: Towards a Sociology of Childbirth* (New York: Schocken, 1980), 34–35.

104. Barbara Katz Rothman, *Giving Birth: Alternatives in Childbirth* (New York: Penguin, 1982), 34–49.

105. Tess Cosslett, *Women Writing Childbirth: Modern Discourses of Motherhood* (Manchester: Manchester University Press, 1994), 2, 48–49.

106. Sandra Bryant, "Nursing Aspects and Organization for Perinatal Care," *Clinics in Perinatology* 3, no. 2 (1976): 493–496.

107. Patricia H. Ellison et al., "Electronic Fetal Heart Monitoring, Auscultation, and Neonatal Outcome," *American Journal of Obstetrics and Gynecology* 164, no. 5, pt. 1 (1991): 1281–1289.

108. Committee on Obstetric Practice, "Fetal Distress and Birth Asphyxia" (committee opinion, American College of Obstetricians and Gynecologists, Washington, D.C., April 1994).

109. Michael K. Lindsay, "Intrauterine Resuscitation of the Compromised Fetus," *Clinics in Perinatology* 26, no. 3 (1999): 569–584.

110. Roger K. Freeman, "Evaluation of Monitoring Techniques in Pregnancy," in Sachs et al., *Reproductive Health Care for Women and Babies,* 293–304. I am taking this comment at face value, although I have wondered whether it was meant tongue-in-cheek, since it was based on the relatively high mortality rates of infants in the first day of independent life, many of which are known to be due to birth defects, very-low birthweight, and other factors not related to the birth process.

111. Edward J. Quilligan, "The Obstetric Intensive Care Unit," *Hospital Practice* 7, no. 6 (1972): 61–69.

112. Anja Hiddinga and Stuart S. Blume, "Technology, Science, and Obstetric Practice: The Origins and Transformation of Cephalopelvimetry," *Science, Technology, and Human Values* 17, no. 2 (1992): 154–179.

113. Watson A. Bowes, "Monitoring the Term Fetus: Cesarean Section Deliveries," in *The Term Newborn Infant: A Current Look* (Columbus, Ohio: Ross Laboratories, 1991), 14–19.

114. Richard H. Paul, "Electronic Fetal Monitoring and Later Outcome: A Thirty-Year Overview," *Journal of Perinatology* 14, no. 5 (1994): 393–395.

115. Javier Cifuentes et al., "Mortality in Low Birth Weight Infants According to Level of Neonatal Care at Hospital of Birth," *Pediatrics* 109, no. 5 (2002): 745–751.

Nine Managing Birth

1. Avedis Donabedian, "An Examination of Some Directions in Health Care Policy," *American Journal of Public Health* 63, no. 3 (1973): 243–246.

2. J. Warren Salmon, "The Health Maintenance Organization Strategy: A Corporate Takeover of Health Services Delivery," *International Journal of Health Services* 5, no. 4 (1975): 609–624; Pamela Doty, *Guided Change of the American Health System* (New York: Human Sciences Press, 1980), 74.

3. John E. Kralewski and Roice D. Luke, "The Group Practice of Medicine: Some Implications for Health Planning," in *Papers on the National Health Guidelines: The Priorities of Section 1502* (Rockville, Md.: U.S. Health Resources Administration, 1977), 45–55.

4. Robert M. Heyssel et al., "Decentralized Management in a Teaching Hospital," *New England Journal of Medicine* 310, no. 22 (1984): 1477–1480.

5. Robert F. Jones, *Academic Medicine: Institutions, Programs, and Issues* (Washington, D.C.: Association of American Medical Colleges, 1997), 8–9.

6. Daniel F. O'Keeffe and Jay Mayes, "Managed Obstetrical Care," *Clinical Obstetrics and Gynecology* 40, no. 2 (1997): 414–419.

7. John Kennell et al., "Medical Intervention: The Effect of Social Support during Labor," *Pediatric Research* 23, no. 4, pt. 2 (1988): 211A. Doulas might become more acceptable if research confirms preliminary work suggesting that their presence is more effective than active management of labor in reducing cesarean section use.

8. Kenneth A. Krieg, "Obstetrics/Gynecology Network Development," *Clinical Obstetrics and Gynecology* 40, no. 2 (1997): 446–452; Maryann Szostak-Ricardo, "Survival of the Specialist: Creating a Specialty IPA," *American Medical News,* June 9, 1997, 13–14; Arnold W. Cohen, "Perinatologists and Managed Health Care: Friend or Foe?" *Seminars in Perinatology* 21, no. 6 (1997): 457–463.

9. Kevin Grumbach, "Specialists, Technology, and Newborns—Too Much of a Good Thing," *New England Journal of Medicine* 346, no. 20 (2002): 1574–1575.

10. A. C. Bachmeyer, "Selecting and Organizing the Medical Staff," *Modern Hospital* 42, no. 4 (1934): 59–62.

11. Joseph S. Coyne, ed., "Financial Strategies of MIOs in Price-Competitive Markets," *Topics in Health Care Financing* 11, no. 2 (1984).

12. Elvoy Raines, "Hospital Risk Management for Perinatal Care: Theory and Practice," *Journal of Perinatology* 8, no. 2 (1988): 96–100; Jim Langabeer, "Competing on Price: The Economics of Managed Competition," *Academic Medicine* 71, no. 11 (1996): 1244–1246.

13. Robert B. Fetter and Jean L. Freeman, "Diagnosis Related Groups: Product Line Management within Hospitals," *Academy of Management Review* 11, no. 1 (1986): 41–54; James X. Reynolds, "Using DRGs for Competitive Positioning and Practical Business Planning," *Health Care Management Review* 11, no. 3 (1986): 37–55; James C. Folger and E. Preston Gee, *Product Management for Hospitals: Organizing for Profitability* (Chicago: American Hospital Publishing, 1987), 43–45.

14. Robert C. Newbold, "Notes on a Management Information System for United Health Services," June 22, 1983, MS included in packet for a conference on "The Management and Financing of Hospital Services," London, December 11–13, 1986.

15. Harold E. Smalley and John R. Freeman, *Hospital Industrial Engineering: A Guide*

to the Improvement of Hospital Management Systems (New York: Reinhold, 1966), 59, 177–178, 181–183, 282, 291; Donald M. Berwick, A. Blandon Godfrey, and Jane Roessner, *Curing Health Care: New Strategies for Quality Improvement* (San Francisco: Jossey-Bass, 1990), 29, 32.

16. Harry B. Wolfe, Magdi Iskander, and Tom Raffin, "A Study of Obstetrical Facilities," in George K. Chacko, ed., *The Recognition of Systems in Health Services* (Arlington, Va.: Operations Research Society of America, 1969), 369–392.

17. Glenn Laffel and David Blumenthal, "The Case for Using Industrial Quality Management Science in Health Care Organizations," *JAMA* 262, no. 20 (1989): 2869–2873; B. Jon Jaeger, Arnold D. Kaluzny, and Curtis P. McLaughlin, "TQM/CQI: From Industry to Health Care," in Curtis P. McLaughlin and Arnold D. Kaluzny, eds., *Continuous Quality Improvement in Health Care* (Gaithersburg, Md.: Aspen, 1994), 11–32.

18. Jeffrey D. Horbar, "The Vermont-Oxford Neonatal Network: Integrating Research and Clinical Practice to Improve the Quality of Medical Care," *Seminars in Perinatology* 19, no. 2 (1995): 124–131; T. Allen Merritt et al., "Clinical Practice Guidelines in Pediatric and Newborn Medicine: Implications for Their Use in Practice," *Pediatrics* 99, no. 1 (1997): 100–114; David A. Bergman, "Evidence-based Guidelines and Critical Pathways for Quality Improvement," *Pediatrics* 103, no. 1, supp. (1999): 225–232.

19. Mark R. Chassin, "Part 3: Improving the Quality of Care," *New England Journal of Medicine* 335, no. 14 (1996): 1060–1063; Zeses C. Roulidis, Hallie K. DeChant, and Kevin A. Schulman, "Resource Utilization Control Processes as Indicators of Quality in Managed Care Organizations: A Proposal," *American Journal of Medicine* 103 (1997): 146–151.

20. Kenneth M. Ludmerer, *Time to Heal: American Medical Education from the Turn of the Century to the Era of Managed Care* (New York: Oxford University Press, 1999), 365–375.

21. Joseph C. Gambone and Robert C. Reiter, "Quality Improvement in Women's Health Care," in Thomas R. Moore et al., eds., *Gynecology and Obstetrics: A Longitudinal Approach* (New York: Churchill Livingstone, 1993), 27–36; Susan Paul Johnson and Curtis P. McLaughlin, "Measurement and Statistical Analysis in CQI," in McLaughlin and Kaluzny, eds., *Continuous Quality Improvement in Health,* 70–101; Jean-Christophe Luthi, Mary S. Dolan, and David J. Ballard, "Evidence-Based Healthcare Quality Management in Obstetrics and Gynecology," *Clinical Obstetrics and Gynecology* 41, no. 2 (1998): 348–358. A challenging alternative medical view that predated the thrust of the IQMS movement held that clinical variation was acceptable because "much of medical knowledge is ambiguous and because few services are absolutely necessary" (John M. Eisenberg, *Doctors' Decisions and the Cost of Medical Care* [Ann Arbor, Mich.: Health Administration Press, 1986], 5).

22. Joseph B. DeLee, "The Use of Solution of Posterior Pituitary in Modern Obstetrics," *Journal of the American Medical Association* 115, no. 16 (1940): 1320–1326.

23. William J. Dieckmann and Morris S. Kharasch, "Solution of Posterior Pituitary Sulfonate (Pit-sulfonate) in Labor," *American Journal of Obstetrics and Gynecology* 44 (1942): 820–832.

24. Duncan E. Reid, "The Treatment of Prolonged Labor with Posterior Pituitary Extract," *American Journal of Obstetrics and Gynecology* 52 (1946): 719–734.

25. G. W. Theobald, H. A. Kelsey, and J. M. B. Muirhead, "The Pitocin Drip," *Journal of Obstetrics and Gynaecology of the British Empire* 63, no. 5 (1956): 641–662.
26. Nicholson J. Eastman, "Pituitary Extract in Uterine Inertia: Is It Justifiable?" *American Journal of Obstetrics and Gynecology* 53, no. 3 (1947): 432–441.
27. Robert E. Hall, "Standard Practices at Sloane Hospital: The Management of the Induction of Labor," *Bulletin of the Sloane Hospital for Women* 7 (1961): 55–58.
28. Harry Fields, John W. Greene, and Kaighn Smith, *Induction of Labor* (New York: Macmillan, 1965), 164, 169, 174, 180. Data covered 1950–1963. All elective inductions were performed on private patients; indicated induction added another 2 percent.
29. Dean V. Coonrod, R. Curtis Bay, and Glen Y. Kishi, "The Epidemiology of Labor Induction: Arizona, 1997," *American Journal of Obstetrics and Gynecology* 182, no. 6 (2000): 1355–1362. Russel K. Laros in discussion.
30. R. B. Fetter and J. D. Thompson, "The Simulation of Hospital Systems," *Operations Research* 13, no. 5 (1965): 689–711.
31. Kenneth R. Niswander and Myron Gordon, *The Women and Their Pregnancies* (Washington, D.C.: National Institute of Neurological Diseases and Stroke, 1972), 352–358. Data covered 1959–1965. Oxytocin use among black women in the same hospitals was considerably lower. The full title of the study was the "Collaborative Study of Cerebral Palsy, Mental Retardation and Other Neurological and Sensory Disorders of Infancy and Childhood." Its assumption that the named neurological disorders often originated in problems in the childbirth process, while useful to the development of obstetrics, was ultimately not upheld.
32. American College of Obstetricians and Gynecologists, *National Study of Maternity Care* (Chicago: American College of Obstetricians and Gynecologists, 1970), table IV-12.
33. Ronald R. Rindfuss, Steven L. Gortmaker, and Judith L. Landinsky, "Elective Induction and Stimulation of Labor and the Health of the Infant," *American Journal of Public Health* 68, no. 9 (1978): 872–877.
34. W. N. Hubbard, "Welcome Address," *Journal of Reproductive Medicine* 9, no. 6 (1972): 249 and whole issue.
35. Proceedings from the Brook Lodge Symposium on Prostaglandins, *Journal of Reproductive Medicine* 9, no. 6 (1972): 249–477.
36. Linda M. Davies and M. F. Drummond, "Management of Labour: Consumer Choice and Cost Implications," *Journal of Obstetrics and Gynaeology* 11, supp. 1 (1991): S28–S33; Charles E. L. Brown, Andrew J. Satin, and Kenneth J. Leveno, "The Economic Advantages of Measured Change in Health Care: An Example from Obstetrics," *Obstetrics and Gynecology* 84, no. 5 (1994): 893–895; Arthur S. Maslow and Amy L. Sweeny, "Elective Induction of Labor as a Risk Factor for Cesarean Delivery among Low-Risk Women at Term," *Obstetrics and Gynecology* 95, no. 6, pt. 1 (2000): 917–922.
37. Kieran O'Driscoll, Reginald J. A. Jackson, and John T. Gallagher, "Prevention of Prolonged Labour," *British Medical Journal* 2 (1969): 477–480; Kieran O'Driscoll and Declan Meagher, *Active Management of Labour* (London: W. B. Saunders, 1980), 3. O'Driscoll called midwives "nurses," thus obfuscating their capacity to perform as responsible birth attendants.
38. Kieran O'Driscoll, "Abolition of Prolonged Labour: Impact of Active Management on Delivery Unit Practice," *Proceedings of the Royal Society of Medicine* 65 (1972): 697–698.

39. Kieran O'Driscoll and Declan Meagher, with Peter Boylan, *Active Management of Labour: The Dublin Experience* (London: Mosby, 1993), 34.
40. Kieran O'Driscoll, John M. Stronge, and Maurice Minogue, "Active Management of Labour," *British Medical Journal* 3 (1973): 135–137; O'Driscoll and Meagher, *Active Management of Labour*, 39–40, 107.
41. O'Driscoll, Stronge, and Minogue, "Active Management of Labour," 135–137. O'Driscoll held that active management was appropriate only for primiparae.
42. Peter C. Boylan, "Active Management of Labor: Results in Dublin, Houston, London, New Brunswick, Singapore, and Valparaiso," *Birth* 16, no. 3 (1989): 114–118.
43. Emanuel A. Friedman, "Primigravid Labor: A Graphicostatistical Analysis," *Obstetrics and Gynecology* 6, no. 6 (1955): 567–589.
44. Emanuel A. Friedman, *Labor: Clinical Evaluation and Management,* 2d ed. (New York: Appleton-Century-Crofts, 1978), 18–20.
45. Emily Martin, *The Woman in the Body: A Cultural Analysis of Reproduction* (Boston: Beacon Press, 1987), 56–59.
46. Friedman, "Primigravid Labor: A Graphicostatistical Analysis," 567–589.
47. Emanuel A. Friedman, "The Introduction of Objectivity to the Study of Abnormal Labor," *Bulletin of the Sloane Hospital for Women* 10 (1964): 121–127; Pai Wen Sheen and Robert H. Hayashi, "Graphic Management of Labor: Alert/Action Line," *Clinical Obstetrics and Gynecology* 30, no. 1 (1987): 33–41.
48. Emanuel A. Friedman, "Synthetic Oxytocin: Critical Evaluation in Labor and Post Partum," *American Journal of Obstetrics and Gynecology* 74, no. 5 (1957): 1118–1124.
49. Ann Oakley, *The Captured Womb: A History of the Medical Care of Pregnant Women* (Oxford: Basil Blackwell, 1984), 110.
50. Marjorie Tew, *Safer Childbirth? A Critical History of Maternity Care* (London: Chapman and Hall, 1990), 155–156.
51. Roger Hadley and Don Forster, eds., *Doctors as Managers* (London: Longman, 1993), 63–69, 103–104.
52. Robin Dowie, *Patterns of Hospital Medical Staffing: Obstetrics and Gynaecology* (London: HMSO, 1991), 8, 32.
53. Alison Macfarlane and Miranda Mugford, *Birth Counts: Statistics of Pregnancy and Childbirth, Tables* (London: Her Majesty's Stationery Office, 1984), 245, 537. Scotland also had a higher proportion of academic obstetric units.
54. Alison Macfarlane et al., *Birth Counts: Statistics of Pregnancy and Childbirth, Volume 2—Tables* (London: Stationery Office, 2000), 529. Earlier figures pertain to England and Wales, later ones to NHS hospitals in England.
55. Preston V. Dilts and James E. Wade, "Criteria for Selecting an Infusion Device," *Contemporary Ob/Gyn* 16, special issue, "Technology 1981" (1980).
56. J. G. Francis, A. C. Turnbull, and F. F. Thomas, "Automatic Oxytocin Infusion Equipment for Induction of Labour," *Journal of Obstetrics and Gynaecology of the British Commonwealth* 77, no. 7 (1970): 594–602.
57. J. D. Hamlett, "A New Electronic Pump for Oxytocin Infusion," *British Journal of Clinical Practice* 26, no. 2 (1972): 69–72; M. P. M. Richards, "Innovation in Medical Practice: Obstetricians and the Induction of Labour in Britain," *Social Science and Medicine* 9 (1975): 595–602; Brian Alderman, "Factors Influencing Planned Delivery," *Clinics in Obstetrics and Gynaecology* 2, no. 1 (1975): 19–47.

58. Qtd. in Ann Cartwright, *The Dignity of Labour? A Study of Childbearing and Induction* (London: Tavistock, 1979), 2.

59. Cartwright, *Dignity of Labour,* 18–23.

60. I. Chalmers, J. G. Lawson, and A. C. Turnbull, "Evaluation of Different Approaches to Obstetric Care: Part I," *British Journal of Obstetrics and Gynaecology* 83, no. 12 (1976): 921–929, and "Evaluation of Different Approaches to Obstetric Care: Part II," 83, no. 12 (1976): 930–933.

61. Department of Health and Social Security, *Hospital In-patient Enquiry: Maternity Tables, 1977–1981* (London: Her Majesty's Stationery Office, 1986), 15, 56. Figures for England and Wales.

62. Sarah Robinson, Josephine Golden, and Susan Bradley, *A Study of the Role and Responsibilities of the Midwife* (London: Chelsea College, University of London, 1983), 141.

63. Anne Fleissig, "Mothers' Experiences of Induction of Labour," *Journal of Obstetrics and Gynaecology* 11, supp. 1 (1991): S11–S15.

64. John M. Beazley and Asim Kurjak, "Influence of a Partograph on the Active Management of Labour," *Lancet* 19, no. 2 (1972): 348–351.

65. John M. Beazley, "The Active Management of Labor," *American Journal of Obstetrics and Gynecology* 122, no. 2 (1974): 161–168.

66. Mark Hackett, "Developing Consultant Care on Delivery Suite," *Health Manpower Management* 24, no. 6 (1998): 229–233.

67. Macfarlane et al., *Birth Counts: Volume 2—Tables,* 4, 479, 485, and 495.

68. J. S. Scott, "Dublin Deliveries," *British Medical Journal* 282, no. 6269 (1981): 1064.

69. J. Garcia, S. Garforth, and S. Ayers, "Midwives Confined? Labour Ward Policies and Routines," *Research and the Midwife Conference Proceedings* (1986): 2–30.

70. Division of Obstetrics and Gynaecology, *Annual Clinical Report: 1985* (Harrow, U.K.: Northwick Park Hospital, 1986), 69.

71. Marc J. N. C. Keirse, "Augmentation of Labour," in Iain Chalmers, Murray Enkin, and Marc J. N. C. Keirse, eds., *Effective Care in Pregnancy and Childbirth* (Oxford: Oxford University Press, 1989), 951–966; Murray Enkin et al., "Effective Care in Pregnancy and Childbirth: A Synopsis," *Birth* 28, no. 1 (2001): 41–51.

72. Charles Montacute, *Costing and Efficiency in Hospitals: A Critical Survey of Costing as an Aid to the Management of Hospitals* (London: Oxford University Press, 1962), xi.

73. F. N. Garratt, "The Maternity Services: A Problem of Management," *Royal Society of Health Journal* 90, no. 3 (1970): 164–168.

74. Gordon Marnoch, *Doctors and Management in the National Health Service* (Buckingham, U.K.: Open University Press, 1996), 21–22.

75. Ray Brooks, ed., *Management Budgeting in the NHS* (Keele, U.K.: Health Services Manpower Review, 1986), 37.

76. Christopher Pollitt, "Beyond the Managerial Model: The Case for Broadening Performance Assessment in Government and the Public Services," *Financial Accountability and Management* 2, no. 3 (1986): 155–170.

77. A. Szczepura, M. Mugford, and J. A. Stillwell, "Information for Managers in Hospitals: Representing Maternity Unit Statistics Graphically," *British Medical Journal* 294 (1987): 875–880.

78. House of Commons, *Perinatal and Neonatal Mortality* (London: Her Majesty's Stationery Office, 1980), 1:29.

79. Marnoch, *Doctors and Management in the National Health Service,* 51–58.

80. North West Thames Regional Health Authority, *Regional Strategy: Towards a Strategy for Maternity and Neo-Natal Services* (London: North West Thames Regional Health Authority, 1984); M. Mugford and J. Stilwell, "Maternity Services: How Well Have They Done and Could They Do Better?" in A. Harrison and J. Gretton, eds., *Health Care UK, 1986* (Cambridge: Burlington Press, 1986), 53–64.

81. Wendy Savage, *A Savage Enquiry: Who Controls Childbirth?* (London: Virago, 1986).

82. London Hospital, "Annual Obstetric Report, 1982" (MS, London Hospital, London, 1982).

83. Michael Drummond, Jonathan Cooke, and Tom Walley, "Economic Evaluation under Managed Competition: Evidence from the U.K.," *Social Science and Medicine* 45, no. 4 (1997): 583–595.

84. Department of Health, *Changing Childbirth* (London, Her Majesty's Stationery Office, 1993), 70.

85. Garcia, Garforth, and Ayers, "Midwives Confined?" 2–30.

86. Robinson, Golden, and Bradley, *Study of the Role and Responsibilities of the Midwife,* 155–168.

87. John MacVicar et al., "Simulated Home Delivery in Hospital: A Randomised Controlled Trial," *British Journal of Obstetrics and Gynaecology* 100, no. 4 (1993): 316–323; Josephine M. Green et al., *Continuing to Care: The Organization of Midwifery Services in the UK: A Structured Review of the Evidence* (Hale, Cheshire, U.K.: Books for Midwives Press, 1998).

88. David J. Hunter, "The Changing Roles of Health Care Personnel in Health and Health Care Management," *Social Science and Medicine* 5 (1996): 799–808.

89. Tracey Vanner and Jason Gardosi, "Intrapartum Assessment of Uterine Activity," *Baillière's Clinical Obstetrics and Gynaecology* 10, no. 2 (1996): 243–257.

90. Geoffrey Chamberlain, Philip Steer, and Luke Zander, eds., *ABC of Labour Care* (London: BMJ, 1999), 25. Authors claimed, however, that a cervical dilation rate of less than 0.5 cm/hr (half of O'Dricoll's speed limit) was the more commonly accepted criterion for acceleration.

91. Stavros Petrou, Jane Henderson, and Cathryn Glazener, "Economic Aspects of Caesarean Section and Alternative Modes of Delivery," *Best Practice and Research: Clinical Obstetrics and Gynaecology* 15, no. 1 (2001): 145–163.

92. Rudolf Klein, ed., *Implementing the White Paper: Pitfalls and Opportunities* (London: King's Fund, 1998), 33, 37, 70.

93. Brown, Satin, and Leveno, "Economic Advantages of Measured Change in Health Care," 893–895.

94. Gina Kolata, "New York Is First State Trying to Curb Caesareans," *New York Times,* January 27, 1989, 1, 12; Julie A. Gazmararian and Jeffrey P. Koplan, "Economic Aspects of the Perinatal Hospital Stay," *Clinics in Perinatology* 25, no. 2 (1998): 483–498.

95. Anne G. Castles, Arnold Milstein, and Cheryl L. Damberg, "Using Employer Purchasing Power to Improve the Quality of Perinatal Care," *Pediatrics* 103, no. 1, supp. E (1999): 248–254.

96. Community and Organization Research Institute, *1984–1988 Maternal and Child Health Data Base: Descriptive Narrative* (Santa Barbara, Calif.: Community and Organization Research Institute, 1992), 188–190.

97. Eugene W. J. Pearce, comment to Michael L. Socol et al., "Reducing Cesarean Births at a Primarily Private University Hospital," *American Journal of Obstetrics and Gynecology* 168, no. 6, pt. 1 (1993): 1748–1758.

98. Henk W. Jongsma and Jan G. Nijhuis, "Critical Analysis of the Validity of Electronic Fetal Monitoring," *Journal of Perinatal Medicine* 19, nos. 1–2 (1991): 33–37.

99. Carl A. Sirio and Dwain Harper, "Designing the Optimal Health Assessment System: The Cleveland Quality Choice (CHQC) Example," *American Journal of Medical Quality* 11, no. 1 (1996): S66–S69.

100. Krieg, "Obstetrics/Gynecology Network Development," 446–452.

101. Nicholas A. Hanchak, "A Performance-based Compensation Model for Obstetricians/Gynecologists," *Clinical Obstetrics and Gynecology* 40, no. 2 (1997): 437–445.

102. Luis Sanchez-Ramos, Rebecca I. Moorehead, and Andrew M. Kaunitz, "Cesarean Section Rates in Teaching Hospitals: A National Survey," *Birth* 21, no. 4 (1994): 194–196.

103. Robin S. Richman, "Managed Care in Obstetrics," *Current Opinion in Obstetrics and Gynecology* 8 (1996): 329–332; D. Oberer and L. Aukerman, "Best Practice: Clinical Pathways for Uncomplicated Births," *Best Practices and Benchmarking in Healthcare* 1, no. 1 (1996): 43–50.

104. Committee to Study Medical Professional Liability and the Delivery of Obstetrical Care, *Medical Professional Liability and the Delivery of Obstetrical Care* (Washington, D.C.: Institute of Medicine, 1989), 1:118.

105. Stephen M. Shortell et al., "Physician Involvement in Quality Improvement: Issues, Challenges, and Recommendations," in David Blumenthal and Ann C. Scheck, eds., *Improving Clinical Practice: Total Quality Management and the Physician* (San Francisco: Jossey-Bass, 1995), 205–228.

106. James P. Thompson, "Forcep Deliveries," *Clinics in Perinatology* 22, no. 4 (1995): 953–972.

107. U.S. General Accounting Office, *A Review of Research Literature and Federal Involvement Relating to Selected Obstetric Practices* (Washington, D.C.: U.S. Government Printing Office, 1979), 36; Sally C. Curtin and Melissa M. Park, "Trends in the Attendant, Place, and Timing of Births, and in the Use of Obstetric Interventions: United States, 1989–97," *National Vital Statistics Reports* 47, no. 27 (1999): table 9; Stephanie J. Ventura et al., "Births: Final Data for 1999," *National Vital Statistics Reports* 49, no. 1 (2001): 15.

108. Bruce L. Flamm, Donald M. Berwick, and Andrea Kabcenell, "Reducing Cesarean Section Rates Safely: Lessons from a 'Breakthrough Series' Collaborative," *Birth* 25, no. 2 (1998): 117–124.

109. Stephen A. Myers and Norbert Gleicher, "A Successful Program to Lower Cesarean-Section Rates," *New England Journal of Medicine* 319, no. 23 (1988): 1511–1516.

110. Mary T. Koska, "Reducing Cesareans—A $1 Million Trade-Off," *Hospitals* 63, no. 5 (1989): 26.

111. Peter Boylan et al., "Effect of Active Management of Labor on the Incidence of Cesarean Section for Dystocia in Nulliparas," *American Journal of Perinatology* 8, no. 6 (1991): 373–379.

112. Kimberly D. Gregory et al., "Using the Continuous Quality Improvement Process to Safely Lower the Cesarean Section Rate," *Joint Commission Journal on Quality Improvement* 25, no. 12 (1999): 619–629.

113. Fredric D. Frigoletto et al., "A Clinical Trial of Active Management of Labor," *New England Journal of Medicine* 333, no. 12 (1995): 745–750.

114. José A. López-Zeno et al., "A Controlled Trial of a Program for the Active Management of Labor," *New England Journal of Medicine* 326, no. 7 (1992): 450–454; Trisha Woollcott, "The Active Management of Labor," *New England Journal of Medicine* 327, no. 5 (1992): 358.

115. Mortimer G. Rosen, *Management of Labor: Physician Judgment and Patient Care* (New York: Elsevier, 1990), 1, 151.

116. Maternal and Newborn Health / Safe Motherhood Unit, *Care in Normal Birth: A Practical Guide* (Geneva: World Health Organization, 1996), 23.

117. Susan I. DesHarnais and Curtis P. McLaughlin, "Clinical Quality, Risk Adjustment, and Outcome Measures in Academic Health Centers," in William F. Minogue, ed., *Managing in an Academic Health Care Environment* (Tampa: American College of Physician Executives, 1992), 87–113; David Plocher et al., "Introduction to Advanced Care Management and Its Implementation," in Peter R. Kongstvedt and David W. Plocher, eds., *Best Practices in Medical Management* (Gaithersburg, Md.: Aspen, 1998), 1–17.

118. Nicolas V. Simon, Kenneth P. Heaps, and Charles H. Chodroff, "Improving the Processes of Care and Outcomes in Obstetrics/Gynecology," *Joint Commission Journal on Quality Improvement* 23, no. 9 (1997): 485–497.

119. Frank J. Zlatnik, "Elective Induction of Labor," *Clinical Obstetrics and Gynecology* 42, no. 4 (1999): 757–765; Deborah A. Wing, "Elective Induction of Labor in the U.S.A.," *Current Opinion in Obstetrics and Gynecology* 12, no. 6 (2000): 457–462.

120. Dean V. Coonrod, R. Curtis Bay, and Glen Y. Kishi, "The Epidemiology of Labor Induction: Arizona, 1997," *American Journal of Obstetrics and Gynecology* 182, no. 6 (2000): 1355–1362.

121. Sally C. Curtin and Melissa M. Park, "Trends in the Attendant, Place, and Timing of Births, and in the Use of Obstetric Interventions, 11; Joyce A. Martin et al., "Births: Final Data for 2000," *National Vital Statistics Reports* 50, no. 5 (2002): 58. The figures included multiparae, on whom active management was less likely to be used. The percentage is in terms of live births. Racial differences were higher for induction (20 percent for whites and 15 percent for blacks in 1998) than they were for acceleration (18 percent and 16 percent, respectively). Birth certificate data reported only 2 percent of births with both induction and augmentation, a figure that seems too low.

122. Stacy T. Seyb et al., "Risk of Cesarean Delivery with Elective Induction of Labor at Term in Nulliparous Women," *Obstetrics and Gynecology* 94 (1999): 600–607. The study population included term nulliparae (women who had not previously given birth) with singleton pregnancies and no planned cesarean section.

123. John D. Yeast, Angela Jones, and Mary Poskin, "Induction of Labor and the Relationship to Cesarean Delivery: A Review of 7,001 Consecutive Inductions," *American Journal of Obstetrics and Gynecology* 180, no. 3, pt. 1 (1999): 628–633. The 44 percent induction rate pertained to singleton births only.

124. Patrick S. Ramsey, Kirk D. Ramin, and Susan M. Ramin, "Labor Induction," *Current Opinion in Obstetrics and Gynecology* 12, no. 6 (2002): 463–473.

125. Watson A. Bowes, "Clinical Aspects of Normal and Abnormal Labor," in Robert K.

Creasy and Robert Resnik, eds., *Maternal-Fetal Medicine: Principles and Practice* (Philadelphia: W. B. Saunders, 1994), 527–557.

126. Wing, "Elective Induction of Labor in the USA," 457–462.

127. Marge Morris and Joseph C. Gambone, "Making Continual Improvements to Health Care," *Clinical Obstetrics and Gynecology* 37, no. 1 (1994): 137–148; Marc Berg, *Rationalizing Medical Work: Decision-Support Techniques and Medical Practices* (Cambridge, Mass.: MIT Press, 1997), 53.

128. Paul E. Plsek, "Quality Improvement Methods in Clinical Medicine," *Pediatrics* 103, no. 1, supp. E (1999): 203–214.

129. Jo Murphy-Lawless, *Reading Birth and Death: A History of Obstetric Thinking* (Bloomington: Indiana University Press, 1998), 223.

Ten   Conclusion

1. Patricia H. Werhane, "The Ethics of Health Care as a Business," *Business and Professional Ethics Journal* 9, nos. 3–4 (1990): 7–20; Diane M. Duffy, "Market Model Fails: Linkages between Health Policy and Performance Outcomes in Western Industrial Countries," *Journal of Health and Human Services Administration* 21, no. 3 (1999): 278–309.

2. Roger M. Battistella, "Hospital Receptivity to Market Competition: Image and Reality," *Health Care Management Review* 10, no. 3 (1985): 19–26.

3. Malik M. Hasan, "Sounding Board: Let's End the Nonprofit Charade," *New England Journal of Medicine* 334, no. 16 (1996): 1055–1057.

4. Robert Martinsen, "The History of Bioethics: An Essay Review," *Journal of the History of Medicine and Allied Sciences* 56, no. 2 (2001): 168–175.

5. Susan D. Horn, "Comments on 'Is the Spirit of Capitalism Undermining the Ethics of Health Services Research?'" *HSR: Health Services Research* 28, no. 6 (1994): 678–683.

6. Dan E. Beauchamp, "Public Health as Social Justice," *Inquiry* 8 (1976): 3–14.

7. Gavin Mooney and Alistair McGuire, "Economics and Medical Ethics in Health Care: An Economic Viewpoint," in Gavin Mooney and Alistair McGuire, eds., *Medical Ethics and Economics in Health Care* (Oxford: Oxford University Press, 1988), 19.

8. Sheryl Burt Ruzek, "Access, Cost, and Quality of Medical Care: Where Are We Heading?" in Sheryl Burt Ruzek, Virginia L. Olesen, and Adele E. Clarke, *Women's Health: Complexities and Differences* (Columbus: Ohio State University Press, 1997), 183–230.

9. Camilla Stivers, "Reframing Health Policy Debate: The Need for Public Interest Language," *Administration and Society* 19, no. 3 (1987): 309–327.

10. Glenn Porter, *The Rise of Big Business, 1860–1910* (New York: Thomas Y. Crowell, 1973), 98; Carol C. Gould, *Rethinking Democracy: Freedom and Social Cooperation in Politics, Economy, and Society* (Cambridge: Cambridge University Press, 1988), 5.

11. H. Tristram Engelhardt and Michael A. Rie, "Morality for the Medical-Industrial Complex: A Code of Ethics for the Mass Marketing of Health Care," *New England Journal of Medicine* 319, no. 16 (1988): 1086–1089.

12. Stephen S. Mick, "Themes, Issues, and Research Avenues," in Stephen S. Mick

and Associates, *Innovations in Health Care Delivery: Insights for Organization Theory* (San Francisco: Jossey-Bass, 1990), 1–19.

13. Patricia Benner and Judith Wrubel, *The Primacy of Caring* (Menlo Park, Calif.: Addison-Wesley, 1989), 6.

14. Jean Watson, *Nursing: The Philosophy and Science of Caring* (Boston: Little, Brown, 1979), 8, 52.

15. Carol Gilligan, *In a Different Voice* (Cambridge: Harvard University Press, 1982); Renee C. Fox, "The Evolution of American Bioethics: A Sociological Perspective," in George Weisz, ed., *Social Science Perspectives on Medical Ethics* (Dordrecht: Kluwer, 1990), 201–217.

16. Virginia Held, *Feminist Morality: Transforming Culture, Society, and Politics* (Chicago: University of Chicago Press, 1993), 66; Joan C. Tronto, "Care as a Political Concept," in Nancy J. Hirschmann and Christine Di Stefano, eds., *Revisioning the Political: Feminist Reconstructions of Traditional Concepts in Western Political Theory* (Boulder: Westview Press, 1996), 139–156.

17. John Friedmann, "Feminist and Planning Theories: The Epistemological Connection," in Scott Campbell and Susan S. Fainstein, eds., *Readings in Planning Theory* (Cambridge, Mass.: Blackwell, 1996), 467–470.

18. Norman Daniels, "Health-Care Needs and Distributive Justice," in John D. Arras and Nancy K. Rhoden, *Ethical Issues in Modern Medicine* (Mountain View, Calif.: Mayfield, 1989), 501–509; Len Doyal and Ian Gough, *A Theory of Human Need* (New York: Guilford Press, 1991), 110.

19. Susan Sherwin, *No Longer Patient: Feminist Ethics and Health Care* (Philadelphia: Temple University Press, 1992), 86.

20. Herbert E. Klarman, "Planning for Facilities," in Eli Ginzburg [*sic*], ed., *Regionalization and Health Policy* (Washington, D.C.: U.S. Department of Health, Education, and Welfare, 1977), 25–36.

21. Hugh W. Long, "Investment Decision Making in the Health Care Industry: The Future," *Health Services Research* 14, no. 3 (1979): 183–205.

22. Frank Cerne, "Cash Kings," *Hospitals and Health Networks* 69, no. 7 (1995): 51–52, 54.

23. W. Richard Scott et al., *Institutional Change and Healthcare Organizations: From Professional Dominance to Managed Care* (Chicago: University of Chicago Press, 2000), 2.

24. Paul J. DiMaggio and Walter W. Powell, "The Iron Cage Revisited: Institutional Isomorphism and Collective Rationality in Organizational Fields," in Walter W. Powell and Paul J. DiMaggio, eds., *The New Institutionalism in Organizational Analysis* (Chicago: University of Chicago Press, 1991), 63–82.

25. Haven Emerson, C. Rufus Rorem, and Louis S. Reed, "The Problem of Medical Care: A Statement and Analysis of the Deficiencies of the Present Economic Organization of Medicine," part of a Confidential Report to the Executive Committee, Committee on the Costs of Medical Care, November 23, 1931, 24, Countway Library of Medicine Historical Collection, Boston.

26. Joseph A. Califano, "The Health-Care Chaos," *New York Times Magazine,* March 20, 1988, 44, 46, 56–58.

27. Jonathan B. Kotch et al., eds., *A Pound of Prevention: The Case for Universal Maternity Care in the U.S.* (Washington, D.C.: American Public Health Association, 1992).

28. Women's Institute for Childbearing Policy, *Childbearing Policy within a National Health Program: An Evolving Consensus for New Directions* (Roxbury, Vt.: Women's Institute for Childbearing Policy, 1994), 1, 5, 11.

29. John M. Eisenberg and Andrea Kabcenell, "Organized Practice and the Quality of Medical Care," *Inquiry* 25, no. 1 (1988): 78–89.

30. Christine L. Malcolm and Mayumi Fukui, "Specialty Service Contracting," *Topics in Health Care Financing* 20, no. 2 (1993): 68–75.

31. Committee on Ethics, "Commercial Ventures in Medicine: Concerns about the Patenting of Procedures" (committee opinion, American College of Obstetricians and Gynecologists, Washington, D.C., November 1993).

32. Philip Cole and Joyce Berlin, "Elective Hysterectomy," *American Journal of Obstetrics and Gynecology* 129, no. 2 (1977): 117–123.

33. Curtis P. McLaughlin, "Systems Analysis for Health," in Alan Sheldon, Frank Baker, and Curtis P. McLaughlin, eds., *Systems and Medical Care* (Cambridge, Mass.: MIT Press, 1970), 230–267.

34. T. Flint Porter and Michael W. Varner, "Using Evidence-based Medicine to Optimize Cesarean Section Outcomes," *Clinical Obstetrics and Gynecology* 40, no. 3 (1977): 542–547.

35. Dolores L. Burke, *Physicians in the Academic Marketplace* (New York: Greenwood Press, 1992), 30.

36. Stephen J. Heinig et al., "The Changing Landscape for Clinical Research," *Academic Medicine* 74, no. 6 (1999): 726–745.

37. David Dranove, *The Economic Evolution of American Health Care* (Princeton: Princeton University Press, 2000), 110.

38. Roger Hite, "Catholic HealthCare West: Documenting Operational Improvement," in Peter Boland, ed., *Redesigning Healthcare Delivery: A Practical Guide to Reengineering, Restructuring, and Renewal* (Berkeley: Boland Healthcare, 1996), 331–360.

39. Joint Commission on Accreditation of Healthcare Organizations, *The Measurement Mandate: On the Road to Performance Improvement in Health Care* (Oakbrook Terrace, Ill.: Joint Commission on Accreditation of Healthcare Organizations, 1993), 32.

40. Lawrence D. Brown, "Competition and the New Accountability: Do Market Incentives and Medical Outcomes Conflict or Cohere?" in Richard J. Arnould, Robert F. Rich, and William D. White, eds., *Competitive Approaches to Health Care Reform* (Washington, D.C.: Urban Institute Press, 1993), 223–244, quoting William D. White.

41. Carl A. Sirio and Dwain Harper, "Designing the Optimal Health Assessment System: The Cleveland Quality Choice (CHQC) Example," *American Journal of Medical Quality* 11, no. 1 (1996): S66–S69.

42. Jeffrey B. Gould, "Vital Records for Quality Improvement," *Pediatrics* 103, no. 1, supp. E (1999): 278–290.

43. H. David Banta and Stephen B. Thacker, "Historical Controversy in Health Technology Assessment: The Case of Electronic Fetal Monitoring," *Obstetrical and Gynecological Survey* 56, no. 11 (2001): 707–719.

44. David J. Hunter, "The Changing Roles of Health Care Personnel in Health and Health Care Management," *Social Science and Medicine* 43, no. 5 (1996): 799–808.

45. Steven Quay, "New Tools for Biotech Product Development," *Biotechnology* 13

(1995): 319–320; Dranove, *Economic Evolution of American Health Care,* 99–100; Martin F. Shapiro, "Is the Spirit of Capitalism Undermining the Ethics of Health Services Research?" *HSR: Health Services Research* 28, no. 6 (1994): 661–672.

46. Carolyn Hughes Tuohy, *Accidental Logics: The Dynamics of Change in the Health Care Arena in the United States, Britain, and Canada* (New York: Oxford University Press, 1999), 127.

47. Michael M. Davis and C. Rufus Rorem, *The Crisis in Hospital Finance and Other Studies in Hospital Economics* (Chicago: University of Chicago Press, 1932), 170.

48. Wesley C. Mitchell, "The Social Sciences and National Planning" (1935), reprinted in Findlay Mackenzie, ed., *Planned Society: Yesterday, Today, Tomorrow* (New York: Prentice-Hall, 1937), 108–127. Mitchell also believed in economic planning, however.

49. Michael Walzer, *Spheres of Justice: A Defense of Pluralism and Equality* (New York: Basic Books, 1983), 75, 65; Harmon L. Smith and Larry R. Churchill, *Professional Ethics and Primary Care Medicine: Beyond Dilemmas and Decorum* (Durham: Duke University Press, 1986), 93.

50. Carole Pateman, *Participation and Democratic Theory* (Cambridge: Cambridge University Press, 1970), 14–15; Anne Phillips, *Engendering Democracy* (University Park: Pennsylvania State University Press, 1991), 15–16.

51. Gould, *Rethinking Democracy,* 183–186.

52. Sandra Morgen, *Into Our Own Hands: The Women's Health Movement in the United States, 1969–1990* (New Brunswick: Rutgers University Press, 2002), 71–72.

53. J. K. Gibson-Graham, *The End of Capitalism (As We Knew It): A Feminist Critique of Political Economy* (Cambridge, Mass.: Blackwell, 1996), 148–152.

54. Alberto Guerreiro Ramos, *The New Science of Organizations: A Reconceptualization of the Wealth of Nations* (Toronto: University of Toronto Press, 1981), xi.

55. Joy A. de Beyer, Alexander S. Preker, and Richard G. A. Feachem, "The Role of the World Bank in International Health: Renewed Commitment and Partnership," *Social Science and Medicine* 50 (2000): 169–176.

Index

academic medical centers: and business model, 3; capital intensity of, 61; clinical departments of, 14, 29; competitive advantages of, 73, 160; and corporate funding, 165; history of, 19, 25–26; and integrated systems, 79; as perinatal centers, 88; as regional managers, 81, 96; and regional organization, 15, 76–77, 80, 95; and standard medical care, 84

academic practice plans: and business model, 16; and corporate organization, 138–139; and family medicine, 105; and industrial quality management, 141; history and growth of, 28, 66, 75, 77; and integrated systems, 79; intensive care units of, 122–124, 131–132, 137; and regional organization, 76, 96; and revenue generation, vii; and socioeconomic discrimination, 154

acceleration of labor. *See* labor acceleration

accounting methods and principles, 67, 81

active management of labor: congruency with managed care, 153; cost efficiency of, 144; and economic organization, 137; history of, 16, 143, 147–151; and mechanical model of birth, 135; and redefining labor, 145; scientific evidence of, 153

Adair, Fred Lyman, 44, 48

Aetna U.S. ʟealthcare, 152

Alabama, 93

Allegheny system, 79

ALPHA Center for Health Planning, 73, 80

alternative birth centers (ABCs), 110–111

Alternatives to Medical Control (Romalis), 10

American Academy of Dermatology, 115

American Academy of Family Physicians, 106

American Academy of Pediatrics, 41, 124

American Association for Study and Prevention of Infant Mortality, 56

American Business System, The (Cochran), 7

American College of Obstetricians and Gynecologists: and allied health personnel, 107, 132; and cesarean section, 152; and elective induction, 154; and fetal distress, 135; and hospital privileges, 105; national maternity care survey, 86, 92; and practice guidelines, 41, 92, 118; and routine hysterectomy, 164

About the Author

Barbara Bridgman Perkins works as an independent scholar. She holds a master's degree (ABD) in Medical Sciences / Pathology from Harvard University and a Ph.D. degree in Health, Society, and Policy from the Union Institute & University. She has worked in electron microscopy at the Howe Laboratory of Ophthalmology and the Beth Israel Hospital in Boston, adolescent pregnancy research at the Child Welfare League, research and teaching at the Scripps Foundation Gerontology Center at Miami University, and health planning at the Alameda-Contra Costa Health Systems Agency as well as the Washington State Health Coordinating Council. She was an early member of the Boston Women's Health Book Collective, which wrote *Our Bodies, Ourselves,* and has published broadly on health care organization in scholarly journals across several disciplines. She lives in Olympia and Seattle, Washington, with her husband, John H. Perkins; they have a son, Ivan B. Perkins.